Philosophical Issues in Psychiatry IV

International Perspectives in Philosophy and Psychiatry

Series editors: Bill (K.W.M.) Fulford, Lisa Bortolotti, Matthew Broome, Katherine Morris, John Z. Sadler, and Giovanni Stanghellini

VOLUMES IN THE SERIES:

Portrait of the Psychiatrist as a Young Man: The Early Writing and Work of R.D. Laing, 1927–1960
Beveridge

Mind, Meaning, and Mental Disorder 2e
Bolton and Hill

What is Mental Disorder?
Bolton

Delusions and Other Irrational Beliefs
Bortolotti

Postpsychiatry
Bracken and Thomas

Philosophy, Psychoanalysis, and the A-Rational Mind
Brakel

Unconscious Knowing and Other Essays in Psycho-Philosophical Analysis
Brakel

Psychiatry as Cognitive Neuroscience
Broome and Bortolotti (eds.)

Free Will and Responsibility: A Guide for Practitioners
Callender

Reconceiving Schizophrenia
Chung, Fulford, and Graham (eds.)

Darwin and Psychiatry
De Block and Adriaens (eds.)

Oxford Handbook of Philosophy and Psychiatry
Fulford, Davies, Gipps, Graham, Sadler, Stanghellini, and Thornton

Nature and Narrative: An Introduction to the New Philosophy of Psychiatry
Fulford, Morris, Sadler, and Stanghellini (eds.)

Oxford Textbook of Philosophy and Psychiatry
Fulford, Thornton, and Graham

The Mind and its Discontents
Gillett

The Abraham Dilemma
Graham

Is evidence-based psychiatry ethical?
Gupta

Thinking Through Dementia
Hughes

Dementia: Mind, Meaning, and the Person
Hughes, Louw, and Sabat (eds.)

Talking Cures and Placebo Effects
Jopling

Philosophical Issues in Psychiatry II: Nosology
Kendler and Parnas (eds.)

Philosophical Issues in Psychiatry III: The Nature and Sources of Historical Change
Kendler and Parnas (eds.)

Philosophical Issues in Psychiatry III: The Nature and Sources of Historical Change
Kendler and Parnas (eds.)

Discursive Perspectives in Therapeutic Practice
Lock and Strong (ed.)

Schizophrenia and the Fate of the Self
Lysaker and Lysaker

Embodied Selves and Divided Minds
Maiese

Responsibility and Psychopathy
Malatesti and McMillan

Body-Subjects and Disordered Minds
Matthews

Rationality and Compulsion: Applying action theory to psychiatry
Nordenfelt

Diagnostic Dilemmas in Child and Adolescent Psychiatry
Perring and Wells (eds.)

Philosophical Perspectives on Technology and Psychiatry
Phillips (ed.)

The Metaphor of Mental Illness
Pickering

Mapping the Edges and the In-between
Potter

Trauma, Truth, and Reconciliation: Healing Damaged Relationships
Potter (ed.)

The Philosophy of Psychiatry: A Companion
Radden

The Virtuous Psychiatrist
Radden and Sadler

Addiction and Weakness of Will
Radoilska

Autonomy and Mental Disorder
Radoilska (ed.)

Feelings of Being
Ratcliffe

Experiences of Depression: A study in phenomenology
Ratcliffe

Recovery of People with Mental Illness: Philosophical and Related Perspectives
Rudnick (ed.)

Values and Psychiatric Diagnosis
Sadler

The Oxford Handbook of Psychiatric Ethics
Sadler, Van Staden, and Fulford

Disembodied Spirits and Deanimated Bodies: The Psychopathology of Common Sense
Stanghellini

One Century of Karl Jaspers Psychopathology
Stanghellini and Fuchs

Emotions and Personhood
Stanghellini and Rosfort

Essential Philosophy of Psychiatry
Thornton

Naturalism, Hermeneutics, and Mental Disorder
Varga

The Healing Virtues: Character Ethics in Psychotherapy
Waring

Empirical Ethics in Psychiatry
Widdershoven, McMillan, Hope and Van der Scheer (eds.)

The Sublime Object of Psychiatry: Schizophrenia in Clinical and Cultural Theory
Woods

Alternate Perspectives on Psyciatric Validation: DSM, ICD, RDoC, and Beyond
Zachar, St. Stoyanov, Aragona, and Jablensky (eds.)

Philosophical Issues in Psychiatry IV
Classification of Psychiatric Illness

Edited by

Kenneth S. Kendler and Josef Parnas

OXFORD
UNIVERSITY PRESS

OXFORD
UNIVERSITY PRESS

Great Clarendon Street, Oxford, OX2 6DP,
United Kingdom

Oxford University Press is a department of the University of Oxford. It furthers the University's objective of excellence in research, scholarship, and education by publishing worldwide. Oxford is a registered trade mark of Oxford University Press in the UK and in certain other countries

First Edition published in 2017

Impression: 1

Published in the United States of America by Oxford University Press
198 Madison Avenue, New York, NY 10016, United States of America

British Library Cataloguing in Publication Data
Data available

Library of Congress Control Number: 2016963453

ISBN 978–0–19–879602–2

Printed in Great Britain by
Ashford Colour Press Ltd, Gosport, Hampshire

Preface

All the chapters of this book began as talks given at a conference held in Copenhagen, Denmark, on September 9–11, 2015. The conference was organized and chaired by the editors of this volume, Kenneth S. Kendler (KSK) and Josef Parnas (JP).

The conference itself was a stimulating three-day experience. Each talk was followed by a formal commentary and then an open give-and-take with the audience and other speakers, who were rarely shy about raising hard questions. So each speaker coming to the meeting agreed to present a paper of their own, comment formally on another, and write them both up for publication.

As with the earlier volumes in this series (Kendler and Parnas 2008, 2012, 2015), we have sought to capture the interactive nature of the meeting through the organization of this volume. In addition to a general introduction, written by KSK, each individual paper has an introduction (written by KSK or JP) and a discussion. Hopefully, this will provide readers with a sense of the give and take of the actual meeting.

In working on a book like this, we have naturally accumulated debts. Our greatest sense of gratitude goes to the contributors to the volume. Their enthusiasm and willingness to make the effort to connect across disciplinary boundaries was vital to the success of this venture. We got many compliments during the meeting about the quality of individual contributions and the thought-provoking nature of the discussions. The conference was funded by Psychiatric Services of the Capital Region of Denmark. The Center for Subjectivity Research is also acknowledged for financial and institutional support.

As in years past, we owe a special thanks to Jill Opalesky with her wonderful organizational skills and perpetual good cheer. She was central to all aspects of this project, from the invitation of the speakers, to establishing the schedule, to helping run the meeting itself (always a hectic experience), to aiding the too frequently distracted editors to keep straight all the submitted chapters and comments through their multiple revisions. We also want to express our appreciation to Helene Stephensen, MA, and Merete Lynnerup for their invaluable managerial and administrative assistance. Doctor Lars Siersbæk Nilsson is gratefully acknowledged for helping to prepare some manuscripts.

We have in all the previous volumes of this series ended this preface with these words which describe the experience of organizing this conference and editing this volume: "This project was, to use the philosophical term, emergent—in the end, the sum was much more than the individual parts." We are pleased to say that, again this time, this accurately described our experience and hope that you, the readers, will agree with us as you work your way through this volume.

Contents

Part III **Epistemic iteration**

Section 10 **Epistemic iteration in scientific taxonomies**

Section 11 **Problems in the validation of psychiatric diagnoses**

Section 12 **Personality disorders in DSM-5**

Section 13 **The progressive validation of medical and psychiatric disorders**

Contributors

Professor Paul S. Appelbaum, Columbia University and New York State Psychiatric Institute, USA.

Professor Derek Bolton, Institute of Psychiatry, Psychology and Neuroscience, King's College London, UK

Professor Denny Borsboom, University of Amsterdam, The Netherlands

Professor John Campbell, University of California, Berkeley, USA

Professor Hasok Chang, University of Cambridge, UK

Professor Michael B. First, Columbia University and New York State Psychiatric Institute, USA

Professor Stephan Heckers, Vanderbilt University, USA

Professor Paul Hoff, University of Zurich, Switzerland

Professor Kenneth S. Kendler, Virginia Commonwealth University, USA

Professor Dominic Murphy, University of Sydney, Australia

Professor Josef Parnas, University of Copenhagen, Denmark

Georg Repnikov, University of Sydney, Australia

Professor Kenneth F. Schaffner, University of Pittsburgh, USA

Professor Miriam Solomon, Temple University, USA

Professor Dan J. Stein, University of Cape Town, South Africa

Assistant Professor Kathryn Tabb, Columbia University, USA

Professor Eric Turkheimer, University of Virginia, USA

Annick Urfer-Parnas, University of Copenhagen, Denmark

Professor Peter Zachar, Auburn University at Montgomery, USA

Introduction

A good way to start this introduction is to share the editors' first organized thoughts about the contents of this volume, contained in the introductory letter sent to the prospective attendees of the conference in Copenhagen on which this volume is based:

> *Conference Content*:
> This is the fourth conference in the series on theoretical and conceptual issues in psychiatry. This time, we are returning to the seminal issue of Psychiatric Nosology particularly in light of the revision processes recently completed for DSM-5 and still in progress for ICD-11, as well as the launch of the Research Domain Criteria (RDoC) project by the NIMH.
>
> *The conference topics*:

1. *The nature of psychiatric illnesses* and the way we define them—how do we set the limits of what is a psychiatric disorder? We want to ground this discussion in practical examples from DSM or ICD.
2. The problem of criteria "*reification*" (i.e. converting ideas, concepts, and abstractions into really existing objects). What reification is (and is it one thing or several) and why it occurs is a worthy topic of sustained consideration. It is generally accepted that diagnostic criteria *only index* (signal) disorder but *do not constitute them*, but in practice this rule is not always followed despite concerns about reification.
3. The "epidemics" of individual psychiatric disorders—what social and biomedical factors contribute to "popularity" of individual disorders? Consider PTSD, borderline personality, autism spectrum, multiple personality disorder.
4. *The definition of individual symptoms or signs*. How to consider the nature (ontology) of a symptom, its individuation, potentially constitutive relations to other phenomena? Discuss in the context of a specific phenomenon, e.g. hallucinations.
5. A critique of the concept of epistemic iteration, esp. in light of the experience in DSM-5 with the Scientific Review committee. Epistemic iteration as applied to psychiatric nosology refers to an historical and scientific approach that requires that each change to a nosologic construct be required to show its empirical superiority to that which came before. Can such a model work for psychiatric disorders? What are its key limitations?
6. The problem of *scientific authority*. Why should the APA or the World Health Organization get to develop diagnosis criteria? What gives them the authority?

7. Can we, and if so how, actually move from descriptive to etiologically based diagnoses?
8. To review the advantages and disadvantages of moving from a model in which we revise our diagnostic manuals every 10-15 years to a living document model.

While like all plans of mice and men, the conference did not entirely adhere to these goals, the correspondence ultimately was relatively high. I now want to provide a broad overview of this volume, which contains 16 main chapters, and a corresponding number of introductions and discussions. As noted above, of the four volumes in this series, this is the second to focus on psychiatric nosology. Why return to this topic?

This question can be briefly answered. Psychiatric nosology raises a range of intriguing issues which can be examined from empirical, clinical, theoretical and philosophical perspectives. These are just the sort of fertile topics that fit well into a conference that seeks to explore the interface between psychiatry and philosophy. Furthermore, psychiatric nosology is important and has practical impact out in the world.

So the topic is a fruitful one given our efforts to help build the philosophy of psychiatry as a rigorous and relevant field. The best way to do so is to bring together individuals with expertise in a substantive area of psychiatry and in the relevant philosophical literature. That is not too hard to do for nosologic questions—witness the interest this has generated in philosophers such as Miriam Solomon and Hasok Chang who are rather new to the field of psychiatry.

Philosophical issues in nosology are also easy to ground in the real world. While the metaphysical reaches of the mind–body problem can generate endless fascinating questions, there can often arise, in such inquiries, the feeling of floating free of the shackles of the clinical reality in which most psychiatrists live and work (or any kind of reality for that matter). Not so with problems of nosology. In particular, our conference was grounded in the experiences of the revision of DSM-5 (in which four of our participants played a major role—Drs. Stein, First, Appelbaum, and Kendler) and the subsequent shaping of the next iteration of the DSM revision process under the watchful eye of our concluding speaker, Dr. Paul S. Appelbaum.

What are the kinds of chapters you will read in the book? (I will review them using my own idiosyncratic scheme rather than following the order in which the papers appear in the book). Three of them represent thoughtful analysis of key DSM-5 efforts. Stein reviews, from a conceptual perspective, the efforts of the Anxiety Disorder Work Group, particularly in the area of obsessive-compulsive and related disorders. By and large, this was a successful effort that raise a series of important conceptual issues about the nature and basis of change. By contrast, Zachar provides an overview of what was probably the most controversial and painful episode in the entire DSM-5—the unsuccessful attempt to dramatically revise the personality disorder criteria. Drawing from an oral history project, he outlines the conceptual issues that contributed to this failure, provided a fascinating behind the scenes view of the process. Solomon focuses on a more delimited but also important event—the demise of the category of Asperger's disorder. She raises issues rarely heard in the halls of the DSM-5 process. In particular, what responsibility, if any, do the revisers of a nosology have to the patients whose categories they are changing or, in the case of Asperger's disorder, eliminating?

Kendler's chapter also focuses on an important episode in DSM history but from a much earlier era. He reviews the separation of panic disorder from the broader category of anxiety neurosis in the pre-DSM-III days and compares the success of that effort with a paradigmatic diagnostic division in general medicine—the separation of juvenile (or type 1) diabetes from adult-onset (or type 2) diabetes. This review is in the service of asking what might be gained by viewing the process of validation of psychiatric disorders from an historical (aka diachronic) rather than cross-sectional (aka synchronic) perspective.

While these chapters looked backward on nosologic successes and failures, the final chapter, by Appelbaum, looks forward, clearly outlining the framework that will govern DSM revisions for the foreseeable future under the supervision of the "DSM Steering Committee." As readers will see, the framework is substantially different from that used in prior revisions.

Two chapters are from leading thinkers in psychology on the continually challenging question of the nature of psychiatric categories. In rather different ways, both of the them approach this question from a measurement or "psychometric" perspective. Borsboom reviews the increasingly influential network models of psychiatric illness and how this approach challenges some of the fundamental assumptions about their nature and etiology—in particular the common factor model in which symptoms are seen as manifestations of a latent disease liability. Turkheimer reviews the question of "mapping" of psychopathology from the perspective of measurement theory in psychology. He is particularly interested in the question of the degree to which a given diagnostic category is something "natural" in the world or a construct of our own making. He will introduce readers to the pithy but quite informative phrase "meaningful but arbitrary" or MBA for short. A number of his comments will remind some readers of the classical realism versus pragmatism (aka instrumentalism) debate in the philosophy of science

Campbell's chapter takes on the validation of psychiatric disorders from a quite different, and more critical, philosophical perspective. In particular, he worries that our inability to ground our validation efforts in a "world out there" (as might occur if we had a definitive biological test or a clear understanding of etiology) is fundamentally crippling. The field of psychiatry, he argues, works with an amputated and deficient version of a full validation model. Part of his concern stems, he argues forcibly, from a confusion in the field as to whether the criteria for psychiatric disorders index or constitute the disorders themselves.

Several papers focused on aspects of the concept of epistemic iteration and its possible relevance as a guiding principle for revisions of psychiatric nosology. The chapter by Chang, the originator of the concept of epistemic iteration, provides a background to its development, a charming review of the problems of classificatory changes in the "hard sciences" (so that we working in psychiatry should not feel we are the only ones with such troubles), and a concerted plea for an incorporation of scientific pluralism into the iterative process. How to balance a pluralism that will maximally stimulate the scientific enterprise but not confuse the world of "official medical practice" is a challenge. He also reviews the hard problem of "local minima" (aka box canyons) in an iterative landscape, suggesting that they may not be as problematic as first thought.

Schaffner and Tabb take on the issue of how, in psychiatry, we might move from the descriptive to the etiological. While we all want to move from our focus on symptoms and signs to a grounding of our nosology in causal biological stories, their approach is cautionary. They conclude that a complete reduction of psychiatric disorders is not plausible within any realistic time frame (or ever). But, they suggest, more proximal goals of parts of an etiologic story (a "patchy" reductionism) are a more viable aim.

The book contains three chapters which explore relevant conceptual, historical, and cultural aspects of psychiatric disorders. Bolton provides an incisive critique of the nature of the relationship in psychiatry between "disorder" and "disability." He argues that, unlike what might occur in traditional medical disorders, for psychiatric disorders it is not easy and probably unwise to separate "illness" on the one hand from "disability" on the other. First gives a scholarly overview of the problems of psychiatric "epidemics," outlining the substantial difficulties associated with determining whether changes in reported prevalence for a disorder represent true changes in the frequency of the disorder versus a range of other confounding factors. Murphy examines the question of culture-bound syndromes, what they mean and how they can inform us about how culture shapes the presentation of psychiatric disease. With the increasing internationalization of psychiatric research, these questions are taking on a new urgency including, for example, molecular genetic studies which are now assessing and hoping to jointly analyze major psychiatric disorders as they occur among all the major human ethnic groups.

Hoff attempts to put the problem of reification of psychiatric diagnosis into its philosophical and historical context. He contrasts the naturalistic (or realist) view of Kraepelin and the more nominalist perspective that we might expect to be associated with the use of operationalized criteria in the more recent editions of the DSM. However, he cautions against the rise of "uncritical" reification of DSM (and ICD) categories that incorrectly assumes that they represent natural kinds.

One chapter digs deeply into the phenomenology of psychiatric illness. Parnas explores auditory–verbal hallucinations (AVH) in detail as a basis for an exploration of a range of relevant philosophical issues. He is critical of the current use of operationalized diagnostic criteria and the lack of appreciation in both clinical and research studies of the subtlety and contextualization of key psychiatric symptoms, of which AVH is a good example. This chapter serves as a reminder of the depth of the descriptive psychopathologic literature we have in psychiatry which, in the world dominated by DSM manuals, is rarely taught and even more rarely read.

In what is, along with Appelbaum's contribution, the most forward-looking chapter in this book, Heckers—a leading biological psychiatrist and journal editor—attempts to envision how the science of psychiatry will move forward over the coming years. Given his major interest in psychotic disorders, his chapter is largely an exposition and evaluation of the dominant Kraepelinian paradigm that has had its greatest impact in the areas of severe psychiatric illness. Hecker reviews the major critiques of Kraepelin. In a final section, entitled "Where do we go from here?," he ranges across a variety of possible directions but in the end substantially endorses the continued fertility of the Kraepelinian paradigm.

As I hope I have convinced you, this book provides a rich intellectual repast where serious scholars from several parts of the field of psychiatry, in particular clinicians, historians, and nosologists, join with psychologists and philosophers of varying orientations to struggle with a wide range of key issues in psychiatric nosology. Our goal was to stimulate cross-disciplinary dialog with the conviction that the best work in the philosophy of science comes for such interactions. We hope that you will agree that our organizing efforts, fulfilled in the devoted work of our diverse contributors, have met those goals.

Part I

Nature of psychiatric illness

Section 1

Clinical significance and disability in psychiatric illness

Chapter 1

Introduction to "Clinical significance, disability, and biomarkers: Shifts in thinking between DSM-IV and DSM-5"

Kenneth S. Kendler

In this clearly articulated essay, the clinical psychologist and philosopher of psychiatry Derek Bolton addresses the question of whether it is possible or advisable to separate the concept of mental (or psychiatric) illness from illness-associated disability. I might frame the problems as follows. Can we understand illness to be one thing that may or may not be accompanied by some disability—defined by the DSM as "impairment in social, occupational, or other important areas of functioning"—or is such disability part and parcel of the illness concept?

As I often do when confronting such issues, I first try to take some clear examples from general medicine. I can have a pea-sized astrocytoma (aka brain cancer) growing away in my frontal cortex. With such a small tumor, it is likely that I could have no discernable symptoms and disability for some time. Eventually, if it keeps growing it will cause both local and possibly general dysfunction but that could take years. Few would want to argue that a pea-sized cancer is not an illness. So, can I have a medical illness with no disability? Yes.

Let me take a subtler issue. Imagine two people with very similar bad osteoarthritis of the hip. Their X-rays look very similar and show terrible joint degeneration. There is moderate to severe pain. One of these patients, Bill, is an owner of a small grocery store. He bears the pain and has no discernable impairment in function. He doesn't take long walks like he used to, but no "important area of functioning" is impaired. The other patient, Harold, is more sensitive to pain. He worked as a postman and found it too difficult to do his daily rounds. Although he was offered a position sorting mail, he applied for and was granted disability due to the arthritis. Do we wish to argue that Bill does not have an illness—because he has no disability—while Harold does?

Let's move to psychiatric illness. Let me provide four cases adapted from my prior clinical work.

> Jerry was a rather socially isolated 46-year-old man working as a vice-president for an important advertising firm. He was referred by the company president. I was told

that despite quite good work performance, he had disturbed some of his colleagues by talking about "odd things." He was told to "go get a psychiatric evaluation." He presented as well groomed and articulate, and denied drug use or any other problems in psychological functioning. He said he was an introvert with a low sex drive and he was comfortable with his rather limited social life. He then looked embarrassed and said "There is something more." He went on to describe a bizarre delusional belief. He was in communication with extraterrestrial powers. Every morning he assumed a special posture and received "rays" emanating from outer space that helped keep him healthy and well prepared for the events of the day. He knew this was an unusual belief but was convinced of its reality. He had no other symptoms that I could discern.

Alice was a anxious 23-year-old recent college graduate. She was driven to see me by her mother and described herself as housebound. Classic panic attacks had begun about 5 months ago after she graduated from college and began looking for a job. They were at first largely "out of the blue." The attacks were classic with typical features and at their worst occurred 3 or 4 times a week. Over a course of about 6 weeks, she had moved back in with her parents and refused to leave the house unaccompanied. She described a lifelong passive-dependent personality pattern with low self-esteem and low assertiveness.

John was a 52-year-old truck driver who's wife had recently died from breast cancer. A friend had told him that he thought he had panic attacks and should go see a psychiatrist. Indeed, since his wife's death, he described classic panic attacks—very similar in frequency and intensity to those reported by Alice. Like Alice's, they mostly occurred without clear precipitants. John, however, had refused to alter his behavior in the least. He described several times needing to pull his truck over to the side of the road and wait till the panic attack passed. He once panicked in an elevator and he described "white-knuckling it" hoping the others did not notice. He said "I'll be darned if I am going to let my nerves get the better of me, Doc."

Sally was a 37-year-old housewife I was asked to evaluate for depression. In my review with her, I asked about phobic fears. She said that for her entire life, she had been scared of the dark. Her house had a basement where they stored food and other household goods. If she had to, she would go down there herself but would tremble. Mostly, she would get one of her children or her husband to go down for her. There were no other practical effects of her fear of the dark. She slept with the lights off.

What can these four scenarios teach us about the possible relationship between disability and psychiatric illness? Let us start with the simplest case. I did not give Sally a diagnosis of phobia. Fears of the dark are common. She has no appreciable disability. I saw it as a normal variation, not an illness.

But I did diagnose Jerry as "Psychotic disorder not otherwise specified." Was I correct? I could find no appreciable illness-related disability. Yes I would to this day be uncomfortable with calling him psychiatrically well. I would not consider such beliefs to reflect "normal variation."

Then what about John and Sally? In both cases I gave a diagnosis of panic disorder. They met the symptomatic criteria. Sally got the extra diagnosis of agoraphobia. Their stories echo those of Bill and Harold—a similar pathological process (osteoarthritis or panic disorder) but very different functional outcomes (disability versus no substantial impairment). (Of note, the frequency of panic attacks in both John and Sally were considerably reduced in frequency by medication.)

At one level I am inconsistent. Why does Sally not get a diagnosis and Jerry does, in that each had some symptoms (fear of the dark and delusions of alien influence) but no objective impairment? My defense is that irrational fears are really common and probably part of the human condition but beliefs about aliens are not. Is this a defensible position and how could such a line be clearly drawn? What kinds of psychiatric syndromes are "inherently" disordered versus require accompanying disability to achieve the status of a disorder?

So, I hope I have introduced the readers to some of the conundrums of the association between psychiatric illness and disability. Bolton provides a strong argument for an inherent link between the two. He argues that the basic function of the mind–brain modules involved in psychiatric illness are to "regulate action in the outside world" just as the cardiovascular system is to provide nutrients and take away waste products in the body as a whole. His line of argument might reach different conclusions than I did in the cases of Jerry and John. One way to think about Jerry's case is to ask whether developing broadly realistic models of how the world actually works is an important function of our central nervous system (I am obviously here not talking about religious beliefs accepted by one's subculture). Jerry's central nervous system is not doing that. Is that enough of an impairment to call him ill? (Note that Bolton treats this issue toward the end of his essay when he asks whether we might "have conditions that seem 'inherently' pathological even though in the absence of functional impairment.")

I hope reading this introduction, Bolton's essay, and the response can stimulate readers—both those with and without clinical experience of their own—to ponder these questions. I hope they will try out Bolton's line of argument to see how well it fits their intuitions about this difficult issue, which is of both practical and considerable theoretical interest.

Chapter 2

Clinical significance, disability, and biomarkers: Shifts in thinking between DSM-IV and DSM-5

Derek Bolton

The fifth edition of the *Diagnostic and Statistical Manual of Mental Disorders* (DSM-5, American Psychiatric Association 2013) follows its definition of mental disorder, slightly changed from the fourth edition (DSM-IV, American Psychiatric Association 1994), with this paragraph headed "criterion for clinical significance" (p. 21):

> There have been substantial efforts by the DSM-5 Task Force and ... WHO [the World Health Organization] *to separate the concepts of mental disorder and disability (impairment in social, occupational, or other important areas of functioning).* In the WHO system, the ... ICD [International Classification of Diseases] covers all diseases and disorders, while the International Classification of Functioning, Disability and Health (ICF) provides a separate classification of global disability ... *However, in the absence of clear biological markers or clinically useful measurements of severity for many mental disorders, it has not been possible to completely separate normal and pathological symptom expressions contained in diagnostic criteria* ... Therefore, a generic diagnostic criterion requiring distress or disability has been used to establish disorder thresholds, usually worded "the disturbance causes clinically significant distress or impairment in social, occupational, or other important areas of functioning ... (italics added)

My main topic is the first italicized sentence, the effort to separate the concepts of mental disorder and "disability," understood here as impairment in social, occupational, or other important areas of functioning. I will present a line of thought suggesting that this is a mistake, that the concepts are bound together, and that—referring to the second italicized sentence in the above quote—they are so regardless of the presence or absence of biomarkers.

By way of background, the concept of "clinical significance" has played an important role in the DSM characterization of mental disorder. It also figures—as "clinically recognizable"—in the *International Classification of Diseases* (ICD) definition (ICD-10; World Health Organization 1992). The concept is not much explained, but generally it has been intended as a severity measure or as a threshold marker for clinical attention (see, e.g., Spitzer and Williams 1982, p. 19). It is recognized on the other hand that disability—or distress and/or disability—is a function of many fuzzy psychosocial variables such as distress tolerance, character factors, motivation, social support, environmental contingencies, or task demands. Biomedicine, by contrast, offers precise markers for the presence or absence and for severity of disease. However, in the absence of appropriate biomarkers for diagnosing and setting thresholds for mental disorders (Charney et al. 2002), DSM-5 retained distress or social impairment associated with clinical syndrome as a generic diagnostic criterion.

As is well known the tension here has resulted in something of a parting of ways between the National Institute of Mental Health (NIMH) and DSM approaches. After a few decades of research on the biological bases of mental disorders, the outcome in short was this:

- No biomarkers for mental disorders (ICD/DSM major depression, schizophrenia, etc.)

The straightforward conclusion was this:

- Bad news for the biomarking paradigm in psychiatry, more broadly for psychiatry aspiring to the clarity and success of biomedicine.

But a less obvious conclusion gradually appeared, a more radical diagnosis of the problem:

- * Bad news for mental disorders—*that is, as defined by the DSM and ICD.*

This second option, inferring from poor correlation between psychiatric conditions and biological correlates, that the psychiatric conditions are poorly defined, is the one adopted in the NIMH's Research Domains Criteria Framework (RDoC) project. Here for example is Tom Insel's blog on the eve of DSM-5 publication (Insel 2013):

> Unlike our definitions of ischemic heart disease, lymphoma, or AIDS, the DSM diagnoses are based on a consensus about clusters of clinical symptoms, not any objective laboratory measure. In the rest of medicine, this would be equivalent to creating diagnostic systems based on the nature of chest pain or the quality of fever ... Patients with mental disorders deserve better. NIMH has launched the Research Domain Criteria (RDoC) project to transform diagnosis by incorporating genetics, imaging, cognitive science, and other levels of information to lay the foundation for a new classification system ... But it is critical to realize that we cannot succeed if we use DSM categories as the "gold standard." The diagnostic system has to be based on the emerging research data, not on the current symptom-based categories. Imagine deciding that EKGs were not useful because many patients with chest pain did not have EKG changes. That is what we have been doing for decades when we reject a biomarker because it does not detect a DSM category. We need to begin collecting the genetic, imaging, physiologic, and cognitive data to see how all the data—not just the symptoms—cluster and how these clusters relate to treatment response.

This line of thought invokes the tension that found its way into the DSM-5's cautious approach to "clinical significance" quoted at the start of this chapter, tension between finding biomarkers for disorders and characterizing disorders by clinical symptoms, which, in the case of mental disorders, typically involve impairments in social functioning. I will argue that while there may be some tension here, we are not faced with a choice between the one and the other, and especially, it is not possible to disentangle diagnosis of mental disorder from impairments in social functioning.

In 2009 *World Psychiatry* published an important forum on these issues with the title: "The role of functional impairment in the diagnosis of mental disorders: toward ICD-11 and DSM-V." The target article by Üstün and Kennedy (2009) had the title "What is 'functional impairment'? Disentangling disability from clinical significance", and there was a reply by Narrow et al. (2009), "DSM-V perspectives on disentangling disability from clinical significance."

In their target article Üstün & Kennedy (2009) argue that the disease/disorder construct is not the same as the functional impairment construct, that therefore they should be rated separately, and that functional impairment should not be used either in the diagnosis of disease, or in setting a threshold, or as a measure of severity. They present this view in the case of physical disorders, and argue that it applies no less to mental disorders. In their commentary Narrow and colleagues (2009) outline the benefits of including a functional impairment criterion in diagnosis, including better identification of persons using mental health services or with more severe symptoms. They go on to agree, however, that the DSM does not sufficiently distinguish symptom severity from impairments of social functioning and look forward to more consistency between the DSM and WHO approaches. But they add an important caveat, referring to improving assessments of symptom severity and disability (Narrow et al. 2009, p. 89):

> However, this exercise [improving assessments of symptom severity and disability] is somewhat dependent on the extent to which the symptom criteria themselves are already liberated from elements that are better seen as activity limitations. Contrary to Üstün and Kennedy's assertion, this is not a minor issue limited to occasional disorders such as residual schizophrenia. The DSM-IV and the ICD-10 criteria for research both have many examples of activity limitations serving as symptoms. In the ICD-10, personality disorders, substance dependence, hyperkinetic disorders, and conduct disorder all have substantial components of activity limitations in their symptom criteria. It is unclear at this point whether symptom criteria for these disorders can be fully "cleansed" of their activity limitations components. Ideally, more specific assessments would target the impaired mental processes that underlie these activity limitations. The development and implementation of such assessments will depend largely on the state of the existing science and technology as well as the practical limitations of implementation in routine clinical settings.

I think Narrow and colleagues are right to see a problem here for the Üstün & Kennedy proposal to disentangle mental disorder from activity impairments. Here is a line of thought suggesting the two really cannot be disentangled. Because the context here is partly to align characterization of mental disorder with physical disorder, especially conditions that are reasonably well understood in biomedicine, I illustrate the line of thought for cardiovascular disease.

Cardiovascular disease covers numerous problems, many related to atherosclerosis, which inhibits blood flow, raising risk of thrombus and of embolus, which block blood flow and hence oxygen supply to cells, hence cardiac arrest or stroke, with more or less permanent damage due to cell death. The crucial point for the present purpose is that this model of disease *is closely linked to the model of what the cardiovascular system (CVS) is for: delivering nutrients and oxygen to all cells in the body and removing waste products.* The model of the disease process essentially draws on the failure of a normal function. In brief, the disease process involving atherosclerosis is a 'disease process' *because* it disrupts (or raises the risk of disruption of) normal CVS function such as supplying oxygen to cell tissue for cell respiration—resulting in more or less catastrophic outcomes.

The general point I suggest is this: *system dysfunction (e.g., in cardiovascular disease) is defined in terms of "disability," (in scare quotes), by which I mean here: failure to achieve normal outcomes in its environment.* In the CVS, this means failure to transport enough oxygen (and other nutrients like glucose) to cells for them to survive and prosper. The general point draws on the fact that internal bodily organs or systems operate in environments to achieve certain outcomes, and organ or systemic dysfunction cannot be conceptually disentangled from downturn in achieving those outcomes. This is intended as a general point, applying to all internal systems: the CVS, the gut, the liver, the immune system, and so on. We can expect it to apply also to the central nervous system (CNS).

To see how the general point in the preceding paragraph, assuming for the sake of argument that it valid or at least plausible, applies to the CNS, we need first a characterization of the system is supposed to do—its normal function. The CNS is involved in the regulation of, processing efferent and afferent information about several broad kinds of "environment": first, inner organs and systems, for example the CVS; second, balance and orientation of the whole body; and third, activity in the outside world. It is this latter—*regulating action in the outside world,* outside the body—which is the special characteristic of the CNS for the present purpose. Of course "action in the outside world" is an indefinite concept, but let us suppose we can roughly identify broad headings of "important" activities, important from some point of view but including survival, such as obtaining food, water, shelter, and, given that we are social beings, many kinds of social activities such as work, education, childcare, cooperation with kin and non-kin. Application of the general point outlined in the preceding paragraph would then read something like this: *the concept of disorder or disease in the functioning of those parts or subsystems in the CNS which regulate activity in the outside world cannot be conceptually disentangled from downturn in achieving some of these "important" functional outcomes, including but not only social.*

This formulation refers to the biological CNS and its various parts and circuits. We don't get to "mental disorder" except by an additional move which runs something like this: concepts of mind (attention, memory, beliefs, emotions, decision) refer at least and probably mainly to the activities of the person in the outside world, and is a way of referring to CNS functions regulating those activities. This is an approximation but close enough to let the argument go through to the conclusion that "mental disorder" cannot be conceptually disentangled from downturn in "important person-level activity outcomes", including but not only social. The logic here is meant to be the same as for the cardiovascular disease: it makes no more sense to disentangle social impairments from mental disorder than it does to disentangle failure to supply sufficient nutrients to maintain cell survival from cardiovascular disease.

For this reason I believe Üstün & Kennedy in their 2009 article misunderstood the different role that social impairments have in relation to mental disorders compared with their role in physical diseases. By all means social impairments can be disentangled from diseases of internal systems, because it not part of, e.g., normal CVS functioning to regulate social behaviors, such as emotional responsiveness (except via the autonomic nervous system), or indeed any behaviors of the whole body in the external environment. But because "the mind"—instantiated in ways we poorly understand in CNS structures and circuits—does regulate these functions, its dysfunctions cannot be disentangled in that way. The CVS and the CNS are different, they do different things, and different functions and outcomes are at stake when they don't work well enough.

This argument does not at all counterindicate investigation of biomarkers, central to the RDoC project; it runs independent of this issue. There may be biomarkers, e.g., for depression, or a subtype of depression, or a supratype of emotional negativity, but this would not change the fact that mental disorder is conceptually linked to downturn in social functioning, any more than biomarkers for atherosclerosis count against the conceptual linkage between cardiovascular disease and failure to maintain oxygen transport for cell respiration, for example. In this sense the DSM-5 apology for its clinical significance criterion, quoted at this beginning of this chapter, and the conclusion of the paper by Narrow and colleagues cited above, both to the effect that we have to keep the social impairment criterion in play to diagnose mental disorder *because we have not yet found biomarkers*, are misconceived. Biomarkers for mental disorders, as and when discovered, would mark biological processes that have a specific functional characteristic: they cause, or raise risk for, downturn in social, occupational, or other important areas of functioning.

Having argued that mental disorder is conceptually linked to downturn in social functioning it is necessary now to recognize the fact that the two *are somewhat distinct also*. I will consider three important kinds of qualification: first, empirical research assessing the two phenotypes separately; second, cases of impairment without disorder; and third, cases of mental disorder without impairment.[1]

The effect of adding impairment as a diagnostic criterion for mental disorder was investigated by Foley and colleagues on a large sample of the Virginia Twin

---

[1] I am grateful to Professor Kendler for drawing my attention to such cases in his comments on an earlier draft.

Registry taking major depression as example (Foley et al. 2003). They assessed DSM-III-R lifetime major depression and then subsequently and separately associated functional impairment. It was found that while the genetic risk factors for major depression and associated functional impairment are substantially correlated, they are not identical. The authors speculated that risk factors specific for associated functional impairment would index personal characteristics, such as personality, coping skills, and perceived support, and contextual features, such as education, marital history, and socioeconomic status.

Given the above line of argument that mental disorder cannot be conceptually disentangled from functional impairment, how would such findings be interpreted? The first point to make is that an *adequacy condition* of any theory is that the extent of correlation between mental disorder and impairment is an open question and amenable to empirical study. In effect this rules out defining mental disorder in terms of impaired social functioning, which would have the correlation equal to 1 a priori. The line of argument in this paper is not like this: the point is not to define mental disorder as social disorder. The argument does however rule out a priori a correlation of 0 or anything much less than "a lot." The a-priori nature of the requirement of a substantial correlation would show up as a response to an empirically found low correlation to the effect: "well, whatever phenotype you are assessing here is not helpfully called a mental disorder, pathology, but is apparently just a population variant."

The position being argued for, however, can—and wants to— accommodate the option of a correlation between mental disorder and social impairment of less than 1, though not too much less. The general theoretical reason is that while systemic dysfunction has to (by definition, according to the argument presented here), involve some failure, or risk of failure, to achieve normal outcomes in its environment, *how much* failure, short-term or longer-term, how much restoration or compensation of function—is another matter. The extent of failure of function is partly dependent on factors independent of the original dysfunctional process within the system, including relevant states of its environment and relevant interactions with other systems. In the case of major depression these independent factors might include personal characteristics and contextual features of the sort cited by Foley and colleagues.

Again the relevant points can be made in relation to medical conditions such as cardiovascular disease. Any condition of the CVS warranting the name pathology has to be associated "often" with failure of normal function and poor outcomes, e.g., failure of oxygen delivery to cells sufficient to maintain cell respiration leading to cell damage or death; otherwise it is no more than a (harmless) population variant. Nevertheless, at the same time, the extent of poor outcomes resulting from failure of normal function will depend on several additional factors. The extent of cell damage will be partly a function of the disease process itself, including the severity of atherosclerosis and the size of embolus. However, the extent of cell damage will also depend on further factors, either inside the CVS, such as the pattern of vasculature that could provide additional blood flow to the tissue through other blood vessels, or outside the CVS, such as the sites affected, and persistence of disruption to brain functioning will depend on further factors again, such as spontaneous recovery and compensatory mechanisms.

The general point is that bodily systems interact with their environment regulating certain outcomes, often interacting with other systems. A disease process by definition, it is being argued, involves some failure to achieve (or risk of failure to achieve) normal outcomes—but the extent of the failure depends not only on factors in the disease process but also on factors in the environment and in interacting systems.

This general point relates to the problem of reduction of disease to a single primary cause. If a normal function of a biological system is carried out by only that one system, then failure of that function will be reducible to processes within that one system. For example, insofar as it is only the CVS that delivers oxygen to cells, failure to achieve that function, failure of oxygen delivery to cells, is attributable only to—and in this sense is reducible to—cardiovascular dysfunction, a cardiovascular disease process such as atherosclerosis. In many cases, however, and this may be the general rule, biological functions are controlled by interacting subsystems, with the effect that achievement of a particular function is not a matter of processes in any one system, but may be affected by many interacting systems. This is likely to the case for the CNS regulation of whole-person activity in the external environment. This typically involves many systems acting at once and interacting, systems such as those involved in perception, attention, memory, motivation, and motor planning. In these circumstances, downturn in a particular activity such as work may be caused by many kinds of systemic dysfunction—in memory or attention, say—or may emerge from unfortunate complex interaction between systems. In this case failure of function will not reduce to processes always in the same system—the causal processes will be heterogeneous. But further, in the case of the CNS regulating activity in the outside world, we also have to take into account processes and systems in the outside world, not only in the internal biology. Processes and systems in the outside world, as well as internal processes and systems, make a difference to whether or not, or the extent to which, activities in the outside world are achieved well enough. For example, excessive task demands jeopardize task fulfillment, while access to social support promotes success, as does access to resources that come with higher socioeconomic status.

I said above that the proposed conceptual linkage between mental disorder and functional impairments would prohibit finding zero linkage in "most cases." Nevertheless there are kinds of case where the two constructs seem to dissociate. One kind of case might be fear of heights, which in some situations is clearly normal and not pathological. How would the view proposed here deal with this? Criteria for judging pathology are complex and include downturn in functioning as emphasized here but also deviance from some presumed statistical or "natural design" norms (see, e.g., Bolton 2008). Fear of heights, let's suppose, comes in as normal in relation to these presumed norms, and yet it can cause functional impairments, for example for a person living or working in a high building. It is important here that the examples of tasks underpinning the attribution of impairment and hence pathology are in "important" areas, such getting in and out of the house and working. Fear of bunjee jumping and other extreme sports probably wouldn't count; unless the person were a professional at such an activity and wanted to get back to it after an accident. Generally the concept delivered by the impairment criterion is *need to treat* (need for healthcare attention)—and this usually, but does not always, coincide with intuitions around norms determining attribution of *disorder* and its cognates.

In other kinds of case we have conditions that seem "inherently" pathological even in the absence of functional impairment; for example, in a man with a complex delusional system who has no appreciable impairment. Our intuition of "inherent" pathology in such cases may arise from some presumed statistical or "natural design" norm, or it may arise from the accumulated experience especially in the clinic of *very high correlations between* delusional systems and impairments. The line of thought presented here favors the impairment criterion as critical to the pathology attribution. If there are no activity limitations, and if we do not draw on background convictions (however evidenced) of increased risk/likelihood of activity limitations—then grounds for disorder attribution are undermined and we have only *difference* left. The view being proposed here imposes high standards of tolerance of diversity.

I conclude with a reference to the work that I believe underpins the approach being proposed here. Readers may recall that in response to the question posed in the 1970s as to whether homosexuality should remain classified as a mental disorder, the American Psychological Associaion established a task force to provide principled advice. The principles arrived at found their way into the DSM-III definition of mental disorder, then into DSM-IV, though I fear they have been somewhat obscured in the DSM-5 and especially in the ICD approach as described by Üstün & Kennedy (2009) discussed previously. Here is the key point, in Spitzer and Williams (1982, p. 16):

> Spitzer concluded that, with the exception of homosexuality, and perhaps some of the other "sexual deviations," they all regularly caused subjective distress or were associated with generalized impairment in social effectiveness or functioning. *It was argued that the consequences of a condition, and not its etiology, determined whether the condition should be considered a disorder* . . . It was proposed that the criterion for a mental disorder was either subjective distress or generalized impairment in social effectiveness (italics added).

References

American Psychiatric Association (1994). *Diagnostic and Statistical Manual of Mental Disorders*, 4th edn. Washington, DC: American Psychiatric Association.

American Psychiatric Association (2013). *Diagnostic and Statistical Manual of Mental Disorders*, 5th edn. Washington, DC: American Psychiatric Association.

Bolton, D. (2008). *What is Mental Disorder? An essay in philosophy, science and values.* Oxford: Oxford University Press.

Charney, D., Barlow, D., Botteron, K., et al. (2002). Neuroscience research agenda to guide development of a pathophysiologically based classification system. In D.J.

Kupfer, M.B. First, and D.A. Regier (eds.) *A Research Agenda for DSM-V*, pp 31–84. Washington, DC: American Psychiatric Association.

Foley, D.L., Neale, M.C., Gardner, C., et al. (2003). Major depression and associated impairment: same or different genetic and environmental risk factors? *American Journal of Psychiatry*, **160**, 2128–2133.

Insel, T. (2013). Director's Blog: Transforming diagnosis. At http://www.nimh.nih.gov/about /director/2013/transforming-diagnosis.shtml. Retrieved December 3, 2015.

Narrow, W., Kuhl, E., and **Regier, D.** (2009). DSM-V perspectives on disentangling disability from clinical significance. *World Psychiatry*, **8**, 88–89.

Spitzer, R.L. and **Williams, J.B.** (1982). The definition and diagnosis of mental disorder. In W.R. Grove (ed.), *Deviance and Mental Illness*, pp. 15–31. Beverly Hills, CA: Sage.

Üstün, B and **Kennedy, C.** (2009). What is functional impairment? Disentangling disability from clinical significance. *World Psychiatry*, **8**, 82–85.

World Health Organization (1992). *The ICD-10 Classification of Mental and Behavioural Disorders: Clinical Descriptions and Diagnostic Guidelines.* Geneva: World Health Organization.

Chapter 3

Distinguishing but not dissociating psychiatric disorder and impairment in functioning: Bolton, Hume, and sentiment

Peter Zachar

David Hume (1739/2000) argued that our ideas about moral goodness and badness are constituted by feelings of approval and disapproval. According to Hume, moral evaluations depend on *sentiment* and cannot be derived from reasoning alone. Sentiments are subjective. One way Hume expressed this claim was to write that

> [It is] not contrary to reason to prefer the destruction of the whole world to the scratching of my finger. [It is] not contrary to reason for me to choose my total ruin, to prevent the least uneasiness of [a] person wholly unknown to me (p. 267).

In Hume's larger philosophical program, our understanding of fact is also supported by subjective experience. Hume claimed that a *feeling of connection* between cause and effect helps constitute our experience of a mind-independent world and of facts. The feeling of connection is a secondary quality—or a vivid psychological impression. Although belief and assent in the factual has a subjective aspect, the feelings involved are not those of approval or disapproval.

Hume was trying to understand how we can believe in a mind-independent world on the basis of experience alone. According to him, our experience of cause and effect connects us to a past and a future that are beyond the present mental moment. This leads us to automatically expect that the present is like the past and the future will be like the present. The concepts of "mind-independence" and of "fact" share in this feature of being beyond what we happen to be experiencing now.

The distinction between objective facts and subjective values has traditionally been part of the motivation for disentangling mental disorder from impairment in social and occupational functioning (or disability). To claim that someone's functioning is impaired is to make a normative statement about what they *should* be able to do. Letting impairment define mental disorder, however, is to potentially reduce psychiatric diagnoses to assertions of disapproval.

One of the attractions of biomarkers is that they are objective indicators of a disorder—and not matters of disapproval. In theory biomarkers are in closer proximity to an underlying pathological process than symptoms—which some thinkers consider to represent surface features (Hyman 2010, Insel 2013). Hence the search for biomarkers has been deemed an important goal for establishing an objective, fact-based psychiatric nosology. Lacking biomarkers, however, the *Diagnostic and Statistical Manual of Mental Disorders* (DSM) uses symptom counts, degree of functional impairment, and subjective distress to (1) establish a threshold between the normal and the abnormal and (2) assess degree of severity.

A less metaphysical yet clinically compelling reason for disentangling mental disorder from impairment in functioning is to enrich our understanding of impairment. For instance, two people can have the same level of back pain but not be equally impaired. One of them may succumb to the pain and experience important activity limitations. The other might persevere and maintain functioning despite the pain. The same can be the case with depression and anxiety. Temperament, motivation, and degree of social support all moderate functioning in the presence of a psychiatric disorder (Foley et al. 2003, Sartorius 2009). According to this line of thought, conceiving of impairments in functioning as inherent features of psychiatric disorder is to misunderstand, even simplify them.

Given the above considerations, the usefulness of distinguishing between psychiatric disorder and functional impairment should not garner much controversy. One of the virtues of Bolton's chapter is to also show that it is a mistake to set ourselves the goal of completely dissociating them.

According to Bolton, the function of the central nervous system (CNS) is to regulate action in the external world. Therefore, it is not possible to identify a failure of normal CNS function in the absence of activity limitations. Very importantly, discovering biomarkers will not eliminate the role of impairment in our understanding of psychiatric dysfunction because any biomarker is only a "marker" of a psychiatric dysfunction if it indexes some kind of activity limitation.

If this is the case, how can it be, as suggested above, that someone can have a diagnosable psychiatric disorder but not experience either occupational or social impairment? For any putative psychiatric dysfunction, we are more confident in labeling it dysfunctional if there is either an unexpected decline in functioning (as in psychosis), or a failure to develop and mature in typical ways (as in autism). All individuals, however, possess a combination of vulnerabilities and resources. Psychiatric symptom clusters are part of this larger network. With the right supply of resources, some people can, with effort, maintain functioning despite having a diagnosable disorder. However, the *potential* for impairment seems to be an inherent feature of the concept of psychiatric dysfunction.

Yet, the goal of immunizing our menu of psychiatric disorders from biased value judgments about what is normal and what is impaired remains worthwhile. One way to think about this is to ask whether evaluative statements about what someone *should* be able do can be translated into non-normative language composed of factual statements. The usual strategy among philosophers is to propose a theory of natural functioning. For example Christopher Boorse (1977, 2014) claims that a natural function is

- the statistical average functioning in some group (presumably a factual issue) that
- makes a positive contribution to survival or reproduction (also a matter of statistical probabilities).

For Boorse, a dysfunction refers to an internal state that interferes with natural functioning—or reduces functional ability. Although we are strongly inclined to elaborate upon these objective dysfunctions with normative language involving "should" and "should nots," according to Boorse we need not do so.

Once you fix a norm for some natural function, then whether or not that norm is met can become a matter of fact (Putnam 1987). One criticism of norm fixing is to question the considerations used to select a norm (Ereshefsky 2009, Kingma 2013). Another problem is that even if the discipline agreed to fix survival or reproduction as the normative standards, those concepts remain obscure enough to be elaborated upon in different ways. For instance, if the natural function of sex is to have children, one might be inclined to consider being gay or lesbian as dysfunctional. If the natural function of sex is also to promote intimacy and pair-bonding, then not. In fact, the discovery that gay sex is not invariably compulsive and lacking in pleasure, but contributes to the establishment of lasting intimacy, was an important factor in its being removed from the DSM (Bayer 1987, Zachar and Kendler 2012).

The natural function approach is aspirational. It has very little to do with the factors that have actually been used to make disorder attributions in psychiatry. Unfortunately, some factors we do rely upon can make attributions of psychiatric disorder subject to all kinds of normative assumptions.

Taking inspiration from Hume, one factor we rely on is sentiment. For instance, a feeling on the part of the person with a "disorder" or their friends and family that something has gone awry is part of the phenomenology of many psychiatric disorders. As Bolton (2013) said elsewhere, a feeling that impairment or distress has become unmanageable is often what motivates people to seek professional help. Such feelings could be considered secondary qualities, not with respect to experiences of facticity or of moral evaluation, but with respect to the experience of psychiatric disorder. The strength of such feelings may partly underlie opposition to Szasian claims about mental illness being a myth.

This tentative supposition needs more work, both conceptually and empirically. The initial feeling might be more akin to puzzlement or confusion. The feeling that things are not as they should be is not a moral "should." Feelings of approbation may occur in due course, and the awry can become the "wrong." When this transition occurs, it can occasion worries about psychiatry being a tool for moral disapproval.

All kinds of cultural, religious, political, and ethical norms can feed into an impression that something has gone awry. This can result in value judgments biased with respect to these norms, such as seeing homosexuality, masturbation, or attempting to escape from slavery as mental diseases (Cartwright 1851/2004, Socarides 1973, Engelhardt 1974,). It is even likely that future generations will come to see some of our current judgments about the abnormal as inappropriately biased as well.

Horwitz and Wakefield (2007, 2012) have suggested that because certain aspects of psychological normality are universal, people have a shared capacity to detect psychological dysfunction. In places they suggest that we share cognitive mechanisms for detecting failure of natural functions. Less elaborately, one could just say that people across the world develop similar, habitual expectations about what is normal, and these expectations result in some shared impressions about things going awry.

About the importance of improving upon our initial impressions with conceptual analysis, Horwitz and Wakefield are on target. One would also hope that conceptual analysis can refine and improve upon our impressions. For instance, we may be biased not to accept variation as normal—both variation between individuals and between environments. Scientifically informed conceptual analysis in particular can teach us that the different and the confusing is not necessarily the disordered.

References

Bayer, R. (1987). *Homosexuality and American Psychiatry: The politics of diagnosis.* Princeton, NJ: Princeton University Press.

Bolton, D. (2013). What is mental illness? In K.W.M. Fulford, M. Davies, R.G.T. Gipps, et al. (eds.) *The Oxford Handbook of Philosophy and Psychiatry*, pp. 434–450. New York: Oxford University Press.

Boorse, C. (1977). Health as a theoretical concept. *Philosophy of Science*, **44**, 542–573.

Boorse, C. (2014). A second rebuttal on health. *Journal of Medicine and Philosophy*, **39**, 683–724.

Cartwright, S.A. (1851/2004). Diseases and physical peculiarities of the negro race. In A.L. Caplan, J.J. McCartney, and D.A. Sisti (eds.) *Health, Disease, and Illness*, pp. 28–39. Washington, DC: Georgetown University Press.

Engelhardt, H.T., Jr. (1974). The disease of masturbation: values and the concept of disease. *Bulletin of the History of Medicine*, **48**, 234–248.

Ereshefsky, M. (2009). Defining health and disease. *Studies in History and Philosophy of Biological and Biomedical Sciences*, **40**, 221–227.

Foley, D.L., **Neale, M.C.**, **Gardner, C.O.**, **Pickles, A.**, and **Kendler, K.S.** (2003). Major depression and associated impairment: Same or different genetic and environmental risk factors? *American Journal of Psychiatry*, **160**, 2128–2133.

Horwitz, A.V. and **Wakefield, J.C.** (2007). *The Loss of Sadness: How psychiatry transformed normal sorrow into depressive disorder.* New York: Oxford University Press.

Horwitz, A.V. and **Wakefield, J.** (2012). *All We Have To Fear: Psychiatry's transformation of natural anxieties into mental disorders.* Oxford: Oxford University Press.

Hume, D. (1739/2000). *A Treatise of Human Nature.* Oxford: Oxford University Press.

Hyman, S.E. (2010). The diagnosis of mental disorders: The problem of reification. *Annual Review of Clinical Psychology*, **6**, 155–179.

Insel, T. (2013). Director's Blog: Transforming diagnosis. Retrieved from http://www.nimh.nih.gov/about/director/2013/transforming-diagnosis.shtml.

Kingma, E. (2013). Naturalist accounts of mental disorder. In K.W.M. Fulford, M. Davies, R.G.T. Gipps, et al. (eds.) *The Oxford Handbook of Philosophy and Psychiatry*, pp. 363–384. New York: Oxford University Press.

Putnam, H. (1987). *The Many Faces of Realism*. Peru, IL: Open Court.

Sartorius, N. (2009). Disability and mental illness are different entities and should be assessed separately. *World Psychiatry*, **8**, 86–86.

Socarides, C.W. (1973). Homosexuality: Findings derived from 15 years of clinical research. *American Journal of Psychiatry*, **130**, 1212–1213.

Zachar, P. and **Kendler, K.S.** (2012). The removal of Pluto from the class of planets and homosexuality from the class of psychiatric disorders: A comparison. *Philosophy, Ethics, and Humanities in Medicine*, 7, 4.

Section 2

Psychometric models in psychiatric nosology

Chapter 4

Introduction to "The hard question in psychiatric nosology"

Josef Parnas and Kenneth S. Kendler

Dr. Eric Turkheimer is a clinical psychologist, psychometrician, behavior geneticist, and a theoretician well known for provocative and fertile insights into a wide range of psychological, genetic, and measurement questions. He has a good grasp of the clinical phenomenon of psychopathology but has also managed to stay out of the fray surrounding the *Diagnostic and Statistical Manual of Mental Disorders* (DSM) and so is in an excellent position to provide this thought-provoking commentary.

His essay, while demanding, will pay-back careful reading. In it, Turkheimer examines the basic principles and criteria according to which we try to classify mental disorders. At each step, he tries to illuminate to what extent a given classificatory object is something "natural" or a construct of our own cognitive activity.

This essay raises more points than we can hope to note in this brief introduction. Here is a selection of what readers will confront. Turkheimer introduces a lovely term, "MBA"—*meaningful but arbitrary.* It well captures a lot of what people ask about in the DSM. Why is the duration of major depression set at 2 weeks—why not 1, 3, or 4? Why do you need 5 out of 9 symptoms for major depression but only 2 out of 11 for alcohol use disorder? In each case there is a rationale, but we often do not have strong arguments as to why specifically "here" but not "there." We now have a quick, succinct answer—"it's MBA."

Turkheimer talks about maps. Mostly he is interested in the big picture in the DSM—how do different disorders relate to one another? In DSM-5 jargon, this was called the "meta-structure" question. Compared to the thousands of hours of debate about specific diagnostic criteria for individual disorders or the inclusion or exclusion of newly proposed categories, quite modest amounts of time were taken up by meta-structure issues in DSM-5. Indeed, meta-structure questions in DSM-5 were removed from the purview of the Scientific Review Committee. This was decided by the DSM-5 leadership as they wanted to have the freedom to align the DSM-5 structure as much as possible with that of the 11th edition of the *International Classification of Diseases* (ICD-11). Empirical issues were a secondary concern for them.

For us, reading this essay highlights the differences in culture between the world of medicine—where we see things in binary categories (ill vs. well, admit to the hospital or send home, treat or not treat)—and the world of psychology with its long tradition of quantitative scale scores (think IQ, MMPI, or EPQ) and the associated increasingly sophisticated psychometric theories. One of us (KSK) has been in thousands of hours of DSM discussions and can report that the amount of time in those meetings that involved psychometric issues is well below 1%. As we see in this essay, Paul Meehl was the rare individual—with no parallel major figure in psychiatry—who lived in both psychometric and clinical arenas and worked hard to try to reconcile them.

One of the several sobering points of this essay is the problem of the indeterminacy of factor analysis. Not being deeply trained in the history of this method, one of us (KSK) recalls in his early exposure thinking that all you had to do was click on one of the variety of rotations (Varimax was the most popular in those days) and bingo—factor loadings appear. Only much later did it become clear that it was not that simple at all. Indeed, whatever rotation you pick it reflects another example of MBA.

Although it is not openly noted, we cannot avoid seeing an underlying philosophical thread running through this essay—the classic realism vs. pragmatism (or instrumentalism) debate in the philosophy of science. Are diagnostic categories real things out there in the world or practical tools we develop because they help us decide on treatment, predict prognosis, or correlate well with our MRI scans? Using more of Turkheimer's language, are the divisions between our diagnoses all MBA—where the lines are chosen because they work for us in a practical sense, not because they reflect some critical features of nature? Or, are there taxons out there in the world that we need to be smart enough to try to detect given all the inevitable messiness involved? There is, in our view, a healthy tension between these two views of the underlying nature of psychiatric disorders.

Turkheimer's attempt to rethink the basic structures of classification is undoubtedly prompted by the persisting lack of solid findings linking phenotypic dimensions or categories to hypothetical neurobiological substrates. The essential message in Turkheimer's review of the processes of classification is that it is easy to forget that many steps in these processes, such as results from mathematical analysis, do not reflect nature as it truly is. Rather, many pragmatic and other psychological influences have been operating from the start.

Turkheimer generally advocates the view that the reality which we perceive in psychiatry and psychology is always infused with our own cognitive contributions and is not a reality in itself, independent of human subjectivity. Truth and objectivity is a matter of intersubjectivity rather than noumenal reality. This view eliminates a position of strong realism and tempers our reductive enthusiasm. Indeed, Turkheimer would likely argue that the domain of human behavior with its cultural entanglements has a complexity that is likely to defy any simple reductionist project.

Chapter 5

The hard question in psychiatric nosology

Eric Turkheimer

5.1 Introduction

As the chapters in this book will no doubt serve to remind us, nosology represents many things to psychiatry. It is a repository of its history, a crucible for its theories and controversies. Systems of classification crystallize the scientific content of psychiatry at any given moment. Indeed, the very fact of nosological systems—that they exist at all—is emblematic of psychiatry's status as a basic science and branch of medicine. Prior to any of these historical and foundational roles, however, psychiatric classification is an exercise in grouping like with like, an activity referred to as taxonomy, clustering, or cladistics. Taxonomy is a distinct, technical, and well-developed field in biology and statistics. Any given system of psychiatric nosology, in addition to its implicit or explicit commitments to ideas about the genesis of disordered behavior, represents at the same time a set of choices about taxonomic methods per se.

To those of us who work somewhat outside the complex institutional scientific processes that go into producing a *Diagnostic and Statistical Manual of Mental Disorders* (DSM),[1] what often seems most opaque is the ambiguous relationship the process of designing a diagnostic system bears to the actual science, mathematics, and philosophy of classifying syndromes or people. After the reams of scientific studies have been conducted, their findings pored over by the scientific review committees, the recommendations exposed to communities of scientists, practitioners, and consumers, the final decisions about psychiatric nosology are made by committees. The categories that result, with their familiar structure of (for example) seven out of ten criteria required to establish a diagnosis, are nosologically neither fish nor fowl. The DSM, with its understandable focus on conducting the real-world business of psychiatry, often seems unwilling to get bogged down

[1] Throughout this essay I (a clinical psychologist by training) will adopt the convention used throughout the book of referring to the problem at hand as, "psychiatric nosology." Needless to say, psychiatry does not actually own the issue (although it literally owns the DSM); in the long run I would be more comfortable characterizing the problem as the classification of psychopathology.

in the theoretical and technical details of what it is actually up to. The goal of this essay is to examine some of those issues.

5.2 Nature's joints

One metaphor in particular has been used over and over again to describe psychiatry's aspiration to science via nosology: "To carve nature at its [or sometimes, morbidly, her] joints." The image comes from Plato, in a discussion, remarkably, of the nature of love and madness. Plato has Socrates making the rhetorical point that clear conceptual analysis requires what in the modern era has come to be called—considerably less elegantly—lumping and splitting. The lumping principle is

> That of perceiving and bringing together in one idea the scattered particulars, that one may make clear by definition the particular thing which he wishes to explain; just as now, in speaking of Love, we said what he is and defined it, whether well or ill. Certainly by this means the discourse acquired clearness and consistency.

The opposite principle involves carving:

> That of dividing things again by classes, where the natural joints are, and not trying to break any part, after the manner of a bad carver.

Carving nature at its joints has become the defining metaphor of psychiatric nosology, a scientific assumption so ingrained that its implications are never examined. Given a rich but superficial (in the non-pejorative sense suggested by the study of descriptive psychopathology) set of observations of the mentally ill, how can one build a classification structure that reflects and reveals the unobserved internal structures that give the patients their outward appearances? Put that way, the appeal to joint-carving seems obvious, a description not only of nosological methodology but of science itself. Yet many difficult theoretical and statistical problems attend this apparently straightforward metaphor. This essay will examine the nosological problem in light of the contributions of two of the last century's great thinkers about complex human systems, one a methodologist and psychometrician, the other a psychologist and psychopathologist. What they have in common is a concern with exactly when and how nosological systems of psychopathology are constrained by data.

5.3 Maps

"Wait a second," you may say. "Shouldn't the selection of nosological systems be completely determined by scientific data?" Constraining nosological decisions with scientific observations might seem to be the whole point of the exercise, but the answer to the question is no: important parts of nosological systems are indeterminate in the face of scientific data. Figure 5.1 is a map of Virginia.[2] The map

---

[2] This figure and much of this section is based on ideas described in Turkheimer et al. (2008), which in turn leaned heavily on Maraun (1997).

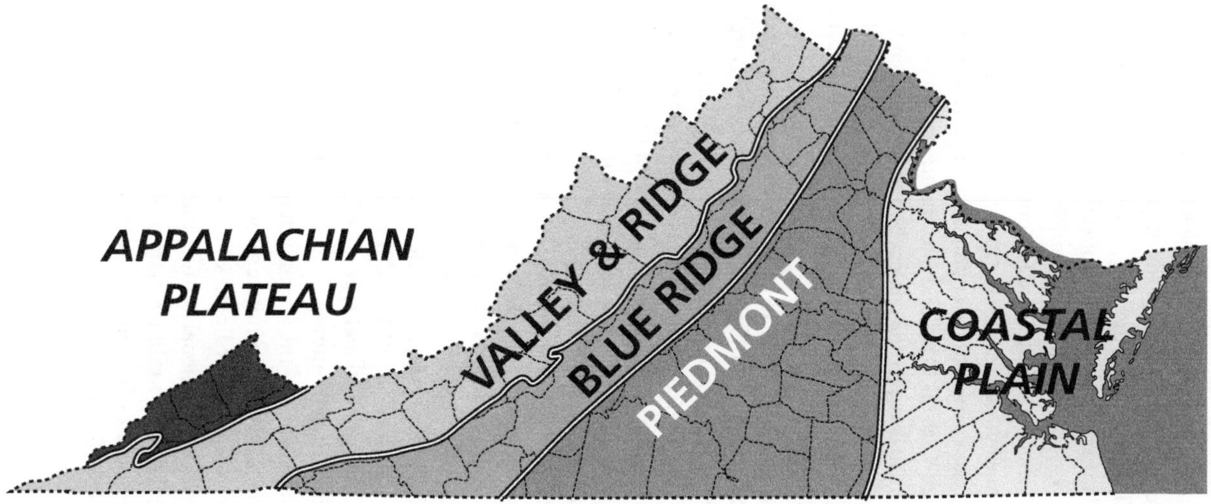

Figure 5.1 A map of Virginia, divided into meaningful but arbitrary (MBA) regions.

divides the state into five geographic regions: Coastal Plain, Piedmont, Blue Ridge, Valley & Ridge, and Appalachian Plateau. What is the scientific status of these regions? They are certainly not imaginary or completely arbitrary: the Coastal Plain region is closer to the Atlantic Ocean than the others, the Piedmont has distinct geological properties, and the Blue Ridge is mountainous. It would be an error in scientific geography to locate the mountains on the Atlantic coast.

As regards other aspects of the map, however, the relations among surface, structure, and data are not so clear. Consider, for example, the location of the line that divides Coastal Plain from the Piedmont. There are reasons the artist drew the line where it is, but those reasons are only partly scientific. The line demarcates—somewhat arbitrarily—a transition between regions that is in fact gradual. It would not occur to us to conduct scientific research to find the correct boundary between Coastal Plain and Piedmont, any more than we would collect geological data to discover the correct boundary between Virginia and North Carolina. To some extent, the line goes where we want it to go, where it is expedient for us to put it. In Turkheimer et al. (2008) we suggested that such lines be called "meaningful but arbitrary," or MBA.[3]

The regional map of Virginia is MBA in another important sense, as well. Obviously, geology is not the only basis for regionalizing Virginia; in fact there is an infinite number of ways to go about it. You could divide the map politically, into counties; or by climate, into hardiness zones for plants. Any such map would be a way of grouping like with like, earning it the M in MBA, but the lines between the regions, demarcating where you can or cannot get azaleas to overwinter, are arbitrary in our non-pejorative sense.

A final aspect of indeterminacy in maps is particularly important to the problem at hand: you do not have to divide maps into regions at all. In fact, if one wished to locate oneself in Virginia with as much precision as possible, the best way would not be to describe a location in terms of regions (I am in the Central Piedmont) but with latitude and longitude. Latitude and longitude are a (spherical, but we will ignore that and think about two-dimensional flat maps) coordinate system for describing a multidimensional space. As I noted they are in some ways more precise than regions in determining specific locations, but in fact they are just as MBA as any regionalization. The Greenwich meridian was not discovered in the bedrock; it was made up by a committee. From a mathematical point of view, there are an infinite number of coordinate systems that would describe multivariate space exactly as well as traditional latitude and longitude.

Whether one prefers a coordinate system or a regionalization depends on the task at hand. Coordinates are good for establishing precise individual locations. They are not so useful for tasks with more of an analog character. Where is tobacco

---

[3] Early readers of this manuscript were concerned that by using the word, "arbitrary" we are denigrating the use of such lines, but that is not at all what we intend. MBA lines depicting boundaries or dimensions are in fact very useful scientifically, as we will see in detail in the remainder of this essay.

grown in Virginia? One might be able to answer this question with a string of coordinates that define, dot-to-dot, lines around areas where tobacco is grown, but it is easier to simply draw analog lines around regions, while recognizing that their precise location is MBA.

5.4 Maps of psychopathology

It would be reasonable for a reader new to this topic to wonder what all the discussion of geographical maps has to do with the classification of psychopathology. The answer is this: nosological systems *are* maps of psychopathology. Given data demonstrating that the manifestation of schizophrenia is more like bipolar illness than either one is like antisocial personality disorder (ASPD), the task of the nosologist is to locate individuals in a virtual space that maintains as closely as possible the observed similarities among individuals. The remainder of this essay is about the relative roles of data, theory, and expedience in this process.

Nosological methods begin with a dissimilarity or distance matrix. In the converse of the example above, we could note that schizophrenia and bipolar illness are both more dissimilar to ASPD than they are to each other. This process can be repeated pairwise for all pairs of disorders (more generally referred to as stimuli), producing the lower half of a square matrix, as illustrated in Table 5.1. The diagonal of the matrix, the identity-dissimilarity of stimuli from themselves, can be reasonably set to zero; one can usually assume that the relations are symmetrical (the dissimilarity of A and B is the same as that of B and A) so the upper triangle of the matrix contains the same information as the lower. The numbers used to represent dissimilarity can take many forms. They might be (an inverse function of) correlation coefficients between symptom checklists for different disorders, or clinician ratings of the similarity or dissimilarity of individuals. The choice of an index of difference is one of the methodological choice points in nosology,

Table 5.1 Distances among ten stimuli

	1	2	3	4	5	6	7	8	9	10
Stimulus 1	0									
Stimulus 2	27.43	0								
Stimulus 3	29.15	9.19	0							
Stimulus 4	150.26	127.67	133.34	0						
Stimulus 5	51.16	31.13	39.15	99.09	0					
Stimulus 6	236.74	227.58	236.35	144.78	197.74	0				
Stimulus 7	38.15	20.62	29.58	112.11	13.02	206.97	0			
Stimulus 8	355.11	328.06	329.53	223.56	308.29	305.85	320.19	0		
Stimulus 9	28.60	2.03	7.54	127.85	32.04	228.90	22.04	327.25	0	
Stimulus 10	55.74	29.84	26.78	117.92	41.14	234.74	39.73	304.56	28.10	0

leading to different forms of classification in ways that will not be emphasized here. (Correlation coefficients, for the initiated, generally lead to factor analysis; more literal distances lead in the direction of methods like multidimensional scaling.)

The goal of nosology is to locate the stimuli on a map in a way that preserves, either strictly or more loosely (another choice point), the dissimilarities in the matrix. Figure 5.2 represents the distances from Table 5.1 on a two-dimensional map, with an outline sketched in to help us see what the stimuli actually represent. We see that a two-dimensional map of cities is a physical representation of the distance matrix among them, and that the distance matrix is no more than the matrices of driving distances that one used to find at the bottom of road maps.

The numerical distances in Table 5.1 are in fact two-dimensional straight-line distances among the cities, so the physical distances in Figure 5.2 reproduce them exactly. Had the numerical distances taken the spherical shape of the Earth into account, however, the three-dimensional city differences could not be perfectly represented on a flat map, and our solution would include error. We learn two important lessons from this. First, error, and the attempt to minimize it, is the crucial criterion for deciding whether we have created a good map. Second, we see that any given set of distances requires a certain degree of dimensionality in order to accurately represent them. Spherical geographic distances are inherently three dimensional, but they can be represented reasonably well in two dimensions. The definition of "reasonable" is up to us, and depends on what we are doing. For driving from Roanoke to Williamsburg, a two-dimensional representation is fine; for an astronomer, not so much. Higher dimensions always fit better, at the price of greater complexity. The art, as opposed to the science, of drawing maps consists in part of finding a useful way to balance dimensionality against complexity on the one hand and error on the other.

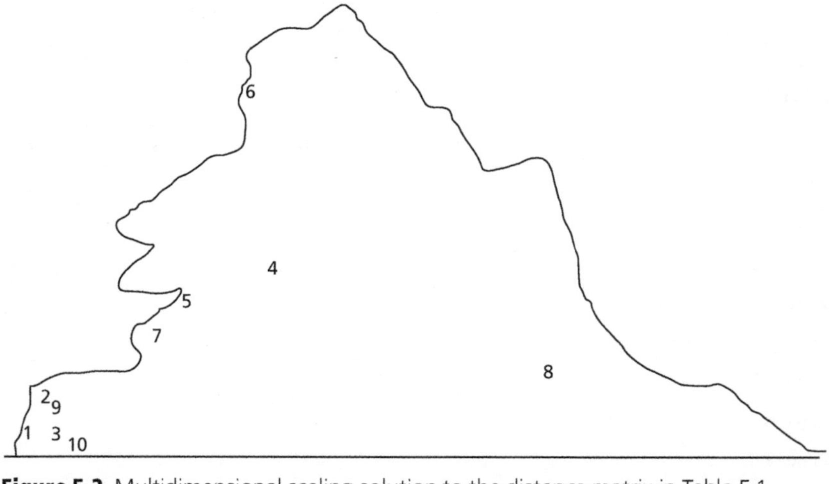

Figure 5.2 Multidimensional scaling solution to the distance matrix in Table 5.1. Stimuli represent cities in Virginia. Note that the map is oriented incorrectly, but that this does not affect the distances between cities.

The reader may have noticed that Figure 5.2 is oriented "incorrectly," with east and west reversed. In terms of reproducing the numerical distance matrix among the cities, however, orientation is arbitrary: north is not really on top, and an inverted map produces exactly the same set of distances. This property, called rotational indeterminacy, is a very important consideration in map creation. In fact, rotational indeterminacy is just another way of talking about the indeterminacy of latitude and longitude that we discussed at the outset. Any grid could be used to locate cities on a two-dimensional map, including grids for which the X and Y axes are not at right angles to each other. A similar arbitrariness, of course, would apply to any attempt to divide the country up into geographical regions: the relative geographical locations of the cities are fixed by their distances, but the exact location of a line dividing the Piedmont from the Mountain region is not.

A summary of the process of empirical map-building emphasizes the distinction between data-driven science and expedience-driven practicality. One uses some method to collect and represent data about the dissimilarity of a set of stimuli. One then investigates how well the resulting distance matrix can be represented in dimensionalities of increasing complexity, starting with one dimension (placing the stimuli on a line) and concluding with dimensionality equal to the number of stimuli. As dimensionality gets lower, and map-interpretation easier, the amount of error will increase. All of these steps are dictated by the data, in terms of the methodological choices the investigator has made. Then, in a transitional step, a decision must be made about the desired dimensionality of the derived map. This step is guided by data, in the empirical trade-off between complexity and error, but the optimal balance of the two is up to the investigator and will depend on the purpose of the analysis. Finally, decisions must be made about whether to represent locations on the map using dimensions (and if so how the dimensions should be located and oriented) or categorical constructions of some kind (and if so where the lines between the categories should be placed). This last step is not constrained by the data at all, at least by data internal to classification problem itself. (One might, for example, make decisions about a particular classification system in terms of feedback about the system's utility in the clinic, but such answers will always be expedient in nature, and will depend on the practical goals embraced by a particular researcher. Also see below.)

5.5 **Thurstone and Guttman**

The foregoing is actually a fairly subversive account of the conduct of multivariate classification procedures. In particular, the distinction between the part of the analysis that is determined by data (selection of a dimensionality for the solution and the positioning of like with like within the solution space) and the part that is not (the drawing of MBA lines to demarcate the space) is not widely maintained in modern practice. The reason is that a partial solution to the rotational indeterminacy problem, proposed by one of the founders of modern factor analysis, L. L. Thurstone (e.g., Thurstone 1940), has become so widely adopted that it is sometimes mistakenly viewed as a necessary part of psychometric methodology.

Simple structure is a criterion for locating the latitude and longitude lines that define a multivariate space. Although there are many numerical means of achieving simple structure, they all come down to drawing the lines so they fall as close as possible to the stimuli in the solution space. More precisely, the goal of simple structure is to produce a solution in which each stimulus has a substantial score on one dimension, and a zero score on the others. The concept is easiest to understand graphically. Figure 5.3 locates a set of points in a two-dimensional space. Where should the lines be drawn? The obvious answer is to draw them through the linear structures of points as they appear in the space. Doing so results in most of the points being located fairly far from zero on one of the axes (these locations are known in factor analysis as "loadings") and fairly close to zero on the others. One can then interpret the meaning of the simple structure dimensions in terms of the stimuli that have high loadings on them.

Although the simple structure procedure may appear natural, it remains MBA in two important senses. The first is that the preference for simple loadings, located close to the axes, is a matter of psychology and not mathematics. Humans find it easier to interpret simple structure dimensions and to conduct computations with a lot of simplifying zeroes, but computers do not care. The second reason simple structure solutions are MBA is empirical: in the real world, it would be very rare for actual data to produce a set of stimuli naturally aligned with an obvious simple structure criterion as is suggested in Figure 5.3 (Pettersson and Turkheimer 2010).

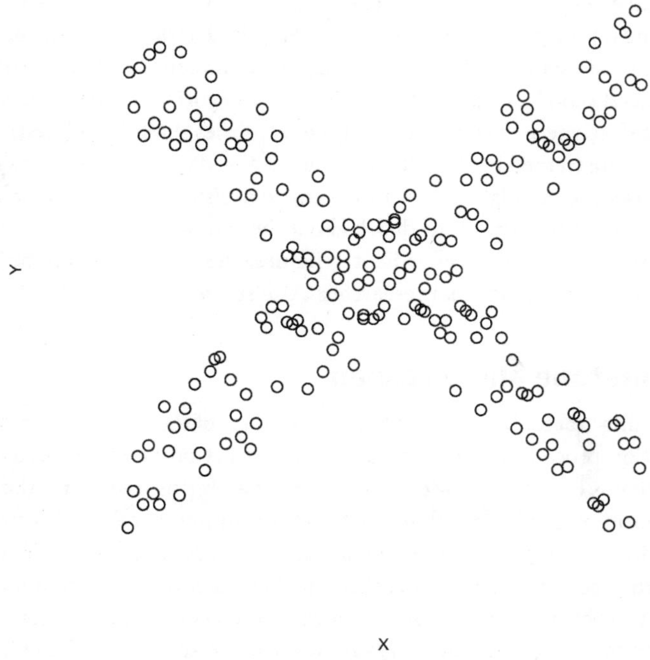

Figure 5.3 A set of stimuli in two-space with clear simple structure.

In fact, for many problems, stimuli wind up fairly uniformly distributed in the solution space, which means that no obvious simple structure solution will conform to them. Nevertheless, there is always some dimensional solution that comes *as close as possible* to providing a simple structure representation of the stimuli, and that solution, whatever it is, will do a perfectly good mathematical job of locating the points in space, because *any* set of dimensions will do a perfectly good mathematical job.

In Thurstone's time, locating simple structure axes was a laborious procedure conducted with pencil and paper or mechanical aids. The difficulty of conducting the analysis served to remind investigators that results often did not conform to simple structure at all, and as a result the wisdom of imposing simple structure was a matter of intense debate among the factor analysts of the middle of the last century. With the explosion of computing power that occurred thereafter, however, that difficulty evaporated, as investigators could rotate solutions to simple structure (or to some imperfect optimization of simple structure in smoothly distributed data) with a press of a button. Slowly but surely, it was forgotten that the resulting dimensions were a post-hoc MBA expedience, not a data-driven realization of a deeper scientific reality.

Another of the great mid-twentieth-century psychometricians, Louis Guttman, developed an alternative to the simple structure methods that came to dominate factor analysis (e.g., Guttman 1954). Guttman (see Figure 5.4) was a major figure in modern psychometrics, and his contributions extend far beyond what can be discussed here. He made important contributions to the mathematics of factor analysis, developed statistical alternatives to factor analysis, created an entire branch of measurement theory (his name is best known in the context of a "Guttman scale" for the measurement of psychological properties), and left an indelible mark on the study of personality and especially intelligence. Here, I want to focus on his

(a) (b)

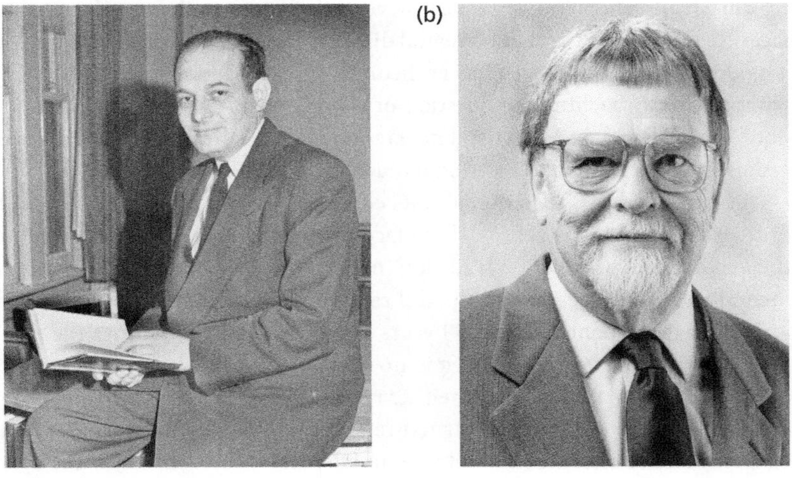

Figure 5.4 Louis Guttman (L) and Paul Meehl (R).
a) Louis Guttman Photo by Anthony Calvacca/New York Post Archives / © NYP Holdings, Inc. via Getty Images.
b) Paul Meehl Photo © University of Minnesota.

contribution to the metatheory of scientific investigation of complex multidimensional properties of human beings, with special attention, of course, on its application to psychopathology. In fact, the whole account of multivariate taxonomy as I have told it here relies heavily on Guttman's theorizing. In particular, the delineation of the role of data in quantifying the dimensionality of data and grouping like with like, as opposed to more contingent matters of line-drawing, is quite distinctly from Guttman.

Once Guttman separated the data-driven estimation of the location of stimuli in a space of some dimensionality from the orientation, division, and dimensionalization of that space, he worked to define a scientific method that focused on the former while conceding the indeterminacy of the latter. The most famous example of his method involves the color wheel (Shephard 1978). If you ask human subjects to rate the similarity of colored stimuli, and then endeavor to locate the matrix of pairwise perceptual distances in a multivariate space, it turns out that they can be located in a two-space, continuously distributed around a circular structure that Guttman called a circumplex. The color-circumplex has no simple structure, and attempting to rotate MBA axes to simple structure does obvious violence to its circularity, even while providing a mathematically acceptable fit. Similarly, Guttman (1991) showed that intelligence test scores have another two-dimensional structure, called a radex, which is a filled-in disk as opposed to an empty circle. In more complex domains of intelligence the radex becomes a three-dimensional cylindrex, and so forth.

Guttman (1982) developed a metatheory, called facet theory, to formalize the process of evaluating scientific hypotheses about multivariate structure. The details of facet theory are beyond the scope of this chapter, and it has never been seriously applied to psychiatric nosology in any event. What interests us here is the reason why psychopathologists have never turned to facet theory. The results of a facet-theoretic investigation of mental disorders would seem oddly incomplete to a modern psychopathologist. Facet theory focuses on the structure of a domain, without even broaching the question of *why* a domain has the structure that it does, especially not in terms of interpretations of MBA dimensions or clusters that are always undermined by rotational indeterminacy.

One can see this distinction and its consequences very clearly in the history of the science of intelligence, where facet theory has been widely deployed. In the classical factor-analytic tradition, upon observing that similarities among mental tests could be reasonably well represented by a single dimension called *g*, investigators spent the next 50 years trying to locate *g* in either the genome or the brain. But for Guttman, *g* is no more than an MBA construct embedded in a multivariate structure, neither requiring nor even permitting biological explanation. The multivariate structure of intelligence *is* intelligence. The goal of Guttman's science was to describe, in falsifiable ways, the structure of multivariate phenomena, but he had no particular commitment to the existence of anatomical joints in that structure, and in the final analysis no interest at all in carving them.

A Guttmanian perspective requires us to remember that any organizing system we may wish to impose on multivariate data is not a scientific given but either a contingent expediency (like latitude and longitude or the boundaries between geographic regions) or a falsifiable empirical hypothesis like simple structure. By extension (and here comes the pill that a scientific psychopathologist will have the most difficulty swallowing), the same logic applies to the assumption that an observed structure of psychiatric symptoms corresponds to a scientifically determined deep structure that explains why the surface characteristics appear as they do. (This idea, clearly, has deep connections to the network models described by Denny Boorsbom (Chapter 11), in which relations among surface characteristics rather than unobserved latent processes explain the structure of multivariate systems. I have reserved my comments on that topic for my discussion of Boorsbom's contribution in Chapter 12 of this volume.)

5.6 The taxometrics of Paul Meehl

Paul Meehl (Figure 5.4), roughly a contemporary of Guttman's, was unquestionably the foremost theoretical psychopathologist ever to emerge from clinical psychology. Meehl's concern with nosology started not with factor analysis, but with the related multivariate procedure of cluster analysis. Cluster analysis is much like factor analysis, but with a more specifically nosological point of view. It begins with the same data: a matrix of pairwise (dis)similarities among a set of stimuli. Rather than trying to locate the stimuli in a k-dimensional space, however, cluster analysis attempts to group the stimuli into clusters while optimizing some criterion of grouping like with like.

The theoretical difficulties underlying factor analysis and cluster analysis, however, are fundamentally the same. Clustering is like simple structure: it is not a necessary property of multivariate data. Most behavioral data do not arrive in what we would recognize as clusters, dense regions separated by relatively open space; complex multivariate data are usually smoothly distributed. But just like simple structure rotations, cluster-analytic procedures will always find an optimal clustering solution, regardless of whether anything resembling actual clustering is present. There is always some solution that produces the best possible clusters, even if it is not what the human eye might recognize as clustering. Finally, even if data *do* have intuitive clusters (like data that do seem to align along simple structure dimensions) the preference for organizing data that way is psychological, not mathematical. Clusters that violate an analog human sense of convenience do just as good a job for an indifferent digital computer.

Meehl had two commitments that Guttman did not. He was a dedicated psychopathologist, and as such was dissatisfied with a blanket conclusion that specifying the outwardly observable structure of psychopathology was a sufficient basis for a science. Surely, the goal of a science of psychopathology was to find the causes of structure, to identify and then to carve psychopathology's joints. Secondly, Meehl was an epistemological realist and a believer in neo-Popperian philosophy of science (Meehl 1978). He was troubled by cluster analysis precisely because it always produced clusters, so the existence of clusters (like the existence of simple structure dimensions) is not a falsifiable hypothesis. Throughout his career, for example, Meehl clung to a single-gene theory of schizophrenia that was, even at the time, obviously incorrect, but was at least falsifiable (Meehl 1962).

What Meehl required, then, was a falsifiable quantitative test of the existence of joints in a multivariate anatomy. To that end he dedicated the second half of his career to what he called taxometrics, or, more specifically, coherent cut kinetics (Meehl 1995). We will skip the statistical details more or less completely, noting only that the method involves examining the joint distributions of multiple indicators of a latent trait. What interests us here is not so much the statistical details of the method, but rather its motivation. Meehl wanted to find natural kinds, what he called "types," or "taxa." And for his search to mean anything, the taxa in question could not be required theoretically to exist, like simple structure and cluster solutions. The object of his search was not MBA expediencies imposed on smooth multivariate data, but on actual structural discontinuities:

> Roughly, then, I mean by a "type" or a "taxon" a class entity having a nonarbitrary basis of categorization, that is, not simply a conjunction of attributes that one might impose conventionally for some useful communicative or administrative purpose [cf. MBA], but a class of persons that really belong together, a classification punchily expressed by the metaphor that we wish, as Plato said, "to carve nature at its joints." (Meehl 1979, p. 566)

He contended, first, that as a practical matter cluster analysis had failed:

> We have here a mind-boggling fact: No accepted entry in psychopathology has owed its initial *discovery* to formal clustering methods, whether those invented by psychologists, biologists, or statisticians. (Meehl 1979, p. 567, emphasis in original).

This is in contrast to non-psychiatric medicine in which widely accepted disease entities abound, many of them discovered before their etiological foundation was fully understood. The standard example, used as a test case for the mathematical methods, was biological sex, which (this being a simpler time) was taken as an obviously dichotomous latent variable (Golden and Meehl 1980). Could one detect an underlying male–female dichotomy in a mixed bag of personality, psychopathology, and attitude scales that each varied continuously with a masculine–feminine dimension? Often, it seemed, one could. The task, then, was to discover whether other observable multivariate forms of behavior—like schizophrenia—with their apparently smooth and continuous shadings from one form into the next, were in fact only the superficial manifestations of a deeper reality with real, carvable joints.

5.7 Conclusions

5.7.1 Psychiatry without taxa

Meehl's statistical work on this topic was complete by the mid 1990s. In the 25 years that have followed, investigators have searched high and low for taxa, but it is not clear that a replicable one has ever been found. There is some evidence for the taxonic structure for the Meehlian construct of schizotypy, but that is hotly contested; recent reviews have detected some evidence for eating disorders or attention deficit disorders, but the overall tone of recent reviews is quite skeptical. What has the apparent absence of latent taxa demonstrated about the nature of psychiatric nosology? In the remainder of this paper I will contend that starting with Meehl himself, its implications have been misconstrued, and that the real consequences of psychiatry without taxa may be more radical than what has been generally acknowledged.

The simplest answer to the question of why taxometrics has failed to find any taxa is that there are no taxa to find. Meehl actually considered the possibility:

> Some believe that the main reason our methods [Meehl is referring to cluster analysis and related methods] haven't been earthshakingly successful in psychopathology is that the model is wrong, that there aren't any entities analogous to measles, mumps and cholera. I don't believe that for the major psychoses, for the psychopath, and for one or two of the neuroses. (Meehl 1979, p. 568)

Meehl did not say why he thought this, but we know that his belief about schizophrenia—that it was under the strong influence of a single dominant gene—was incorrect.

Meehl's position here is a version of the "gloomy prospect" move in behavioral genetics, after a famous passage by Plomin and Daniels (1987), in which they articulated the possibility that the genetics of complex phenotypes might be so complex and non-additive as to resist any attempt to develop coherent genetic explanations. They decided that it could not be true, because the scientific consequences were too awful. In a similar way, Kendler (2013), in the previous volume of this series, developed a thoughtful approach to evaluating when a complex phenotype might or might not comprise a coherent mechanism at a genetic level of analysis, but then pre-emptively dismissed the possibility that such a thing might occur.

5.7.2 Dimensions versus categories

Discussions of the absence of taxa in psychiatry have generally located the problem in the context of an old controversy about whether it is preferable to conduct nosology in terms of diagnostic categories, as has traditionally been the case, as opposed to using models with continuous dimensions to locate behaviors or people in psychopathology space. This, in fact, is how Meehl saw it:

> For me, the purpose of taxometric procedures is [again!] to carve nature at its joints, to identify the real underlying taxonic entities whose conjectured existence motivates a classification rather than a dimensional approach. (Meehl 1979, p. 568)

Traditional nosological systems in psychiatry have always used categories, supported by ad hoc "six out of nine" diagnostic systems, for reasons that mostly have to do with inertia and easy analogy to diagnostic categories in non-psychiatric medicine.

But if taxometric analysis shows that there are no latent categories underlying observed psychiatric symptoms, the argument goes, would it not make more sense to quantify the multivariate space in terms of continuous dimensions, some variety of psychiatric latitude and longitude? Pressure in this direction has mounted during recent revisions of the DSM, originating most strongly from domains outside psychiatry like clinical psychology, with deeper roots in psychometrics, factor analysis, and Meehl. During the DSM-V revision there was a proposal for completely reorganizing the personality disorders using a categorical system, but it was eventually rejected.[4] (For more details about this sad story see Chapter 35 in this book by Zachar.)

The most comprehensive account of the search for psychiatric taxa is by Haslam et al. (2012). They conducted a meta-analysis of 311 results reported in 177 articles. They did find that some taxa were reliably reported, but more frequently in older articles with weaker methodology. Controlling for methodological strength, they estimated that 14% of studies produced evidence for taxa. Such taxa as were found related to schizotypy (a construct that was *created* to be a taxon), drug addiction, and autism. What concerns us here, however, is how the absence of taxa were interpreted. The first sentence of the abstract of Haslam et al. states, "Taxometric research methods were developed by Paul Meehl and colleagues to distinguish between categorical and dimensional models of latent variables." Meehl's intentions notwithstanding, this sentence misstates what taxometric models actually do. A Guttmanian perspective on the organization of multivariate space suggests that it is an oversimplification to view the absence of replicable Meehlian taxa as a victory for dimensions over categories. Dimensions, just like categories, are MBA, impossible to locate decisively on the basis of psychometric data alone. Taxometric models test whether latent distributions are distributed categorically or *continuously*, and the point of the current essay can be summed up as follows: continuous multivariate distributions do not need to be parameterized *dimensionally*. Indeed, they can be parameterized using either MBA categories or MBA dimensions, chosen according to the researcher's intentions, not the data.

Return for a moment to two-dimensional maps of physical space. Geography is literally continuous, but there is no inherent reason to prefer dimensional latitude and longitude over categorical state lines as a method for organizing it; they do different things well and suffer from exactly the same problems of MBA indeterminacy. The existence of meaningful simple structure dimensions is just as much an empirical hypothesis as the existence of real taxonic boundaries, and there is just as little evidence that any such dimensions actually exist in more than an MBA sense.

---

[4] The reasons for the unproductive kerfuffle that broke out over Axis II might be considerably elucidated by the analysis offered here, but that is a topic for another paper.

One influential line of research, for example, has shown that matrices of covariances among symptoms or syndromes of psychopathology can usually be fit reasonably well by factor models in two dimensions, and that these two factors can be rotated to a simple structure aligning with dimensions that can be characterized as "internalization" and "externalization" (Krueger 1999). It does not diminish the importance or apparent generality of this conclusion to note that these dimensions are MBA, dependent for their existence on simple structure criteria that do not compel any particular rotation. It is unlikely, therefore, that such a dimensional model can deliver on Krueger's promise of reducing the arbitrariness and comorbidity inherent in traditional categorical models. If one wanted, one could establish mutually exclusive boundaries in two-space that would eliminate comorbidity by decree; in the same way, one could dimensionalize psychopathological two-space with oblique dimensions that permitted covariance between the dimensions that presumably form the "common substrates" of psychopathology. Internalizing and externalizing are not substrates, with the implication of biological reality. They are dimensions, convenient statistical abstractions. We only think of rotated factors as being more natural than category boundaries because they emerge so effortlessly from the computer programs that rotate them into existence.

Taking Meehl seriously necessitates tackling the hard question of whether observed psychiatric syndromes can be understood as high-level representations of real taxa at lower levels, and leads to a consideration of whether we are asking too much. We have tried and failed to develop crisp biological models so many times that the realistic theorist should recognize by now that it is not going to happen. Depression is not mumps, and notwithstanding Meehl's optimism it is clear by now that schizophrenia is not either. Some modern theorists have abandoned the effort for universal and comprehensive biological accounts of psychiatric entities in favor of more limited models, in which local reductions of circumscribed parts of complex entities can be related to discrete biological events (Schaffner 2006, Kendler 2012). There exist relatively specific genetic, neurological, or otherwise biological events that produce instances of psychosis or affective disturbance, even as they fail to explain the disorders in general. Other syndromes, such as Alzheimer's disease, are occasionally caused by genes of large effect, even if they remain biologically blurry in the population. This line of thinking leads quickly to very difficult questions about the possibilities for reductive theory-building in psychiatry that we cannot address here. For present purposes, the point is that a step back from the possibility of comprehensive explanation entails a step back from decisive determination of nosological systems; indeed, they are the same problem.

One could envision a purely Guttmanian, facet-theoretic science of psychopathology, in which the object of research was not large- or small-scale reduction across levels, but simply specification of multivariate structure as it is found. Turkheimer et al. (2008), for example, described a two-dimensional structure for the personality disorders, and showed how it could be used to synthesize the long-standing opposition between dimensional and categorical diagnostic systems. Such an outcome seems unlikely for major psychopathology, even though the two-factor models of internalizing and externalizing could easily be extended in that direction, if they could be freed from their needless reliance on simple structure rotations. As has already been mentioned, the network models of Boorsbom and colleagues offer some other possibilities.

Another direction in which all of this could lead is the Research Domain Criteria, or RDoC (Cuthbert 2015). In many ways the RDoC approach is the opposite of facet theory: instead of making the surface structure of psychopathology the ultimate object of study, RDoC proposes to ignore it, in favor of inter-level explanations of local phenomena. What facet theory and RDoC have in common is skepticism about the Meehlian project of identifying promising inter-level explanations on the basis of clues in the surface structure. But whereas in facet theory the surface structure was promoted as the answer itself, not something to be explained at a lower level of analysis, from the point of view of RDoC if one can specify empirical reductions the higher-level surface structure no longer matters. This is a longer path than can be embarked on at the end of a long essay, but I will say this: I am sympathetic with the notion that "affective disorder" as a full-blown entity is very unlikely to correspond to a well-specified structure (thinking biologically) in the brain or genome or to a non-arbitrary dimension or taxon (thinking psychometrically). I am less willing to give up on the idea that the observable structure of psychopathology may contain important clues to how the system actually works, and to insist that the widespread failure to identify low-level mechanisms that provide crisp explanations of high-level behavior—RDoC or no RDoC—may well be nature's way of informing us that there *are* no low-level mechanisms, no dimensions and no taxa, to be discovered. Greater interest in the high-level structure of psychiatric phenomenology might be a healthy tonic for the aggressive and unnecessary reductionism that RDoC often seems to entail (Parnas 2015).

5.7.3 **Carving Mother Nature**

In a literal sense, (human) nature has to have joints; we are, after all, not that different from the beasts we butcher, in the kitchen or in the lab. This reminds us, however, that there are no melancholic cows, and that we do not butcher humans. Why not? The genesis of human behavior is more complex than that of cows, and somehow our valuation of that complexity precludes human joint-carving for reasons both scientific and ethical. The persistent and scientifically frustrating absence of deep biological structures that explain human function is explained, in part, by the ethical impermissibility of experimental procedures that might otherwise be used to expose them. Our inability or refusal to carve the joints of human nature is both the curse and the blessing of a science that applies itself to domains lacking ready analogs in lower animals. A good veterinarian might be a pretty good orthopedist and could get by as a neurologist, but a veterinarian could be only the most rudimentary psychiatrist. Subjectively, the surface of human behavior is phenomenology; objectively it is meaning. Commitment to phenomenology and meaning, despite their scientific impenetrability, is the indelible mark of a human science.

References

Cuthbert, B.N. (2015). Research Domain Criteria: toward future psychiatric nosologies. *Dialogues in Clinical Neuroscience*, 17, 89.

Golden, R.R. and **Meehl, P.E.** (1980). Detection of biological sex: An empirical test of cluster methods. *Multivariate Behavioral Research*, **15**, 475–496.

Guttman, L. (1954). A new approach to factor analysis: The radex. In P.F. Lazarsfeld (ed.) *Mathematical Thinking in the Social Sciences*, pp. 258–348. Glenco, IL: Free Press.

Guttman, L. (1982). Facet theory, smallest space analysis, and factor analysis. *Perceptual and Motor Skills*, **54**, 487–493.

Guttman, L. and **Levy, S.** (1991). Two structural laws for intelligence tests.*Intelligence*, **15**, 79–103.

Haslam, N., **Holland, E.**, and **Kuppens, P.** (2012). Categories versus dimensions in personality and psychopathology: a quantitative review of taxometric research. *Psychological Medicine*, **42**, 903–920.

Kendler, K.S. (2012). The dappled nature of causes of psychiatric illness: Replacing the organic–functional/hardware–software dichotomy with empirically based pluralism. *Molecular Psychiatry*, 17, 377–388.

Kendler, K.S. (2013). What psychiatric genetics has taught us about the nature of psychiatric illness and what is left to learn. *Molecular Psychiatry*, **18**, 1058–1066.

Krueger, R.F. (1999). The structure of common mental disorders. *Archives of General Psychiatry*, **56**, 921–926.

Maraun, M.D. (1997). Appearance and reality: Is the big five the structure of trait descriptors? *Personality and Individual Differences*, **22**, 629–647.

Meehl, P.E. (1962). Schizotaxia, schizotypy, schizophrenia. *American Psychologist*, 17, 827.

Meehl, P.E. (1978). Theoretical risks and tabular asterisks: Sir Karl, Sir Ronald, and the slow progress of soft psychology. *Journal of Consulting and Clinical Psychology*, **46**, 806.

Meehl, P.E. (1979). A funny thing happened to us on the way to the latent entities. *Journal of Personality Assessment*, **43**, 564–581.

Meehl, P.E. (1995). Bootstraps taxometrics: Solving the classification problem in psychopathology. *American Psychologist*, **50**, 266.

Parnas, J. (2015). The RDoC program: psychiatry without psyche? *World Psychiatry*, **13**, 46–47.

Pettersson, E. and **Turkheimer, E.** (2010). Item selection, evaluation, and simple structure in personality data. *Journal of Research in Personality*, **44**, 407–420.

Plomin, R. and **Daniels, D.** (1987). Why are children in the same family so different from one another? *Behavioral and Brain Sciences*, **10**, 1–16.

Schaffner, K.F. (2006). Reduction: the Cheshire cat problem and a return to roots. *Synthese*, **151**, 377–402.

Shephard, R. (1978). The circumplex and related topological manifolds. In S. Shye (ed.) *Theory, Construction and Data Analysis in the Behavioral Sciences*, pp. 29–80. San Francisco, CA: Josey-Bass.

Thurstone, L.L. (1940). Current issues in factor analysis. *Psychological Bulletin*, **37**, 189.

Turkheimer, E., Ford, D.C., and **Oltmanns, T.F.** (2008). Regional analysis of self-reported personality disorder criteria. *Journal of Personality*, **76**, 1587–1622.

Chapter 6

Representation and explanation in psychometric modeling

Denny Borsboom

In his provocative contribution, Eric Turkheimer raises the question to what extent common psychometric techniques, like factor modeling or clustering methods, can be assumed to "carve nature at its joints," as the philosopher Plato put it. Turkheimer argues that standard psychometric techniques involve assumptions, conventions, and definitions that introduce an arbitrary component into the models used. These arbitrary components block a straightforward interpretation of the model as representing the empirical world directly. At the same time, the models are clearly meaningful, and contain important empirical information. In an attempt to find a middle position between naive realism and complete conventionalism, Turkheimer introduces the idea that, for instance, factor-analytic solutions should be seen as akin to maps: they tell us how the multivariate space that the data span can be navigated. However, the way in which this space is cut need not involve any real "joints"; that is, a factor used in a factor model to represent a multivariate space need not represent properties or variables that are real in the sense that they refer to something "outside" of the data-analytic procedure; rather, variables that, for instance, "load on the same factor" simply indicate *regions* in the multivariate space.

Turkheimer's concerns, in my view, relate strongly to an essential tension in psychometric modeling. On the one hand, techniques like factor modeling are data-analytic techniques that are simply useful as economic representations of the probability distribution that describes the data. For example, the data spanned by many of the disorders in the fifth edition of the *Diagnostic and Statistical of Manual Disorders* (DSM-5; American Psychological Association 2013) can be reasonably represented by a two- or three-dimensional space (Krueger 1999), or perhaps, at the higher-order level, by a one-dimensional space (Caspi et al. 2014). This is the *representational component* of psychometric models. One the other hand, the latent variables that feature in the models are often taken to identify common causes that determine the distribution of the data, in the sense that they explain *why* certain groups of variables cluster as they do. In this interpretation, the factors extracted in a data analysis may be taken to identify "underlying core psychopathological processes" (Krueger 1999, p. 921): the symptoms of, say, anxiety disorders and mood disorders correlate highly because they both arise from an underlying "internalizing factor." This is the *explanatory component* of psychometric models (see also Haig 2005).

The representational and explanatory components of psychometric models do not necessarily sit well together. The reason for this is that the computational procedures involved in factor analysis, which serve to generate a particular type of representation, often invoke assumptions that are pragmatically dictated and sometimes seem arbitrary relative to the explanatory component. An example that Turkheimer mentions (but there are several others) is Thurstone's (1947) insistence on simple structure, which means that each indicator variable should only load on one particular factor. The assumption of simple structure plays an important role especially, for example, in confirmatory factor analysis (CFA), because it constrains the model to such an extent that it generates testable implications, which can then be used to gauge how well the model fits the data.

Assumptions like simple structure are pragmatically useful, but are in many cases substantively questionable. In the example of personality that Turkheimer discusses, for instance, simple structure often creates problems because indicators often show cross-loadings. In addition, the requirement of simple structure has no substantive justification whatsoever. Another example is the model specification that the latent variables in a model should be orthogonal to each other and that the loadings should be chosen such that they maximize the variance of the loading matrix (a technique known as VARIMAX), which is still routinely made in exploratory factor analyses. From a representational point of view, it is highly useful to extract orthogonal components in this way, as it facilitates the navigation through the multivariate space. However, from an explanatory point of view, it is plainly ridiculous to suppose that latent variables are uncorrelated (i.e., if these latent variables are taken to be substantively meaningful factors that refer to objective properties outside of the model).

Thus, the introduction of pragmatic concerns and mathematically convenient fictions is essential to the representational goal of psychometrics, but it compromises the explanatory goal because it endows the model with properties that are very unlikely to hold in reality. As a result, as the model becomes more parsimonious, identifiable, estimable, and mathematically elegant, it often loses its substantive plausibility: in such cases, substantive plausibility and psychometric tractability do not mutually support each other, but are involved in a trade-off. Because the structure of psychometric models is rarely if ever dictated by psychological theory, but derives either from broad considerations of what good measurement models should look like or from statistical considerations of how to optimally analyze data, this trade-off is the rule rather than the exception.

There are various ways to react to this conundrum. One way is to simply deny the problem, and to assume (without independent justification) that any factors in the data-analytic procedure will by necessity correspond to "something out there." This line of reasoning, which we may call *naive realism*, is quite prevalent in the literature. A typical sign of this style of reasoning is visible when people assume that, because a general factor comes out of a statistical modeling procedure, there must be some underlying reality to it (e.g., it must identify an "underlying process," "psychological construct," "psychopathological mechanism," or a similar enigmatic entity). This style of reasoning categorically clinches to the explanatory function of psychometric models without assessing properly the mathematical constraints under which the model operates, with a very significant risk of reification of factors that have only a statistical reality (e.g., see Gould 1996). Of course, a factor model will always return factors, as a matter of mathematical necessity, and it will do so regardless of the way in which these correlations between observables arise: even the best-fitting factor model does not prove the existence of causally operational latent variables, simply because factor analysis does not need the existence of such latent variables to come up with a factor solution (e.g., see Van der Maas et al. 2006).

A second way to deal with the tension between explanatory and representational goals is to deny that psychometric models have any explanatory component whatsoever. This response, which I have found to be more prevalent among technically oriented psychometricians, puts forward a *purely instrumentalist* interpretation of factors, which are taken to be useful *only* as an economic representation of the data. This is a metaphysically lean position in the sense that it dodges some of the darker philosophical problems in psychometrics relating to the existential status of latent variables and the difficult problem of how to interpret factor models causally (Markus and Borsboom 2014). However, it runs into problems of its own. I read Turkheimer's discussion as leaning toward the instrumentalist idea, and so I think it is useful to discuss instrumentalism in more detail.

Instrumentalism has been an important intellectual force in the philosophy of science (e.g., Toulmin 1953). Its earliest incarnation arose in the midst of the scientific revolution, when Andreas Osiander, who oversaw the publication of Copernicus' book *De revolutionibus orbium coelestium* in 1543, added a preface to the text (controversially, without Copernicus' knowledge). In this preface, he stated that the hypotheses put forward by Copernicus

> [. . .] need not be true nor even probable. [. . .] And if any causes are devised by the imagination, as indeed very many are, they are not put forward to convince anyone that they are true, but merely to provide a reliable basis for computation.

Thus, Osiander essentially said that the cosmological hypotheses encoded in the heliocentric theory were not intended to describe the way the cosmos is actually structured, but simply served to represent the observed data in an economic fashion. If we could put Osiander in a time machine, and drop him in the middle of, say, an International Meeting of the Psychometric Society, he would probably feel right at home, for his description of the status of Copernicus' theory is one that quite nicely matches the way many technically oriented psychometricians think of factor in a factor model: A factor is just a mathematical representation useful to describe the data, and nothing more.

It is not clear whether Copernicus ever saw Osiander's preface, as he died just around the time his book appeared in print. But he would likely not have been amused. For the scientist (in contrast to the statistician or psychometrician), the economic representation of data is not intrinsically interesting, and I think

Copernicus would have objected to the reduction of his cosmological theory to a computational device. Scientific researchers tend to use data representation techniques as a means to a specific end, namely, to get at theories that explain phenomena. Explanation invariably requires the postulation of laws, causes, and hypothetical entities to do the explanatory work, and these treasures are not to be found in data representations. Achieving a parsimonious description of data may thus be a respectable goal for the psychometrician, but it is only a means to an end for most substantive scientists. The instrumentalist conception of psychometric models runs the risk of rendering psychometric models substantively sterile, especially when these models contain latent variables and other *prima facie* explanatory entities. The reason for this is that the primary attractiveness of models with latent variables lies precisely in the fact that they introduce the hypothetical entities (in the form of latent variables) and explanatory resources (in the form of causal relations between latent variables or between latent variables and observables) to explain empirical phenomena (correlation patterns) that the substantive scientist *does* care about.

Further, especially more complicated psychometric modeling exercises like CFA or structural equation modeling (SEM) appear to miss the mark entirely if their primary goal is taken to be data representation. If one wants to know whether the individual differences between people in a multivariate space can be described by scores on one, two, or three dimensions, one should not bother to run a CFA. Rather, one should execute a principal components analysis (PCA), which contains no latent variables, is computationally cheap, and can do the job of data-reduction just as well without introducing all kinds of problematic assumptions. In addition, the theoretical status of principal components is crystal clear: they are weighted composites, formed to represent the data in a particular way—not putative theoretical entities with explanatory power—so the risk of unjustified reification is less pronounced.

Does Turkheimer's approach succeed in articulating a middle ground between the positions of naive realism and pure instrumentalism? That depends. As usual, the devil is in the details, and despite the seductive analogies with maps, Turkheimer is less than fully articulated on the important question of *which* properties of psychometric models should be taken as instances of arbitrary (or, perhaps more appropriately, conventional). Naturally, maps depend on conventions. The organization of a system in terms of orthogonal dimensions of longitude and latitude is clearly conventional, as is the location of the Greenwich meridian, and the measurement unit itself. That is not really the point. What makes our ordinary location map so pragmatically useful is not that it has *no* arbitrary elements, but that we know exactly *which* properties of the map are arbitrary and in which way. We know, for instance, that a map displayed at a 1:100 scale will look exactly the same as a map displayed at a 1:1000 scale, except for its size. We also know that rotating the map will not change Euclidean distances between points on the map, and that the map represents physical distance but not traveling distance, as the latter depends also on the third spatial dimension that is suppressed in the longitude–latitude system.

However, what exactly are the arbitrary properties of a psychometric model like a factor model, and which properties of the model are entirely reflections of the empirical reality studied? I see no clear delineation here, and I think this is one of the major problems in the common use of psychometric models. Clearly, the rotation of the factors is indeterminate, as is the unit in which latent and observed variables are scaled. Simple structure, however, appears to introduce empirical hypotheses, as it has falsifying instances, and does not appear fully conventional to me. At the same time, however, I am not entirely certain of the nature of the empirical hypothesis tested. This also holds for the common assumption that the off-diagonal elements of the error covariance matrix are zero. What exactly are the truth conditions of that assumption in substantive empirical terms? I really do not have a clue, nor do I know whether it matters. And what about the latent variables in the model? Does the conventionalist element of Turkheimer's account involve them too? If so, why keep them in the psychometric model at all—it would seem that easier options are available in the form of hierarchical clustering or PCA? If not, what should such latent variables refer to, if *not* a set of common causes hypothesized to underlie the data? How many consistent interpretations of latent variables are available anyway, and what are they? I know of common cause and behavior domain interpretations (Markus and Borsboom 2014) and more recently of a network interpretation (Epskamp et al. *in press*) but surely there must be more?

These issues bother me, especially in relation to Turkheimer's pessimism regarding the project of establishing an empirically adequate psychiatric nosology and his conclusion that

> [. . .] the point is that a step back from the possibility of comprehensive explanation entails a step back from decisive determination of nosological systems; indeed they are the same problem.

I agree with Turkheimer that the prospects for comprehensive *biological* accounts he discusses are bad—in fact, in my view the current fashionable attempts to found nosology on neurobiology or genetics (e.g., Insel and Cuthbert 2015) are unsupported by the scientific record and based on outdated reductionist ideas on the relation between brain, mind, and behavior. However, it seems much too early to me to give up the hope for a scientifically respectable and empirically adequate nosological system in general. The scientist, in my view, should only settle for conventionalist elements in his or her theoretical framework if these are fully understood and are demonstrably harmless in empirical and societal applications. An example would be the choice of origin in the latitude–longitude system being demonstrably harmless in navigating a ship across the Atlantic.

While it is not clear to me that the arbitrary elements of psychometric models are so well understood, I am quite convinced that the degree of arbitrariness in our current models is far too large. Further, it seems relatively obvious to me that our current clinical diagnostic systems are suboptimal too. As a result, although Turkheimer's demonstration of the arbitrary components in classification systems may be broadly correct, I read the consequences that follow from it somewhat differently. In my opinion, we should not accept arbitrariness in the system unless we cannot avoid it: it is our intellectual duty to strive for an intelligible and theoretically funded classification system that avoids arbitrary classification as much as possible. Examples of such systems include the periodic table of the elements in chemistry, definitions of species on the basis of phylogenetic trees in biology, or classifications of diseases on the basis of root causes in medicine. I do not believe that we have an adequate classification system now, and it seems unlikely to me we would ever arrive at one by merely using factor analysis or statistical clustering. In my view, a scientific classification system requires (or is developed in tandem with) a general theory of the domain it covers. If that is correct, then the reason that we don't have a good classification system now may simply be that we have no general theory of psychopathology.

References

American Psychiatric Association (2013). *Diagnostic and Statistical Manual: Mental Disorders*, 5th edn. Washington, DC: American Psychiatric Association.

Caspi, A., **Houts, R.M.**, **Belsky, D.W.**, et al. (2014). The p factor: One general psychopathology factor in the structure of psychiatric disorders? *Clinical Psychological Science*, **2**, 119–137.

Epskamp, S., **Maris, G.**, **Waldorp, L.J.**, and **Borsboom, D.** (*in press*). Network psychometrics. In P. Irwing, D. Hughes, and, T. Booth (eds.) *Handbook of Psychometrics*. New York: Wiley.

Gould, S.J. (1996). *The Mismeasure of Man*. New York: W.W. Norton.

Haig, B.D. (2005). Exploratory factor analysis, theory generation, and scientific method. *Multivariate Behavioral Research*, **40**, 303–329.

Insel, T.R. and **Cuthbert, B.N.** (2015). Brain disorders? Precisely. *Science*, **348**, 499–500.

Krueger R.F. (1999). The structure of common mental disorders. *Archives of General Psychiatry*, **56**, 921–926.

Markus, K.A. and **Borsboom, D.** (2014). *Frontiers of Test Validity Theory: Measurement, Causation, and Meaning*. London: Routledge.

Thurstone, L.L. (1947). *Multiple Factor Analysis*. Chicago: University of Chicago Press.

Toulmin, S. (1953). *The Philosophy of Science*. London: Hutchinson & Co.

Van der Maas, H.L.J., **Dolan, C.V.**, **Grasman, R.P.P.P.**, et al. (2006). A dynamical model of general intelligence: The positive manifold of intelligence by mutualism. *Psychological Review*, **113**, 842–861.

Section 3

Obsessive-compulsive disorders in DSM-5

Chapter 7

Introduction to "Obsessive-compulsive and related disorders in DSM-5, ICD-11, and RDoC: Conceptual questions and practical solutions"

Kenneth S. Kendler

The author of this informative chapter, Dan Stein, is a psychiatrist and chair of department who has been an active nosologist in the *Diagnostic and Statistical Manual of Mental Disorders* (DSM) and *International Classification of Diseases* (ICD) process and thus can speak with the authority of experience as well as a being contributor on a range of issues at the philosophy–psychiatry interface. In this chapter, he reflects on his DSM-5 experiences working on the "Anxiety, Obsessive-Compulsive Spectrum, Posttraumatic, and Dissociative Disorders DSM-5 Work Group"—quite a mouthful. The aim of this chapter, as he writes, is to "review some of the conceptual questions that emerged during these deliberations, and some of the practical solutions that were put forward." As illustrated by several chapters in this volume, the practice of psychiatric nosology raises a series of fascinating conceptual and philosophical issues. But it is also a real discipline in which real decisions need to be made in real time and taking account of what is often a rather messy process. In this sense, it is a bit like medicine itself. When we see a patient complaining of a problem, we have to do something. We do not have the luxury—as do philosophers—of going off and thinking some more about the problem until things become clear. All the speculation—philosophical or otherwise—about what might be necessary or ideal has to be put, at least partially, to the side, and the best decisions made in real time in the often less than ideal environments where you would always want to know more than you do.

Dr. Stein outlines a series of the weighty issues that had to be confronted by this Work Group, the decisions reached, and some of the rationales for those decisions. They include "how to decide whether any condition is a mental disorder, and of how to draw boundaries between symptoms that meet threshold for the disorder, other mental disorders, and normality." If we pick out one of these decisions—the nosological status of what has come to be called "obsessive-compulsive and related disorders" or OCRDs—you can see the impingement of a wide variety of factors.

These included several kinds of empirical data (imaging studies and family studies in particular), administrative issues (are there too many broad categories in DSM and ICD or does the new alphanumeric code provide the opportunity for more categories?), the importance of international relations (how critical is it for the diagnostic meta-structure of DSM and ICD to be the same?) and clinical utility. His discussion of what belongs in and out of the OCRDs documents the struggle of the Work Group in which he participated with the long-popular concept of the "diagnostic spectrum." How can that framework be accurately instantiated in a diagnostic category like OCRD so that it is informative, data-driven, and not overly broad?

Stein also describes the exigencies of trying to get new psychiatric disorders approved—in particular hoarding disorder, skin picking disorder, and olfactory reference disorder. The group succeeded twice and failed once. For such additions to the DSM, the range of issues to be considered widens even further. Does the syndrome meet the definition of a mental disorder? Is the syndrome sufficiently different from other disorders not to be better considered as a subtype (as hoarding had been of OCD in DSM-IV)? Stein notes the pressures to avoid one kind of public perception often very critical of psychiatry—the "medicalization" of the psychiatric aches and pains of human existence. Stein even touches on the perpetual question of the boundary between psychiatry and neurology in the discussions about the proper placement of Tourette's syndrome.

Through his descriptions, the reader can get a sense of the dialog between the rarefied halls of philosophy and the nitty-gritty world of nosologic decision-making. As he writes "Many conceptual issues were raised and a number of practical ways forward were found." For working nosologists confronting deadlines for the completion of revisions, there is no other choice.

Chapter 8

Obsessive-compulsive and related disorders in DSM-5, ICD-11, and RDoC: Conceptual questions and practical solutions

Dan J. Stein

8.1 Obsessive-compulsive and related disorders in DSM-5 and ICD-11

One of the work groups for the fifth edition of the *Diagnostic and Statistical Manual of Mental Disorders* (DSM-5) was that devoted to anxiety, obsessive-compulsive spectrum, post-traumatic, and dissociative disorders (Stein, Craske et al. 2011, 2014). The name of this work group implies that there are distinctions between these different kinds of disorders, and indeed an early decision was to split the work group into three subgroups, one on anxiety disorders, one on obsessive-compulsive and related disorders (OCRDs), and one on trauma- and stressor-related and dissociative disorders. Given this approach, it is not altogether surprising that DSM-5 and the eleventh edition of the *International Classsification of Diseases* (ICD-11), which had agreed to use the same metastructure, or overall configuration of chapters in the nomenclature, eventually ended up having these sets of conditions classified in separate chapters.

The potential importance of the OCRDs as an independent diagnostic rubric had been proposed for some years, including at one of the research conferences held in preparation for DSM-5 (Hollander et al. 2009). The thrust of this conference was consistent with conceptual approaches then circulating that DSM-5 needed to reflect clearly advances in neuroscience, and that there would be a focus on symptom dimensions (Hyman 2007, Kupfer et al. 2008). Contributors emphasized that OCRDs involved similar neurocircuitry, which helped account for the fact that a spectrum of related disorders and symptoms showed selective responses to specific interventions (Ferrao et al. 2009), an argument consistent with the subsequently published Research Domain Criteria (RDoC) framework (Insel et al. 2010).

This chapter describes some of the deliberations in the subsequently established DSM-5 and ICD-11 work groups on OCRDs (both of which I was fortunate to lead). For example, given that some of the conditions proposed as OCRDs (e.g., hoarding disorder, olfactory reference syndrome, skin picking disorder) were new to the official nomenclature, the DSM-5 work group also grappled in some detail with the perennial conceptual questions of how to decide whether any condition is a mental disorder, and of how to draw boundaries between symptoms that meet threshold for the disorder, other mental disorders, and normality. The aim of this chapter is to review some of the conceptual questions that emerged during these deliberations, and some of the practical solutions that were put forward.

8.2 OCRDs and the metastructure

Two related questions for the DSM-5 work group were:

- Should putative OCRDs be classified together in the nosology, and if so which of these conditions should be included?
- Should obsessive-compulsive disorder (OCD) retain its classification as one of the anxiety disorders, or should it be moved into a different section together with related conditions?

The work group undertook detailed literature reviews of the relevant research, obtained feedback from senior researchers and from the public, and commissioned a re-analysis of data from a family study of OCD. There was also significant interaction, partly via the DSM-5 website of the American Psychiatric Association (APA), with a broader community of advocates and consumers interested in these issues.

A first systematic review argued that OCD should remain part of the anxiety disorders, but that the name should be changed to "anxiety and obsessive-compulsive disorders" (Stein, Fineberg et al. 2010). The rationale was that were sufficiently important overlaps between OCD and other anxiety disorders that there was no need to move OCD out of the chapter on these conditions. At the same time, there were important differences between these conditions, and the new chapter title would clarify this. A second systematic review indicated that OCD had close relationships, but also important dissimilarities, with a number of putative OCRDs including body dysmorphic disorder and trichotillomania (Phillips et al. 2010). These conclusions were based on systematic review of a range diagnostic validators (symptom similarity/diagnostic stability, course of illness/comorbidity, neuronal circuitry, family history/genetic risk factors/environmental risk factors, other biomarkers, temperamental antecedents/personality correlates, cognitive-emotional processing) as well as a consideration of clinical utility. Experts indicated that any chapter on OCRDs should include a relatively narrow range of conditions (Mataix-Cols et al. 2007), and the family data also supported this view (Bienvenu et al. 2012).

Early in the DSM-5 process, it was argued that the 16 DSM-5 and 10 ICD-10 chapters were unwieldy, and that the new metastructure should be more parsimonious. In line with a focus on incorporating neuroscientific knowledge and symptom dimensions, an examination of validating criteria suggested five clusters of disorders (Andrews et al. 2009). However, at some point it became clear that with an alphanumeric classification system, it was possible to have multiple chapters in the nosology. Subsequent versions of the metastructure, decided upon by a joint team of those leading DSM-5 and ICD-11, expanded to include anxiety disorders, OCRDs, and trauma- and stressor-related disorders in separate chapters. While this decision was in line with some empirical evidence covered in the systematic reviews undertaken by the DSM-5 work group on anxiety, obsessive-compulsive spectrum, post-traumatic, and dissociative disorder, including a review arguing for separating out trauma- and stressor-related disorders from anxiety disorders, it could not have occurred if only ten DSM-5 chapters had been available. The DSM-5 work group on anxiety, obsessive-compulsive spectrum, post-traumatic, and dissociative disorders proposed that these chapters be adjacent to one another so as to reflect clinical overlap across these conditions (Stein, Craske et al. 2011, 2014).

One key conceptual question raised by this debate is how to decide whether mental disorder *x* belongs in category or spectrum *y*. In an article written at the start of the DSM-5 deliberations, for a special issue devoted to the relevant nosological debates, I suggested that the answer was in turn related to a number of key debates in philosophy of science and language, and had also increasingly been addressed by the cognitive-affective neuroscience of categorization (Stein 2008a). To some extent, these debates are about whether medicine in general and psychiatric nosology in particular should be conceptualized more as an empirical science along the lines of physics, or whether they are best approached as a humanity concerned with depicting the range of human experience (Schwartz and Wiggins 1985).

Indeed, I have elsewhere suggested that it may be of heuristic value to contrast classical and critical views of disorder, each perspective in turn being based on particular approaches within the philosophy of science and language (Stein 1991, 1998, 2008a, 2013). From a classical perspective, which regards disorders as defined by necessary and sufficient criteria (akin to the way in which physicists or mathematicians might define the category of squares), one can potentially make statements such as disorder *x* belongs in category *y*, precisely because it demonstrates certain necessary and sufficient features *z*. In contrast, from a critical perspective, which emphasizes that what counts as a disorder reflects human practices and values, and so varies from time to time and place to place (just as the category of weeds is contingent upon social context), statements about whether a disorder *x* belongs in category *y* are driven primarily by societal values and interests.

An integrative perspective accepts that categorization reflects societal practices and values, but at the same time emphasizes that scientific debate about diagnostic validity and clinical utility can lead to progress in nosology. Rigorous examination of the underlying structures and mechanisms that account for various symptoms and disorders may lead to better classification. Thus, we may reasonably decide that OCD is not an anxiety disorder, because the underlying psychobiology of OCD and the anxiety disorders is sufficiently different. On the other hand, considerations about clinical utility are also key, particularly given the often rudimentary state of our knowledge of psychobiology. Consistent with a view that psychiatric disorders involve multiple levels of causation and necessitate multiple kinds of intervention (Stein 2009, Kendler 2012), there may be no single criterion for determining whether or not disorder *x* falls within category y_1 or y_2.

Indeed, from an integrative perspective, which acknowledges that classifications are for human purposes, but that there are real underlying psychobiological mechanisms that contribute to symptoms, there are pros and cons to any particular proposed metastructure. In line with this conceptual approach, my colleagues and I have been comfortable in acknowledging that any proposal about whether to include OCRDs in the nosology, and what conditions to list, would allow for quite reasonable counterarguments (Stein, Denys et al. 2009, Stein and Phillips 2014). Given the broader decision to expand the metastructure from a small group of clusters into more than ten, both the DSM-5 and ICD-11 work groups agreed that considerations of diagnostic validity as well as clinical utility favored including the OCRDs construct as a separate chapter, and debate shifted to whether or not specific putative OCRDs should be included (Stein, Fontenelle et al. 2014). At outlined below, DSM-5 and ICD-11 entailed somewhat different objectives and processes, and so come to slightly different conclusions on this score.

8.3 New OCRDs

The DSM-5 work group reviewed the literature on a number of OCRDs that had not previously been included in the nosology: hoarding disorder, skin picking (excoriation) disorder, and olfactory reference syndrome. From a nosological perspective, the questions were in some ways straightforward; should these diagnostic entities be included in DSM-5, and if so then in what chapter? But of course the work group soon found itself having to address the conceptual questions of how to decide whether any condition is a mental disorder, and of how to draw boundaries between symptoms that meet threshold for the disorder, other mental disorders, and normality.

At the start of the DSM-5 process, there was a mandate to explore entirely novel nosological approaches and solutions (Kupfer et al. 2008). However, over time, specific criteria for making changes were established by the DSM-5 task force, and indeed thresholds for change became fairly conservative over time (Kendler 2013). During this process, faced with the question of the threshold for adding new diagnoses to the nosology, members of the OCDRs work group collaborated with others to put forward a proposal about the criteria for mental disorder that should be used in DSM-5 (Stein, Phillips et al. 2010). Our work group's systematic reviews of hoarding disorder, skin picking disorder, and olfactory reference syndrome carefully and rigorously referred back to this proposal.

Some features of the proposal may be worth highlighting. We suggested that a mental disorder is a behavioral or psychological syndrome or pattern that occurs in an individual, that the consequences are clinically significant distress or disability, that it must not be a merely expectable response to common stressors or losses or a culturally sanctioned response to a particular event, that it reflected underlying psychobiological dysfunction, and that it is not primarily a result of social deviance or conflicts with society. In addition, we listed a number of other considerations: the condition had to have diagnostic validity and clinical utility, that no definition specifies precise boundaries for either "medical disorder" or "mental/psychiatric disorder," that diagnostic validators and clinical utility should help to differentiate a disorder from diagnostic "nearest neighbors," and that when considering whether to add a mental/psychiatric condition to the nomenclature, potential benefits should outweigh potential harms (Stein, Phillips et al. 2010).

In the case of hoarding disorder, systematic review found a growing literature indicating that this is a prevalent and disabling condition, with research on diagnostic validators (referred to earlier) pointing out importance differences between hoarding disorder and OCD (Mataix-Cols et al. 2010). The work group's proposal to include this condition as a new entity in the chapter on OCRDs received fairly smooth approval through the Scientific Review Committee (SRC) process. While knowledge of skin picking disorder had also grown substantially since the publication of DSM-IV (Stein, Grant et al. 2010), questions were raised by the SRC about the extent of the available evidence and about the degree to which this condition differed from "near neighbors" such as trichotillomania. Detailed review of the literature was required (Grant et al. 2012), and this eventually persuaded the SRC to include the disorder as an independent entity.

In the case of olfactory reference disorder (ORD), the work group's review argued that there was both sufficient diagnostic validity and clinical utility to include this entity. In particular, patients with ORD are at risk of being treated with high doses of antipsychotics, when some might respond to selective serotonin reuptake inhibitors (Feusner et al. 2010). The SRC, in contrast, ruled that the proposed criteria for ORD should not even be included in the DSM-5 chapter on proposed entities requiring further study. Instead, the work group had to be satisfied with listing the phrase "olfactory reference syndrome" in the section on "Other Specified Obsessive-Compulsive and Related Disorders" as part of the discussion of "jikoshu-kyofu," itself a variant of "taijin-kyofusho," a term that is defined in DSM-5's glossary of cultural concepts of distress.

Some points can perhaps be put forward about this process and the related conceptual issues. First, despite an early call for a "conceptual issues" work group in DSM-5 (Kendler et al. 2008), this was not established. Perhaps understandably, it took some time before the extent to which DSM-5 was going to be a paradigm shift or an iterative improvement was clarified (Kendler and First 2010). Practically speaking, however, there was a delay in addressing the key issue of criteria for change from DSM-IV to DSM-5. The establishment of such criteria, which perhaps necessarily involves discussion of conceptual questions, was arguably much needed in order to optimize careful debate about DSM-5 proposals from the various work groups.

Second, even once these criteria had been established, not all DSM-5 work groups followed them in equal measure. As mentioned, our work group carefully and rigorously addressed the criteria for a mental disorder in our reviews of hoarding disorder, skin picking disorder, and olfactory reference syndrome (Feusner et al. 2010, Mataix-Cols et al. 2010, Stein, Grant et al. 2010). This may be contrasted with, for example, proposals from the work group on sexual disorders, where conditions such as paraphilic coercive disorder were described, with arguably less attention to the relevant conceptual issues (Balon 2012). The definition of mental disorder was itself further revised during the final production of the DSM-5 text, with proofs being exchanged between some of those whom had contributed to the earlier more deliberative process.

Third, a view that DSM-5 would potentially be criticized for medicalization of everyday unhappiness played a key role in our deliberations. Work group members were well aware of the growing literature on disease-mongering (Moynihan et al. 2002), and that leading figures in psychiatry were vociferously emphasizing the negative consequences of specialists putting forward entities that led to "false positive" diagnoses (Batstra and Frances 2012). Hoarding, for example, comprises a set of symptoms that needs to be distinguished from everyday collecting. The work group self-consciously set thresholds for the diagnostic criteria for hoarding disorder so as to ensure that this delineation would neither be problematic, nor perceived to be medicalization of everyday variations. While that is likely a good thing, the notion that medicalization is necessarily a bad thing deserves some interrogation (Stein and Gureje 2004, Sadler et al. 2009, Stein and Giordano 2015).

Fourth, it may be worth noting that little if any of the debate around the OCRD proposals for new disorders centered around the question of whether these entities were not so much disorders, as other forms of deviance (e.g., crimes). I have elsewhere argued that it may be useful to distinguish "typical disorders" (in which there are features such as an external precipitant, and the individual is easily granted the sick role) from "atypical disorders" (in which, for example, the person is to some extent responsible for the relevant symptoms, and where the health intervention includes the setting of boundaries) (Stein 2013). For example, if an individual unexpectedly comes down with acute bacterial pneumonia, he or she will likely be conceptualized as having a medical problem and be given time off work to receive medical care. But if an individual starts to perform poorly at work due to increased alcohol consumption, an employer may well characterize the behavior as simply unacceptable (rather than as a health problem) and consider disciplinary action (rather than referral for medical treatment). This distinction may be helpful in explaining certain phenomena, such as increased controversy concerning the disorder status of atypical conditions such as alcoholism, and greater stigmatization of these conditions. However, the disorder status of the proposed entities was not questioned.

Fifth, it is possible that fortune or timing played a role in the relevant proposals for new disorders. Despite lack of support from some key OCD experts, the proposal for hoarding disorder was considered early in the review process, when thresholds for what constituted sufficient evidence were perhaps still being formed. Skin picking disorder is not a widely known or much discussed entity and it seemed to have relatively little professional support; however, a consumer advocacy group enjoined its membership to respond *en masse* on the APA DSM-5 website in favor of its inclusion in the nomenclature. It seems odd that ORD is barely included in the DSM-5 section on "Specified Obsessive-Compulsive and Related Disorders" (a section was deleted during final proofing), while "obsessional jealousy," a less studied entity (Stein, Hollander et al. 1994), is listed. In contrast, ORD had a relatively smooth passage in the ICD-11 process, and will likely be included in this classification (Veale and Matsunaga 2014). The inclusion of skin picking disorder in DSM-5 perhaps made it easier for the ICD-11 work group to accept this disorder, and indeed to move to the next step of lumping trichotillomania and skin picking disorder as examples of body-focused repetitive behavior disorders (Grant and Stein 2014). To some extent this is perhaps as it should be; nosological revision is a messy business, relying on a range of different views and inputs, and has at best a slow albeit steady path forward (Stein 2007, Kendler 2009).

3.4 Miscellaneous DSM-5, ICD-11, and RDoC debates

In this final part of the chapter, a range of miscellaneous nosological discussions in the DSM-5 and ICD-11 OCRDs work groups, each with conceptual interfaces, are briefly reviewed.

First, there is the question of the importance of the RDoC framework. Although early DSM-5 discussions emphasized the importance of including neuroscience, this focus was apparently insufficient for those committed to translational neuroscience who went on to produce RDoC. By the time the ICD-11 work group met, a good deal had already been published on the framework, and it was being implemented in the scoring of grant proposals to the National Institute of Mental Health. My own sense is that the early decision to have a DSM-5 conference on OCRDs, and the ultimate acceptance of this rubric as an independent chapter, was strongly influenced by this perspective. After all, from a viewpoint such as that of cognitive-behavioral therapy, OCD fits well with the anxiety disorders. But the hypothesis that OCRDs are mediated by corticostriatal circuitry, while anxiety disorders are mediated by the amygdala, was important in underpinning their separation.

Many of the arguments in favor of RDoC seem unassailable. Clearly, translational neuroscience will ultimately shed a good deal of light on psychiatric disorders and their optimal classification. Furthermore the emphasis of RDoC on dimensional measures seems consistent with how psychiatric symptoms are distributed in populations. At the same time, it is important to acknowledge a number of reservations about the RDoC approach to assessing psychopathology (Stein 2014). For one thing, much of the approach is far from new; researchers have attempted to identify biological substrates and intermediate phenotypes underlying mental disorders for many years (van Praag et al. 1990). For another thing, it is not at all clear that we have enough data from neuroimaging studies to distinguish clearly anxiety disorders and OCRDs (which are not yet well studied), nor is it clear that brain imaging is the sole or ideal approach to validating such disorders. After all, it is quite possible that in a hundred years' time, current concepts of neurocircuitry will be considered rudimentary. At the very least, it would seem that RDoC requires supplementation with a range of alternative perspectives (Stein, Lund et al. 2013).

Second, and related to the emphasis of RDoC on endophenotypes (Insel and Cuthbert 2009), there is the question of whether Tourette's syndrome (TS) should be classified as an OCRD. The DSM-5 work group was well aware of the important familial relationships between OCD and TS; in some ways TS is the paradigmatic exemplar of an OCRD (Stein 2000). At the same time, in its review of tic disorders, the DSM-5 work group noted that there is an important difference in the perception of the two conditions by the general public and by the medical profession: tic disorders are considered as a neurological disorder by primary care doctors, patients, and patient support groups, while other psychiatric disorders including OCD, although having a clear brain basis, have not been as consistently perceived by the public or non-psychiatric medical professionals as neurological (Walkup, Ferrao et al. 2010). The DSM-5 work group review therefore argued in favor of not including TS as an OCRD (Walkup et al. 2010).

There are a number of considerations at hand. Even to ask whether TS is a neurological or psychiatric disorder seems to reinforce a mind–body dualism that modern nosology has been attempting to avoid (Spitzer et al. 1992, Stein, Phillips et al. 2010). It seems that TS consumer advocacy groups who wanted to prevent stigmatization of TS by association with psychiatric disorders such as OCD may have influenced the work group view. While this is certainly understandable, a counterargument is that this position does a disservice to patients suffering from OCRDs. It is notable that in the ICD-11 discussions, a pragmatic proposal was found; TS could be classified both in the neurological disorders and in the OCRDs (Woods and Thomsen 2014). It is also worth noting that while advances in TS and OCD genetics (Davis et al. 2013) contributed to this discussion, such data did not straightforwardly lead to any particular decision, in keeping with the complexity of extrapolations from genetics to nosology (Kendler 2006, 2013).

A third issue for the DSM-5 work group on OCRDs was whether OCD in the context of pediatric neuropsychiatric disorder associated with streptococcus (PANDAS), should be reconceptualized in terms of a general medical disorder. There is growing evidence that children exposed to streptococcus can develop acute onset of obsessive-compulsive symptoms, presumably on the basis of an autoimmune reaction (Swedo and Grant 2005). On the other hand, the work group noted that empirical studies to date have not been entirely consistent, and it has been suggested that a range of other etiological factors may be associated with acute onset of psychiatric symptoms in children (Singer et al. 2012).

There is certainly some clinical utility in recognizing that general medical disorders as well as various medications and substances may precipitate psychiatric symptoms. A diagnostic criterion that addresses this differential diagnosis may remind the clinician to check the relevant medical history, and to undertake relevant special investigations. At the same time, this criterion appears to imply that in cases where symptoms are precipitated by a general medical disorder, medications, or substances, there is unicausal etiology. In the case of PANDAS, the DSM-5 work group noted that many psychiatric disorders, including OCD, involve a range of contributing causal factors, and concluded that further work on the diagnostic validity and clinical utility of PANDAS is needed before its formal inclusion as an independent entity in the nomenclature (Leckman et al. 2010).

A fourth issue is that surrounding the so-called clinical significance criterion (Spitzer and Wakefield 1999). In both the DSM-5 and ICD-11 processes, the position was taken that it was important to distinguish the concepts of disorder and disability. From the perspective of translational neuroscience, while disorder and normality fall on a continuum, the differentiation lies in the extent of underlying disruption of psychobiological mechanisms. From the perspective of public mental health and ICD-11, it is important that any particular condition may or may not be associated with disability. However, in the case of anxiety and related disorders, where symptoms clearly lie on a spectrum with normal and even adaptive phenomena, the presence of functional impairment is a key pointer to psychopathology. The DSM-5 work group on OCRDs therefore chose to retain the clinical significance criterion for its disorders, although it did not recommend any relevant changes to the tic disorder criteria (where there is, unusually, no clinical significance criterion) (Walkup et al. 2010). The work group did, however, tinker with various clinical significance criteria; in one of my favorite examples, the work group took issue with the DSM-IV use of one hour of OCD symptoms as an index of clinical significance, and added the phrase "for example" just prior to the measure of "one hour," in order to prevent reification of this threshold.

At the current time, psychiatry has few biomarkers that are helpful in delineating pathology from normality. One set of authors seems certain that such biomarkers will one day be found, and certainly advances in genetic research seem to indicate that risk scores for psychopathology are already within reach or soon will be. At the same time, given that certain symptoms of psychiatric disorders are very pervasive and have adaptive origins, a more skeptical group of authors holds that sensitive and specific biomarkers for common mental disorders are some way off (Nesse and Stein 2012, Stein and Nesse 2015). For now, psychiatry has arguably been at the forefront of medical nosology, clearly detailing how a range of measures (including impairment) can be used clinically as markers of underlying dysfunction (First and Wakefield 2013), and showing how to develop reliable and valid diagnostic criteria for psychiatric and medical disorders when biomarkers are not available (Olesen 1996).

A fifth issue is simply to note how few data-based discussions there were of different possible criteria sets for OCRDs. DSM-IV criteria sets are the most commonly used, and there is often a paucity of alternative criteria. Much of the debate about rewording of diagnostic criteria in the OCRDs work groups was based on clinical experience and commonsense argument, rather than on examination of empirical data. There were, however, some notable exceptions, such as the decision to remove DSM-IV criteria B and C for trichotillomania (Lochner et al. 2011), and the DSM-5 work group on OCRDs undertook a number of field surveys in order to assess alternative criteria sets (Lochner et al. 2012a, 2012b).

The lack of data about alternative diagnostic criteria for psychiatric disorders arguably helps reinforce the reification of the current nomenclature (Hyman 2010). We run the risk of forgetting that our current diagnostic criteria for any particular disorder reflect historical tradition, and represent merely one hypothesis about how best to depict that particular condition. Ongoing attention to this issue is needed, with encouragement of researchers to obtain information that goes beyond the DSM and ICD criteria in order to investigate a greater range of potentially important symptomatology (Kendler 2014).

A sixth issue is subtyping of OCRDs. Some members of the DSM-5 work group argued strongly in favor of subtyping OCD along symptom dimensions. This was consistent with the DSM-5 focus on behavioral dimensions, and there was some evidence on systematic review that different symptom dimensions are characterized by different neurobiological features (Leckman et al. 2010). The counterargument is, however, that diagnostic validity and clinical utility for such an approach is insufficient, and both the DSM-5 and ICD-11 work groups therefore focused rather on a range of other approaches to subtyping OCD. Both work groups have emphasized the value of a tic and an insight specifier, and these are included in DSM-5.

Subtyping is an issue that deserves more conceptual work. There is growing acceptance that psychiatric disorders are not traditional natural kinds (Stein 2008b, 2014, Kendler et al. 2011), but further attention may be needed to the question of how disorder subtypes can optimally reflect the heterogeneity that is apparent when considering either diagnostic validity or clinical utility. With regard to the OCRDs, while a potential concern is that tics can be conceptualized as a comorbid symptom, there is a good deal of support for this specifier in OCD from the perspective of both diagnostic validity and clinical utility. Similarly, the inclusion of a delusional, or no insight, specifier in OCD, body dysmorphic disorder, and hoarding disorder seems to make a great deal of sense (Phillips et al. 2014).

8.5 **Conclusion**

This chapter has reviewed some of the nosological issues tackled by the DSM-5 and ICD-11 work groups on OCRDs. Many conceptual issues were raised and a number of practical ways forward were found. While a range of possible avenues of exploration are opened by this discussion, I would like to close by emphasizing the potential importance of further conceptual work on the constructs of diagnostic validity (Hyman 2010, Kendler et al. 2010) and clinical utility (First et al. 2004, First 2013). It is notable that the DSM-5 process emphasized the importance of diagnostic validity while also acknowledging the relevance of clinical utility (Kupfer and Regier 2011), while ICD-11 emphasized the importance of clinical utility albeit acknowledging that this requires diagnostic validity (Reed and Ayuso-Mateos 2011). This to some extent reflects the fact that DSM-5 remains the pre-eminent nomenclature used in psychiatry research settings, while ICD-11 will be used in primary health care settings by non-specialists.

In some ways, the OCRDs work groups' examination of the diagnostic validity and clinical utility of different proposals is merely a nosological exercise that aims at improving the nomenclature. On the other hand, the self-conscious emphasis on both these constructs during the DSM-5 and ICD-11 revisions arguably reflects an engagement with and acceptance of the key conceptual argument that nosology is both an evidence-based exercise and a values-based one (Wakefield 1992, Fulford et al. 2005, Sadler 2005, Kendler et al. 2010, Zachar and Kendler 2012, Stein, Lund et al. 2013). While some continue to emphasize that clinicians ought to be scientists who understand the pathophysiology of disease, and others stress that clinicians should be humanists who understand suffering and the experience of illness, an integrative approach that appreciates both these aspects of being a good diagnostician and researcher arguably allows a path that avoids both scientism and skepticism, and that provides a conceptual foundation supportive of iterative nosological progress (Stein 1991, 2008b).

References

Andrews, G., **Goldberg, D.P.** **Krueger, R.F.**, et al. (2009). Exploring the feasibility of a meta-structure for DSM-V and ICD-11: could it improve utility and validity? *Psychological Medicine*, **39**, 1993–2000.

Balon, R. (2012). The debate about paraphilic coercive disorder is mostly ideological and going nowhere. *Arch Sex Behav*, **41**, 535–536.

Batstra, L. and **Frances, A.** (2012). Holding the line against diagnostic inflation in psychiatry. *Psychother Psychosom*, **81**, 5–10.

Bienvenu, O.J., **Samuels, J.F.**, **Wuyek, L.A.**, et al. (2012). Is obsessive-compulsive disorder an anxiety disorder, and what, if any, are spectrum conditions? A family study perspective. *Psychological Medicine*, **42**, 1–13.

Davis, L.K., **Yu, D.**, **Keenan, C.L.**, et al. (2013). Partitioning the heritability of Tourette syndrome and obsessive compulsive disorder reveals differences in genetic architecture. *PLoS Genetics*, **9**, e1003864.

Ferrao, Y.A., **Miguel, E.**, and **Stein, D.J.** (2009). Tourette's syndrome, trichotillomania, and obsessive-compulsive disorder: how closely are they related? *Psychiatry Research*, **170**, 32–42.

Feusner, J.D., **Phillips K.A.**, and **Stein D.J.** (2010). Olfactory reference syndrome: issues for DSM-V. *Depression and Anxiety*, **27**, 592–599.

First, M.B. (2013). Diagnostic and statistical manual of mental disorders, 5th edition, and clinical utility. *Journal of Nervous and Mental Disease*, **201**, 727–729.

First, M.B., **Pincus, H.A.**, **Levine, J.B.**,et al. (2004). Clinical utility as a criterion for revising psychiatric diagnoses. *American Journal of Psychiatry*, **161**, 946–954.

First, M.B. and **Wakefield, J.C.** (2013). Diagnostic criteria as dysfunction indicators: bridging the chasm between the definition of mental disorder and diagnostic criteria for specific disorders. *Canadian Journal of Psychiatry*, **58**, 663–669.

Fulford, K.W., **Broome, M.**, **Stanghellini, G.**, and **Thornton, T.** (2005). Looking with both eyes open: fact and value in psychiatric diagnosis? *World Psychiatry*, **4**, 78–86.

Grant, J.E., **Odlaug, B.L.**, **Chamberlain, S.R.**, et al. (2012). Skin picking disorder. *American Journal of Psychiatry*, **169**, 1143–1149.

Grant, J.E. and **Stein, D.J.** (2014). Body-focused repetitive behavior disorders in ICD-11. *Revista Brasileira de Psiquiatria*, **36** Suppl 1, 59–64.

Hollander, E., **Kim, S.**, **Braun, A.**, et al. (2009). Cross-cutting issues and future directions for the OCD spectrum. *Psychiatry Research*, **170**, 3–6.

Hyman, S.E. (2007). Can neuroscience be integrated into the DSM-V? *Nature Reviews Neuroscience*, **8**, 725–732.

Hyman, S.E. (2010). The diagnosis of mental disorders: the problem of reification. *Annual Review of Clinical Psychology*, **6**, 155–179.

Insel, T., Cuthbert, B., Garvey, M., et al. (2010). Research domain criteria (RDoC): toward a new classification framework for research on mental disorders. *American Journal of Psychiatry*, **167**, 748–751.

Insel, T.R. and **Cuthbert, B.N.** (2009). Endophenotypes: bridging genomic complexity and disorder heterogeneity. *Biological Psychiatry*, **66**, 988–989.

Kendler, K.S. (2006). Reflections on the relationship between psychiatric genetics and psychiatric nosology. *American Journal of Psychiatry*, **163**, 1138–1146.

Kendler, K.S. (2009). An historical framework for psychiatric nosology. *Psychological Medicine*, **39**, 1935–1941.

Kendler, K.S. (2012). Levels of explanation in psychiatric and substance use disorders: implications for the development of an etiologically based nosology. *Molecular Psychiatry*, **17**, 11–21.

Kendler, K.S. (2013). A history of the DSM-5 Scientific Review Committee. *Psychological Medicine*, **43**, 1793–1800.

Kendler, K.S. (2013). What psychiatric genetics has taught us about the nature of psychiatric illness and what is left to learn. *Molecular Psychiatry*, **18**, 1058–1066.

Kendler, K.S. (2014). DSM issues: incorporation of biological tests, avoidance of reification, and an approach to the box canyon problem. *American Journal of Psychiatry*, **171**, 1248–1250.

Kendler, K.S., Appelbaum, P.S., Bell, C.C., et al. (2008). Issues for DSM-V: DSM-V should include a conceptual issues work group. *American Journal of Psychiatry*, **165**, 174–175.

Kendler, K.S. and **First, M.B.** (2010). Alternative futures for the DSM revision process: iteration v. paradigm shift. *British Journal of Psychiatry*, **197**, 263–265.

Kendler, K.S., Munoz, R.A. and **Murphy, G.** (2010). The development of the Feighner criteria: a historical perspective. *American Journal of Psychiatry*, **167**, 134–142.

Kendler, K.S., Zachar, P. and **Craver, C.** (2011). What kinds of things are psychiatric disorders? *Psychological Medicine*, **41**, 1143–1150.

Kupfer, D.J. and **Regier, D.A.** (2011). Neuroscience, clinical evidence, and the future of psychiatric classification in DSM-5. *American Journal of Psychiatry*, **168**, 672–674.

Kupfer, D.J., Regier, D.A. and **Kuhl, E.A.** (2008). On the road to DSM-V and ICD-11. *European Archives of Psychiatry and Clinical Neuroscience*, **258** Suppl 5, 2–6.

Leckman, J.F., Denys, D., Simpson, H.B., et al. (2010). Obsessive-compulsive disorder: a review of the diagnostic criteria and possible subtypes and dimensional specifiers for DSM-V. *Depression and Anxiety*, **27**, 507–527.

Lochner, C., Grant, J.E., Odlaug, B.L., and **Stein, D.J.** (2012a). DSM-5 field survey: skin picking disorder. *Annals of Clinical Psychiatry*, **24**, 300–304.

Lochner, C., Grant, J.E., Odlaug, B.L., et al. (2012b). DSM-5 field survey: hair-pulling disorder (trichotillomania). *Depression and Anxiety*, **29**, 1025–1031.

Lochner, C., Stein, D.J., Woods, D., et al. (2011). The validity of DSM-IV-TR criteria B and C of hair-pulling disorder (trichotillomania): evidence from a clinical study. *Psychiatry Research*, **189**, 276–280.

Mataix-Cols, D., Frost, R.O., Pertusa, A., et al. (2010). Hoarding disorder: a new diagnosis for DSM-V? *Depression and Anxiety*, **27**, 556–572.

Mataix-Cols, D., Pertusa A., and **Leckman, J.F.** (2007). Issues for DSM-V: how should obsessive-compulsive and related disorders be classified? *American Journal of Psychiatry*, **164**, 1313–1314.

Moynihan, R., Heath, I., and **Henry, D.** (2002). Selling sickness: the pharmaceutical industry and disease mongering. *BMJ*, **324**, 886–891.

Nesse, R.M. and **Stein, D.J.** (2012). Towards a genuinely medical model for psychiatric nosology. *BMC Medicine*, **10**, 5.

Olesen, J. (1996). The International Headache Society classification and diagnostic criteria are valid and extremely useful. *Cephalalgia*, **16**, 293–295; discussion 295–296.

Phillips, K.A., Hart, A.S., Simpson, H.B. and **Stein, D.J.** (2014). Delusional versus non-delusional body dysmorphic disorder: recommendations for DSM-5. *CNS Spectrums*, **19**, 10–20.

Phillips, K.A., Stein, D.J., Rauch, S.L., et al. (2010). Should an obsessive-compulsive spectrum grouping of disorders be included in DSM-V? *Depression and Anxiety*, **27**, 528–555.

Reed, G.M. and **Ayuso-Mateos, J.L.** (2011). Towards a more clinically useful International World Health Organisation classification of mental disorders. *Revista de Psiquiatría y Salud Mental*, **4**, 113–116.

Sadler, J.Z. (2005). Social context and stakeholders' values in building diagnostic systems. *Psychopathology*, **38**, 197–200.

Sadler, J.Z., Jotterand, F., Lee, S.C., and **Inrig, S.** (2009). Can medicalization be good? Situating medicalization within bioethics. *Theoretical Medicine and Bioethics*, **30**, 411–425.

Schwartz, M.A. and **Wiggins, O.** (1985). Science, humanism, and the nature of medical practice: a phenomenological view. *Perspectives in Biology and Medicine*, **28**, 331–366.

Singer, H.S., Gilbert, D.L., Wolf, D.S.,et al. (2012). Moving from PANDAS to CANS. *Journal of Pediatrics*, **160**, 725–731.

Spitzer, R.L., First, M.B., Williams, J.B., et al. (1992). Now is the time to retire the term organic mental disorders. *American Journal of Psychiatry*, **149**, 240–244.

Spitzer, R.L. and **Wakefield, J.C.** (1999). DSM-IV diagnostic criterion for clinical significance: does it help solve the false positives problem? *American Journal of Psychiatry*, **156**, 1856–1864.

Stein, D.J. (1991). Philosophy and the DSM-III. *Comprehensive Psychiatry*, **32**, 404–415.

Stein, D.J. (1998). Philosophy of psychopharmacology. *Perspectives in Biology and Medicine*, **41**, 200–211.

Stein, D.J. (2000). Neurobiology of the obsessive-compulsive spectrum disorders. *Biological Psychiatry*, **47**, 296–304.

Stein, D.J. (2007). Can the cognitive-affective sciences help us rethink psychiatric nosology? Towards DSM-V and ICD-11. *World Journal of Biological Psychiatry*, **8**, 210–211.

Stein, D.J. (2008a). Is disorder X in category or spectrum Y? General considerations and application to the relationship between obsessive-compulsive disorder and anxiety disorders. *Depression and Anxiety*, **25**, 330–335.

Stein, D.J. (2008b). *Philosophy of Psychopharmacology*. Cambridge, UK: Cambridge University Press.

Stein, D.J. (2009). Is there a mosquito net for anxiety and mood disorders? *Current Psychiatry Reports*, **11**, 264–265.

Stein, D.J. (2013). What is a mental disorder? A perspective from cognitive-affective science. *Canadian Journal of Psychiatry*, **58**, 656–662.

Stein, D.J. (2014). An integrative approach to psychiatric diagnosis and research. *World Psychiatry*, **13**, 51–53.

Stein, D.J. (2014). Psychopharmacology and natural kinds: A conceptual framework. In H. Kincaid and J.A. Sullivan (eds.) *Classifying Psychopathology: Mental Kinds and Natural Kinds*, pp. 65–73. Cambridge, MA, MIT Press.

Stein, D.J., Craske, M.A., Friedman, M.J., and **Phillips, K.A.** (2014). Anxiety disorders, obsessive-compulsive and related disorders, trauma- and stressor-related disorders, and dissociative disorders in DSM-5. *American Journal of Psychiatry*, **171**, 611–613.

Stein, D.J., Craske M.G., Friedman, M.J. and **Phillips, K.A.** (2011). Meta-structure issues for the DSM-5: how do anxiety disorders, obsessive-compulsive and related disorders, post-traumatic disorders, and dissociative disorders fit together? *Current Psychiatry Reports*, **13**, 248–250.

Stein, D.J., Denys, D., Gloster, A.T., et al. (2009). Obsessive-compulsive disorder: diagnostic and treatment issues. *Psychiatry Clinics of North America*, **32**, 665–685.

Stein, D.J., Fineberg, N.A., Bienvenu, O.J., et al. (2010). Should OCD be classified as an anxiety disorder in DSM-V? *Depression and Anxiety*, **27**, 495–506.

Stein, D.J., Fontenelle, L.F. and **Reed, G.M.** (2014). Obsessive-compulsive and related disorders in ICD-11. *Revista Brasileira de Psiquiatria*, **36** Suppl 1, 1–2.

Stein, D.J. and **Giordano, J.** (2015). Global mental health and neuroethics. *BMC Medicine*, **13**, 274.

Stein, D.J., Grant, J.E., Franklin, M.E., et al. (2010). Trichotillomania (hair pulling disorder). skin picking disorder, and stereotypic movement disorder: toward DSM-V. *Depression and Anxiety*, **27**, 611–626.

Stein, D.J. and **Gureje, O.** (2004). Depression and anxiety in the developing world: is it time to medicalise the suffering? *Lancet*, **364**, 233–234.

Stein, D.J., Hollander, E., and **Josephson, S.C.** (1994). Serotonin reuptake blockers for the treatment of obsessional jealousy. *Journal of Clinical Psychiatry*, **55**, 30–33.

Stein, D.J., Lund, C., and **Nesse, R.M.** (2013). Classification systems in psychiatry: diagnosis and global mental health in the era of DSM-5 and ICD-11. *Current Opinion in Psychiatry*, **26**, 493–497.

Stein, D.J. and **Nesse, R.M.** (2015). Normal and abnormal anxiety in the age of DSM-5 and ICD-11. *Emotion Review*, 7, 223–229.

Stein, D.J. and **Phillips, K.A.** (2014). Pros and cons of the new DSM-5 chapter on obsessive-compulsive and related disorders. *Current Psychiatry Reviews*, **10**, 325–329.

Stein, D.J., Phillips, K.A., Bolton, D., et al. (2010). What is a mental/psychiatric disorder? From DSM-IV to DSM-V. *Psychological Medicine*, **40**, 1759–1765.

Swedo, S.E. and **Grant, P.J.** (2005). Annotation: PANDAS: a model for human autoimmune disease. *Journal of Child Psychology and Psychiatry*, **46**, 227–234.

van Praag, H.M., Asnis, G.M., Kahn, R.S., et al. (1990). Monoamines and abnormal behaviour. A multi-aminergic perspective. *British Journal of Psychiatry*, **157**, 723–734.

Veale, D. and **Matsunaga, H.** (2014). Body dysmorphic disorder and olfactory reference disorder: proposals for ICD-11. *Revista Brasileira de Psiquiatria*, **36** Suppl 1, 14–20.

Wakefield, J.C. (1992). The concept of mental disorder. On the boundary between biological facts and social values. *Am Psychologist*, **47**, 373–388.

Walkup, J.T., Ferrao, Y., Leckman, J.F., et al. (2010). Tic disorders: some key issues for DSM-V. *Depression and Anxiety*, 27, 600–610.

Woods, D.W. and **Thomsen, P.H.** (2014). Tourette and tic disorders in ICD-11: standing at the diagnostic crossroads. *Revista Brasileira de Psiquiatria*, **36** Suppl 1, 51–58.

Zachar, P. and **Kendler, K.S.** (2012). The removal of Pluto from the class of planets and homosexuality from the class of psychiatric disorders: a comparison. *Philosophy, Ethics, and Humanity in Medicine*, 7, 4.

Chapter 9

"A messy business": Balancing considerations in revising the psychiatric nosology

Miriam Solomon

9.1 Introduction

Dan Stein offers us a ringside view of multiple considerations that went into recent revisions of just one subsection of psychiatric nosologies (in DSM, ICD-11, and RDoC): the subsection covering obsessive-compulsive and related disorders (OCRDs). These considerations include results from imaging neuroscience, results from animal models, genetic data, results from field studies, clinical data and experience, and patient advocacy. In addition, he finds historical contingency, or arbitrariness, in some of the outcomes. I find the story fascinating and philosophically rich. In my comments, I draw attention to five of the themes and develop them a little further. I conclude with some observations about conservatism in revision of psychiatric nosologies.

9.2 Prematurity of the science

Many psychiatric researchers hoped that the fifth edition of the *Diagnostic and Statistical Manual of Mental Disorders* (DSM-5) would incorporate recent results of genetic and neuroimaging studies, going beyond the "cluster of symptoms" approach that characterized DSM-III and DSM-IV to discern more of the etiology of psychiatric disorders. In the area of OCRDs, there have been intriguing results from neuroimaging. In particular, it looks as if the OCRDs are distinguished from anxiety disorders in that the activation is in the forebrain rather than in the amygdala. These studies, which suggest the anatomic outlines of an etiology (although not the etiology itself) were the basis for classifying the OCRDs separately from the anxiety disorders. However, other empirical results do not support this etiology. For example, cognitive-behavioral therapy and selective serotonin re-uptake inhibitors (SSRIs) are effective treatment modalities for both sets of disorders, and the disorders have considerable comorbidity. These results suggest a common, or at least overlapping, etiology, and could reasonably have been used to resist separating the OCRDs from the anxiety disorders. (The possibility of more than one reasonable conclusion is something I will address in section 9.6.) It is not possible to predict how the different streams of evidence—from neuroimaging, genetics, successful treatment, and comorbidity—will develop over time. At this time, new empirical results justify only provisional and modest changes in nosology.

9.3 Pluralism of nosologies

Although most of the focus is on the DSM, Stein describes the situation for three different nosologies: the DSM-5, the eleventh edition of the *International Classification of Diseases* (ICD-11), and the Research Domain Criteria (RDoC). DSM-5 is the classification produced by the American Psychiatric Association and is intended for both researchers and clinicians; ICD-11 is internationally and clinically oriented; and RDoC is a proposed dimensional framework for research that is designed to lead to identifying biomarkers and causal etiologies for mental disorders. (RDoC was developed with the support of Thomas Insel at the National Institute of Mental Health, and has an uncertain future now that Insel is no longer leading that organization.) No one wants the classification systems to diverge too much, because this would lead to confusion over applying the results of research to clinical practice, and vice versa. But small differences are manageable, and serve as a reminder that our classification systems do not (yet) carve nature at the joints. As an example, olfactory reference disorder is having a better reception in ICD-11 discussions than it had in DSM-5 discussions.

9.4 The role of historical contingency

Classification outcomes are dependent on the timing of the committee discussions, the salience of anecdotal experiences, and the influence of authoritative experts. None of these closely track new evidence, and so the result can be a somewhat arbitrary outcome due to what some philosophers of science call "external factors" (I have called them "non-empirical decision vectors" in Solomon 2001). An example is hoarding disorder, which according to Stein benefited from being discussed early in the DSM process, as well as from the support of an influential member of the Scientific Review Committee.

9.5 Patient advocacy

Tourette's syndrome has traditionally been classified among the OCRDs. Some patients and their advocates have preferred that it be classified as a neurological, rather than a psychiatric, disorder. This is because they do not wish to be affected by the stigma sometimes associated with an OCRD psychiatric diagnosis. Dan Stein points out that in resisting the OCRD diagnosis, these patients and their advocates are implicitly reinforcing stigmatization for those who have OCRD psychiatric diagnoses. (This is what Hilde Lindemann (in Nelson 2001) calls a "hostage taking" identity, and in Chapter 23 in this volume I explore a similar situation with the Asperger's diagnosis.) DSM-5 has gone with the wishes of these patients and their advocates, classifying Tourette's with neurodevelopmental disorders such as attention-deficit hyperactivity disorder (ADHD) and autism. On the other hand, ICD-11 classifies Tourette's in both categories—OCRD and neurodevelopmental disorders. Tourette's has considerable comorbidity with both obsessive-compulsive disorder and ADHD, and has been effectively treated with medications and cognitive-behavioral therapy. Thus there is evidence in favor of keeping the traditional classification.

9.6 **"An integrative approach"**

Dan Stein describes the overall situation when revising psychiatric nosologies as one in which both evidence and values play a role and need to be integrated in an overall decision about any changes. He also uses an overlapping dichotomous classification—which he calls "classical" and "critical"—to describe the joint influences of science (corresponds with "evidence") and pragmatic choices (corresponds with "values"). Another dichotomous classification covering similar (but not the same) same ground is "validity" versus "utility." As a first approximation, I think that framing the situation in terms of the integration of factors that fall into these binaries is helpful. But it is only a first approximation. The binary analyses obscure the fact that often it is empirical/scientific factors that conflict with one another (e.g., results of neuroimaging and results of clinical trials with behavior therapy), as well as pragmatic factors/values that conflict with one another (e.g. some patients' values may conflict with those of some psychiatrists, or some clinical demands may conflict with reimbursement practices). In addition, the three sets of binary categories used—classical/critical, validity/utility, and evidence/values—do not precisely coincide with each other. For example, evidence may tell against a "classical" classificatory scheme, and "values" may conflict with "utility."

Moreover, use of the language of "integration" of different factors relevant to classification does not tell us how the integration is done and in particular whether it is possible to do the integration in more than one way. It is likely that there is often more than one apparently reasonable decision, and unrelated factors (such as belief perseverance, or wish to make an impact, or the influence of powerful individuals) can play a deciding role. This is a problem that is not unique to psychiatry; it comes up in any area of science policy in which the evidence is complex,multimodal, and sometimes contrary (Stegenga 2011). Science and technology studies researchers Harry Collins and Trevor Pinch (1993) have argued that, when we study science and technology, "the mess is the message." Stein is right to note that "nosological revision is a messy business."

9.7 **Conclusion**

Finally, some comments about conservatism. DSM-5 ended up being much closer to DSM-IV than was expected or hoped for. This is in part because evidence for a new nosology has not yet reached critical mass. But it is also because of systematic processes that work against change. Every change to the DSM has costs in terms of education, communication, practice change, administrative overhauls, etc. Projected benefits from making a change need to outweigh the costs. Another factor is that the experts invited to serve on consensus committees typically participate in decisions about more than one classificatory system: for example, there is some overlap between those who serve on DSM committees and those who serve on ICD committees. Stein even mentions the role of a joint team of those leading DSM-5 and ICD-11 in settling on a common "metastructure." The deliberative processes of those committees are thus not independent, and the overlap of experts further reduces any potential for difference. If the processes were independent—and especially if they were concurrent—more difference would be likely.

Kenneth Kendler (2013) has pointed out that that there is one factor working against conservatism: the common desire among people who participate in these work groups to show that they have made a difference. Leaving a nosology the way it was before can make it look as if no work was done (even though much work may have been done). Is this factor an adequate corrective to the systematic processes resisting change?

References

Collins, H. and **Pinch, T.** (1993). *The Golem: What everyone should know about science.* Cambridge, UK: Cambridge University Press.

Kendler, K. (2013). A history of the DSM-5 Scientific Review Committee. *Psychological Medicine*, **43**, 1793–1800.

Nelson, H.L. (2001). *Damaged Identities, Narrative Repair.* Ithaca, NY: Cornell University Press.

Solomon, M. (2001). *Social Empiricism*. Cambridge, MA: MIT Press.

Stegenga, J. (2011). Is meta-analysis the platinum standard of evidence? *Studies in History and Philosophy of Biological and Biomedical Sciences*, **42**, 497–507.

Section 4

Network models of psychiatric disorders

Chapter 10

Introduction to "Mental disorders, network models, and dynamical systems"

Kenneth S. Kendler

Physicians are taught that there are things called diseases. We study many of them in our medical training. Diseases have causes (although we know a lot more about some than others). For some of them we have a pretty well understood pathophysiology. Also, very importantly, they have symptoms and signs that a good clinician should be able to detect on personal examination. For most diseases, they also have expected laboratory results or imaging findings on radiographs or more recently MRI or CT scans. Physicians do not actually learn a lot about what a disease is, from a philosophical or perhaps more exactly ontological perspective. But certainly, the idea is that somehow "the disease" causes the symptoms and signs. If I have coronary artery disease and therefore when I exercise too much and my heart does not get enough blood flow, it gets ischemic (not enough oxygen) and then I get chest pain. If I had an EKG at that moment, it might show expected changes in the ischemic heart muscle. If I am subject to migraine headaches, I might get an odd aura for a few minutes, followed by a pounding one-sided headache with photophobia (desire to avoid light) and nausea. The disease causes the symptoms and signs.

Now in psychiatry, while we know a lot about causes (but there are many of them and typically each contributes only a small bit) and very little about pathophysiology (aside from a few of the "organic" syndromes), the same general idea holds. Our patients have a disorder—schizophrenia or major depression—and we expect them to have certain symptoms (respectively, auditory hallucinations and thought disorder versus sad mood and guilt). If asked "What causes the symptoms?" the most typical response would be "The disease, of course!"

In this provocative chapter, Denny Borsboom, who is a psychometrician by profession and also a substantial contributor to the philosophical literature on problems of measurement, summarizes a rich line of research taking a very different look at the relationship between "diseases" and symptoms. Instead of diseases "causing" symptoms, he hypothesizes that the "disease" is a higher-order syndrome that emerges from a causal network of symptoms. So the cause–effect relationship is not "disorder → symptom" but rather "symptom → symptom." This is quite a conceptual shift and takes some getting used to. However, as Borsboom notes, the idea of symptom → symptom causation is not, in and of itself, unusual. Physicians are well used to pain in one hip, knee, or ankle altering the stride in such a way as to put strain on another joint and eventually cause pain there. Closer to home, it is common sense that a bad night's sleep increases tiredness the next day. Indeed, I was trained that if a depressed patient came in with bad insomnia, the advice was to start them on a particularly sedative antidepressant. So while the antidepressant was taking its usual 2–3 weeks to actually work on the core depressive symptoms, one could expect some immediate improvement in symptoms just from the fact that the patient would sleep better. It tended to work. In schizophrenia, hallucinations often lead to delusions. A women who heard voices commenting on her behavior in every room in her apartment decided that someone must have installed a video system with cameras in every room so they could see what she was doing. We sometimes call these "explanatory delusions."

My approach to these network models is not to get caught up in the question of whether they are "true" and the more typical "disorder → symptom" approach is "false." Rather, a more useful question is, "What can this perspective teach us about psychiatric disorders?" Here, I will emphasize five points that Borsboom will take up in more detail in his informative chapter.

- First, when a network is developed from empirical data, we obtain a quite different perspective on the individual symptoms that can be gotten from their listing in DSM-5. In particular, some of the symptoms are at the center of the network and highly connected with other symptoms. Some, by contrast, sit out on the periphery, rather lonely. This is a quite clinically informative way to think about our disorders.
- Second, some sets of symptoms are very strongly interconnected and others less so. Again, this provides a more "dynamic" view than can be obtained from the static listing of diagnostic criteria.
- Third, these network models give us a way to think about "stress to the system." Imagine a node of possible depressive symptoms. Then an individual (call him Mike) experiences a romantic rejection that produces some key symptoms—sadness, feelings of worthlessness, insomnia. We can see how this leads to a range of dynamic responses in Mike to that "insult."
- This leads to the fourth potential insight—that the "level of connectivity" describes a potentially crucial individual difference in network properties. As Borsboom shows with statistical simulation, but can be easily intuited with a bit of effort, for some people the individual symptoms are highly interconnected. One problem quickly leads to another as the syndrome proliferates through the network. Others are less connected or, to use a recent favorite word, more *resilient*. So in Mike's case high connectivity might result in the onset of loss of appetite, guilt, difficulty concentrating, and loss of interest as he develops toward a depressive episode in the next few days. If, however, Mike had low connectivity, he might be sad, a bit dejected, and have trouble sleeping for a day or two but develop no other symptoms.

- Finally, networks can have a very interested property described by a fancy Greek term: *hysteresis*. This is what can happen when the network reaches and then exceeds a tipping point. Importantly, it often is not symmetrical. That is, stress can push you "over the edge" and a depression develops. But when the stress is relieved, the system can be "stuck" in the depression mode and will not easily revert back to the non-depressed state. Anyone who has worked with patients with classically episodic disorders (schizophrenia, depression, mania, alcoholism) knows what this is like. To the clinician, it feels as if a switch has been thrown. This can often happen very quickly and as a clinician you often have to rapidly mobilize both psychosocial and pharmacological resources to deal with the new situation.

In the latter parts of his essay, Borsboom explores the implications of this network model for some key philosophical/conceptual issues in psychiatry. If the network theory is even approximately true, what does that tell us about the ontological status of psychiatric disorders—that is "what sort of things are psychiatric disorders"? What does it tell us about the role of emergence versus biological (aka neuroscientific) reductionism? At a minimum, this essay should render the reader less secure about the standard "disorder → symptom" causal model of psychiatric illness. More richly, it will provide a platform for a range of potential rich insights into psychiatric matters of both clinical and philosophical relevance.

Chapter 11

Mental disorders, network models, and dynamical systems

Denny Borsboom

11.1 Network approaches to psychopathology

In network approaches to psychopathology, mental disorders are conceptualized in terms of causal networks of symptoms. The network approach originated as an attempt to make sense of the robust patterns of associations that hold among symptoms, without invoking latent disorders as common causes (Borsboom 2008, Borsboom and Cramer 2013, 2015). The basic idea is that clusters of symptoms, which define disorders in diagnostic manuals like the fifth edition of the *Diagnostic and Statistical Manual of Mental Disorders* (DSM-5), do not hang together because they are caused by the same latent disorder, but because they directly influence each other (Cramer et al. 2010, Borsboom and Cramer 2013, Cramer and Borsboom 2015).

The network approach has often been placed in opposition to standard treatments of psychiatric data with latent variable models, in which the covariance between symptoms results from the common influence of a latent variable (Borsboom and Cramer 2013). In the latent variable model, causal relations between symptoms are a nuisance, as they will typically present violations of the axiom of local independence (Cramer et al. 2010, but see also Epskamp et al., *in press*, for alternative views). In the network model, these same relations form the flesh and bones of the disorder. Thus, the network model represents a radically different way of psychometric theorizing about the relation between symptoms and disorders.

Despite this radical difference, however, it should be noted that the main ingredient of the network approach—the pervasiveness of symptom–symptom causation—is not a spectacular new scientific hypothesis but a rather prosaic and down-to-earth phenomenon with which clinicians are quite familiar. In fact, when asked to represent relations between symptoms, clinicians spontaneously construct causal diagrams (Kim and Ahn 2002). In addition, diagnostic systems routinely specify the existence of causal relations between symptoms as diagnostic criteria. For example, frequent hand-washing only counts as a diagnostic criterion for obsessive-compulsive disorder (OCD) if the compulsion is triggered by a corresponding obsession with cleanliness or a persistent feeling of being dirty. Increased arousal only counts as a criterion for post-traumatic stress disorder (PTSD) if it results from the exposure to a traumatic event. Reckless behavior only counts as a criterion for alcohol use disorder if it arises as a result of drinking alcohol. Avoiding public places only counts as symptom of panic disorder if it is caused by the presence of panic attacks, which instill the fear of having such attacks in public. Finally, in cases where no explicit symptom–symptom causation is required for a diagnosis, it is still likely that such causation exists. For major depressive episode, for instance, the symptom of insomnia is likely to causally affect the symptom of fatigue, which in turn can influence the symptom of concentration problems, which could result in the symptoms of depressed mood and self-reproach, which may in turn lead back to insomnia.

Thus, causal relations between symptoms play an essential role in the diagnosis and analysis of mental disorders, both explicitly and implicitly. If such causal relations form vicious circles of feedback, the disorder as whole (i.e., the group of symptoms involved in these causal relations) starts functioning as a non-linear complex system. It is not profitable to analyze such a system is with linear methods. For instance, in a non-linear complex system, very small changes can have detrimental effects if the structure of interactions between symptoms is strong, but may have no effects at all if these interactions are minimal (Scheffer et al. 2009). This makes it very hard to analyze these systems with traditional methods, which tend to isolate particular parts of the system while failing to take into account its functioning as a whole. Network models are more promising candidates for studying this type of complex phenomenon, because they naturally represent the functioning of nodes in relation to other nodes in the network (Kolaczyk 2009 p. 398, Newman 2010).

Connected nodes in a network will show synchronized behavior. This can be seen in many familiar natural phenomena. For instance, birds in a flock may synchronize their flight pattern as a result of low-level local interactions between individual birds. In the network perspective, disorders are analogous to such flocks, as disorders result from the interplay of more tightly connected sets of symptoms. This explains why the symptoms of disorders hang together, but also why survey research on psychopathology shows such high levels of comorbidity (Kessler et al. 2007): patterns of symptom–symptom interaction are unlikely to exactly follow the borders between disorders as laid down in a book like the DSM-V. Unless symptom networks are neatly separated (which the evidence suggests is not the case; Boschloo et al. 2015), *bridge symptoms* that connect different disorders will transfer symptom activation from one disorder to another (Cramer et al. 2010). From a network perspective, therefore, high levels of comorbidity are unavoidable: they do not result from artifacts that arise through measurement imperfections or inadequate definitions of disorders, but from real patterns of connectivity that are inherent to the domain of psychopathology. As such, comorbidity should be seen as a key phenomenon in psychopathology research, rather than as a nuisance.

Although the general idea of symptom networks is quite simple, network models yield a rich trove of unexpected theoretical implications and empirical hypotheses.

Causal interactions between symptoms and vicious circles of reinforcement produce emergent network behavior that bears striking similarities to known features of mental disorders. In the present contribution, I want to flesh out these similarities to provide a general model of mental health and mental disorders, and sketch an image of how mental disorders should be conceptually analyzed. I will focus on three topics: the conceptualization of disorders and health in network models, the question of whether mental disorders are real entities or not, and the question of how we should think of mental disorders as networks in relation to the current waves of biological reductionism in psychiatry and clinical psychology.

11.2 Mental health, external stressors, and disorder states

In the network approach, there are two building blocks of mental disorders: symptoms, and relations between symptoms. Symptoms themselves can be triggered by events within the organism (e.g., developmental changes in anxiety pathways involving the amygdala as a result of genetic risk factors) or by events that take place in the environment (e.g., life events, like losing a spouse or getting fired). Once a symptom is triggered, it increases the probability of other symptoms to which it is causally connected. Causal relations may be understood in the sense of Pearl's (2000) model, which is most naturally compatible with the definition of causal relations in terms of hypothetical interventions (Woodward 2003); if one's network includes a causal connection between symptoms like energy loss and psychomotor retardation, then that means that if (by some natural or experimental intervention) energy loss becomes activated, then that will increase the probability of psychomotor retardation becoming activated as well. Causal relations are not necessarily seen as unidirectional; in the example, motor retardation may also trigger energy loss. As a result, symptoms may engage in feedback interactions.

In typical network modeling efforts (e.g., Van Borkulo et al. 2014) no particular directionality of causation is assumed and the network includes pairwise interactions between symptoms. These patterns of pairwise interaction can be interpreted as a Markov random field (MRF; Kindermann and Snell 1980), which describes structural probabilistic relations between pairs of variables: specifically, if a connection (typically denoted an *edge*) between two nodes is missing, this means the nodes are conditionally independent given the remaining nodes in the network, while if an edge is present, they are conditionally dependent. It should be noted that, although the MRF does not encode directionality of relations between nodes, it is not merely a representation of correlations, because in an MRF each connection is evaluated conditional on the remaining nodes. Instead, it is better to think of the MRF as a representation of partial correlations. A visualization of an MRF that we constructed for a subset of DSM-IV symptoms is represented in Figure 11.1.

Dynamics of symptom networks resemble those of other complex systems in nature, such as ecosystems, social networks, or financial networks (Van de Leemput

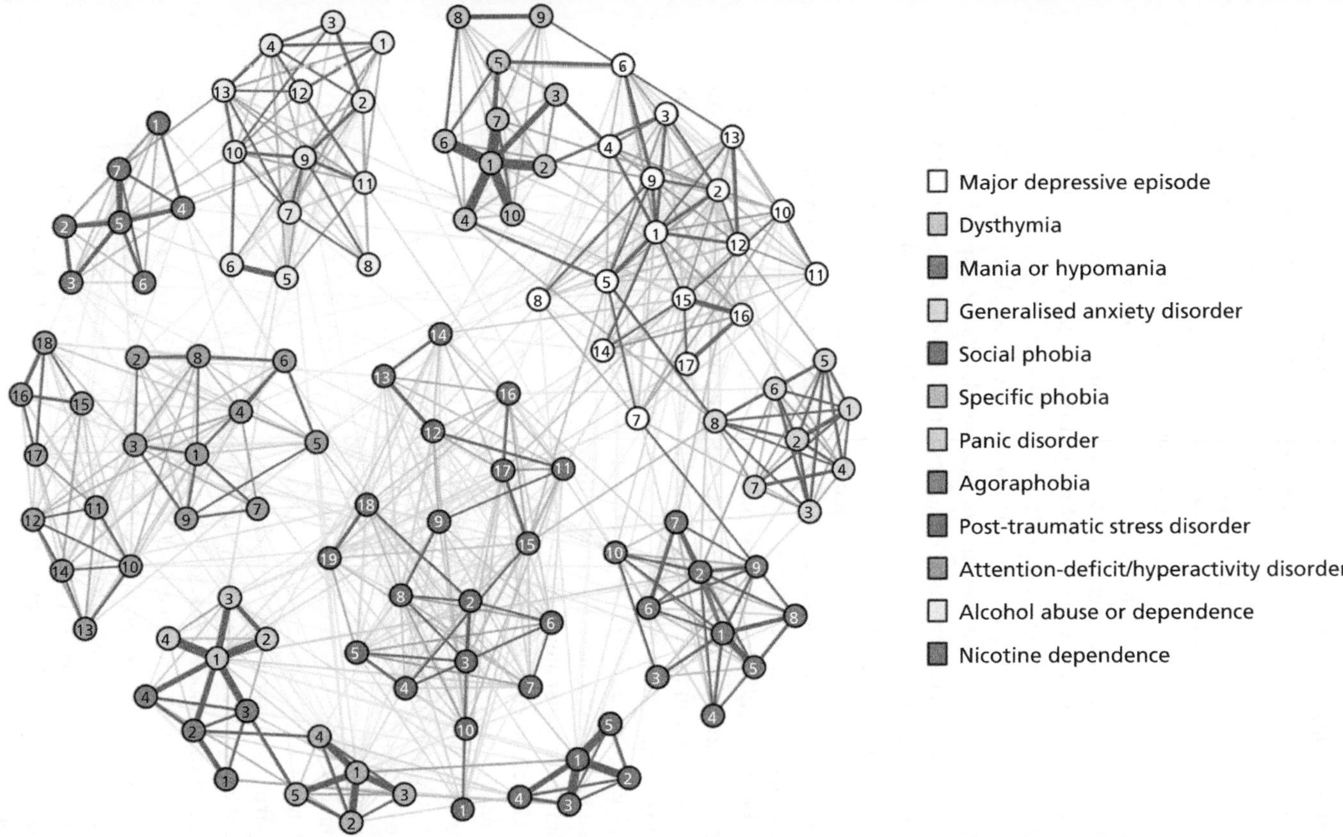

Figure 11.1 Network structure as fitted DSM-IV symptom data from a large community sample (Boschloo et al. 2015), using the R-software package IsingFit (Van Borkulo et al. 2014). Individual symptoms are represented as nodes. The strength of connections between symptoms is estimated using a penalized regression model. In the figure, stronger positive (negative) connections are represented by thicker green (red) edges. Disorders emerge out of the analysis as sets of tightly connected symptoms that tend to synchronize through the connectivity structure. Comorbidity arises as a result of edges that connect symptoms from distinct disorders ('bridge symptoms').

et al. 2014). The basic mechanism in these networks is that external shocks produce activation in a part of the system (e.g., death of a spouse triggers loneliness and depressed mood), which then propagates through the connections in the network (e.g., loneliness and depressed mood may trigger feelings of worthlessness, which in turn cause insomnia, etc.). This is analogous to the way a virus spreads through a population, where affected individuals can infect other individuals in their physical proximity (i.e., to whom they are connected in the network structure).

There are three primary determinants of the dynamics that a network displays in response to external triggers. First, the threshold values of individual nodes, which determine how easily a given node is activated; second, the level of connectivity of the system, which depends on the density and architecture of the network; third, the number and strength of external shocks that impinge on the system, which can be thought of as random perturbations. As a rule, low thresholds, high connectivity, and increased intensity of external shocks each spell bad news in symptom networks. High intensity of random shocks implies that the individual symptoms are under external pressure; low thresholds imply that a person easily develops symptomatology in response to such pressure; high connectivity implies that the activation of particular symptoms easily spreads through the network. We know quite a lot about the structure of the general network of psychopathology symptoms in these three respects.

First, the threshold values of most or all individual symptoms must be typically high (or negative, in an Ising representation; Epskamp et al. *in press*), as most symptoms are known to be rare and symptom distributions are typically heavily skewed to the right (Sturt 1981).

Second, the connectivity of the system must be overwhelmingly positive, in the sense that symptoms tend to aggravate rather than inhibit each other. This can be seen from the fact that almost all coefficients in the MRF for DSM symptoms are positive (Boschloo et al. 2015; see also Figure 11.1). This produces a structure of positive relations between symptoms that factor analysts pick up as a general factor (the *p*-factor; Caspi et al. 2014). The architecture of the relations between symptoms resembles that of a small world, in the sense that most symptoms cluster in groups (which seem to correspond to disorders; Boschloo et al. 2015), but there are also quite a few connections between symptoms from different disorders so that the general "distances" between symptoms in the network are small (Borsboom et al. 2011).

Third, for many disorders we know that external influences impinge on particular parts of the symptom network in a distinguishable pattern; for instance, depressive episodes are often precipitated by adverse life events, but *which* life event triggers the episode seems to determine which particular symptoms are present (Keller et al. 2007, Cramer et al. 2012, Fried et al. 2015a). Depressive symptoms in addition appear to engage in specific and differentiated patterns of statistical and causal associations with external variables (Lux and Kendler 2010, Fried 2015, Fried and Nesse 2015, Fried et al. 2015a, 2015b). It seems safe to assume that the same holds for many other symptoms in psychopathology. If this is correct, then we conceive of external shocks as random events that impinge on particular symptoms or sets of symptoms.

Note that the fact that shocks are considered random within the individual does not mean they are randomly distributed over individuals: some individuals may structurally receive more shocks than others, and this intensity may in fact depend on features of the individual person's network. Also, note that the word "external" here means "external to the network" and not "external to the individual"; for instance, medical conditions that are not part of DSM symptomatology are external in the sense intended here, because they affect the network from outside (e.g., chronic back pain may cause insomnia which may cause fatigue and depressed mood), even though these medical conditions can often be traced to internal physical causes (e.g., a hernia). Thus, "outside the network" does not mean "outside the person."

How easily do these external shocks propagate through the network? It seems likely that individual people will differ in the ease with which symptoms become activated (the model thresholds) and connectivity of the symptoms (model interaction parameters). For instance, Pe et al. (2015) found marked individual differences in time-series networks of individual people, with depressed cases showing increased connectivity among negative mood states; similarly, Van Borkulo et al. (2015) showed that symptom networks of depressed individuals who remit are less strongly connected than networks of those who persist in a depressive episode.

Such differences in the connectivity of symptoms generate dynamics that bear a striking resemblance to known features of mental disorders. If symptom–symptom interactions are not very strong (we have a *weakly connected network*), networks exhibit spontaneous recovery; that is, when a network is perturbed by a random event (say, some symptoms in one's depression network is triggered by the loss of a loved one), the network can show strong symptom activation that resembles a disorder and may actually satisfy diagnostic criteria, but it will spontaneously return to its stable state. In a weakly connected network with realistic settings, this stable state is a situation in which no symptoms are systematically present. These differences in reactivity depending on the connectivity of the system are illustrated in Figure 11.2 with two hypothetical cases of Alice and Bob.

On the basis of this analysis, we may consider a new definition of mental health: *Mental health is the stable state of a weakly connected symptom network.* Mental health is characterized by a resilient symptom network which, if perturbed, quickly returns to its stable state, which is a state in which symptoms are naturally inactive. Note that this definition does *not* equate mental health to the absence of symptoms. Rather it equates mental health to the attractor state of a complex network, which implies absence of symptoms (apart from random variation) but is not identical to it. This is because the implication is not bidirectional: symptoms can be absent even though the system is not healthy. For instance, a system that has high connectivity may nevertheless occasionally visit states in the dynamical landscape in which no symptoms are activated; this can happen as a result of random fluctuations in system behavior. In addition, one can have a situation in which external influences on the system keep symptoms inactive, even though the connectivity between symptoms remains high; one might think of a person with

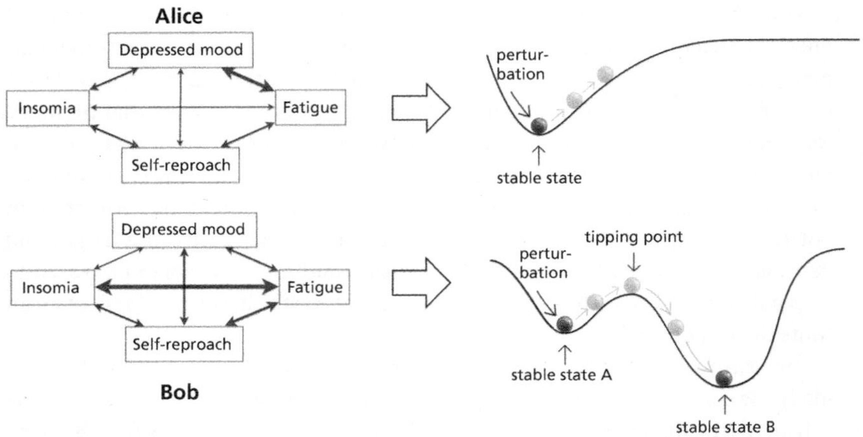

Figure 11.2 *The relation between network structure and disorder dynamics.* Alice's network, which has a weak connectivity profile (left top), gives rise to a single basin of attraction (right top), corresponding to a healthy state. Continued stress (perturbation; force being exerted on the ball from the left) may cause prolonged changes in state (elevated ball), but upon removal of stress the network will return to the healthy state. Bob's more strongly connected network (bottom left) feature alternative stable states (bottom right) and a *tipping point*: If external stress exceeds a given value, then the system collapses to the disordered state, which is itself stable. Thus, the system will maintain the disordered state, even if the stressor is removed.

persistent psychotic episodes, who is momentarily in remission due to medication, but who would revisit the psychotic state as soon as this external factor is removed.

Also note that the definition of mental health given here does not exclude the relevance of positive factors in one's life, or the presence of well-being (the "positive" definition of health; WHO 1948). It is entirely conceivable, and in fact quite likely, that well-being in several domains is a necessary condition for keeping the connectivity of a symptoms network low. If people, for whatever reason, cannot profitably and productively engage in daily life, or cannot maintain rewarding social relations, naturally occurring fluctuations in symptomatology may have much more room to propagate through a problem network.

If mental health is indeed the stable state of a weakly connected symptom network, the question that immediately arises is: how do mental disorders come into being and what are they? In the network model, the patterns of symptom activation that we associate with mental disorders can arise in two ways. First, events external to the network can trigger psychopathology symptoms without these symptoms having increased connectivity. Triggering events may either be environmental stressors (e.g., losing one's job) or may be a function of various abnormalities originating from the body (e.g., chronic pain). Because these effects concern main effects on the symptoms, they lead to elevated symptom levels that are not self-sustaining. For weak levels of symptom–symptom interaction, elevated symptom activation may reach diagnosable levels, and people may be in need of treatment as a result of this, but the network itself is not able to sustain its disordered state by itself. This means that, when stressors are removed, or when symptom level activation is diminished by external interventions (e.g., therapy or medication), the symptoms will return to their resting state: the state of mental health.

A second way in which pathology can arise, which is much more serious and in which mental disorders arise as autonomous phenomena, is through a combination of symptom–symptom interaction and external stressors. Simulations and mathematical derivations show that *highly connected* symptom networks, in which symptoms have increased effects on each other, feature a very different dynamical landscape from weakly connected networks. In highly connected networks, we observe the phenomenon of *hysteresis* (Cramer 2013). Hysteresis is a characteristic of phase transitions, which are characterized by an asymmetry in the route that leads to and from a given state. A familiar example of hysteresis arises when water freezes and melts: although water freezes at 0 degrees Celsius, it only melts at +4 degrees Celsius. Thus, the point at which the system enters an alternative state (e.g., transforming from water to ice) is not the point at which it returns. In a network model, the same phenomenon turns out to occur in highly connected networks: a highly connected network reinforces itself to such a degree that, once it is activated by a given level of stress, removal of the stressor does not lead to recovery. This also means that, in networks that are highly connected, disease status has a non-arbitrary theoretical definition (Table 11.1).

Now, we may occasionally see highly connected networks that are temporarily in a healthy state. Due to the network connectivity, however, this state is unstable and will flip back into disorder upon a small random perturbation. Such networks are, so to speak, in remission, but have increased probability of relapse due to their high vulnerability.

Thus, in the network perspective, both mental health and mental disorders may receive novel theoretical definitions: Mental health is the stable state of a weakly connected network, whereas mental disorders are alternative stable states of highly connected (sub)networks of symptoms. In between these conditions, we find weakly connected networks under stress: these networks exhibit elevated symptom levels, but these are not self-reinforcing to such an extent that the network will autonomously remain in a prolonged disorder state; such conditions may also

Table 11.1. Disease status as a function of network structure and external stressors

		Network structure	
		Weakly connected	Highly connected
Stress level	Low	*Mental health with high resilience*	*Elevated vulnerability (possibly remission status)*
	High	*Elevated Symptomatology*	*Mental disorder*

resemble "reactive" or "psychogenic" disorders in the psychiatric literature, in that they do not primarily result from internal connectivity, but from external shocks. These four situations are depicted in Table 11.1.

11.3 **Are mental disorders real?**

The network model offers a novel approach to answer age-old questions regarding the *ontology* of mental disorders: the question of whether they are real, and, if so, in what sense (Kendler et al. 2011). Classically, the debate on this issue has centered on two extreme positions that could be taken in response to this question. First, the *essentialist* position, which holds that individuals who suffer from, say, depression, share a property that clearly distinguishes them from individuals who suffer from another disorder. This is arguably the classical view in psychiatry, in which psychiatric disorders are seen as fully parallel to medical diseases (Kraepelin 1907). Second, the *constructivist* position, which holds that mental disorders are "merely" labels, which are used to steer policy or execute power over individuals, but may not map onto particular medically homogeneous categories or *natural kinds* (Foucault 1973, Hacking 1999).

Neither of these positions is attractive in the face of the evidence. Essentialism promises that, somewhere beneath the level of symptomatology, disorder types should correspond to some deeper level of reality, much as the overt symptomatology of wound infections betrays the presence of bacteria. Although, in psychiatry, much has been made of attempts to identify similar variables based on neurobiology or genetics, the current evidence suggests that, so far, such attempts have failed to identify *essences* for mental disorders. This is not, of course, to deny that important neurobiological systems are somehow involved in the disorders, but merely to state that no such factors have been shown to operate as a common cause in that way that, say, the presence of spirochetes operates as a common cause in producing the symptoms of what used to be known as general paralysis of the insane (i.e., syphilis; Raju 2006). The same holds for suggestions that locate the essence of disorders in etiology, central psychological mechanisms, or particular environmental circumstances. Instead, the evidence suggests that mental disorders are massively multifactorial in their determinants (Nolen-Hoeksema and Watkins 2011), and lack common pathways from external variables (e.g., gunfire) to overt symptomatology (e.g., fever) via central mechanisms (e.g., the presence of bacteria in a wound).

However weak the evidence for essentialism may be, the purely constructivist position does not convince many scholars either. Although most would admit that, in diagnosis, arbitrary labeling is going on to some extent (e.g., boundaries between disorders like generalized anxiety disorder (GAD) and major depressive disorder (MDD) are so unclear that some cases could receive either diagnosis or both), it is an undeniable fact of the matter that the symptoms associated with disorders do cluster in highly reliable ways. That is, symptoms of GAD and MDD may be hard to separate in individual cases, but this is *precisely because* they correlate so highly; and they do so in many different datasets gathered in many different cultures and in many different temporal periods. In addition, these correlations are markedly higher than, say, the correlation between depressive symptoms and psychotic symptoms. This suggests that, although the current classification schemes may not cut reality precisely at its joints, the allocation of these symptoms to disorders or disorder groups (e.g., internalizing or externalizing) does capture an important objective fact about reality, which transcends purely arbitrary labeling.

Thus, mental disorders seem too real to be fully arbitrary, but do not correspond to neatly identifiable (sets of) essential properties. The network approach may offer an ontological account of disorders that suits the evidence in this respect, as it can explain how disorders may be real *without* corresponding to essentialist properties.

In discussing this, it is important to sharply distinguish between two questions regarding the reality of disorders that are often conflated in the literature. First, the problem of *disorder status*: is there a sharp boundary between healthy and disease status? As has been argued above, in a network model more strongly connected networks may generate objective and discretely separable disease states in the form of attractor states of the network, separated by phase transitions. In this sense, they can be considered as real as anything, even though they do not necessarily correspond to any particular process or property of mind, brain, or genes; instead, they exist as clusters of connected variables or mechanisms (Kendler et al. 2011). The second problem is that of *disorder separation*: how are sets of symptoms (e.g., depression symptoms) distinguished from other sets of symptoms (e.g., anxiety or psychotic symptoms)? With respect to the problem of distinguishing disorders, the network model has been argued to imply that sharp disorder separation is inherently problematic (Cramer et al. 2010). The reason is that, unless networks are entirely isolated, boundaries between disorders are intrinsically fuzzy.

This is illustrated in Figure 11.1, which shows that sets of symptoms that belong to the same disorder are more strongly connected that sets of symptoms that belong to different disorders. Thus, in this particular dataset, symptom clusters do seem to reflect the structure of the DSM. However, at the same time, there is a non-negligible set of relations that connects different disorders to each other, suggesting that these disorders are not neatly separated. In the network model, the excessive level of comorbidity that typically arises in studies using DSM-based interviews has been explained on the basis of this feature. When symptom activation in one area of the network (e.g., depressed mood, feelings of guilt, agitation, which are unique to MDD) causes activation in a related part that is shared with another disorder (e.g., insomnia and fatigue, which are common to GAD and MDD), then this may in itself lead to activation of the symptoms unique to distinct disorder (e.g., anxiety and muscle tension, which are unique to GAD). In this way, symptom activation may spread across the network much like a fire spreads through a forest or an epidemic spreads through a social network.

Thus, at first glance, it seems that the network approach only partly sustains the idea that disorders are distinct. However, it is possible that, if certain areas in the problem network are particularly highly connected in an individual, this may lead that particular part of the network to display discrete boundaries between disorder states—even though the subnetwork that corresponds to the disorder itself is not discretely separated from other disorder networks. That is, even for a system like that depicted in Figure 11.1, distinct disorder states (in the intra-individual sense) are possible as a function of locally strengthened connections between symptoms. Rigorously applying the line of reasoning put forward here, one may then regard the resulting disorder states as being non-arbitrary, and one could define discretely separated disorders indirectly, via the sets of discrete states that they can sustain. In other words, given a network structure, one could identify as many disorders as there are discretely separable attractor states that differ from the healthy state.

It is important to note that discrete states in networks do not necessarily translate into taxometric kinds as traditionally construed in psychometric approaches to clinical psychology (Meehl 1992, Haslam et al. 2012). Classical taxometric kinds are applied to individual differences (each individual belongs to a particular category) whereas the line of reasoning here applies to distinctions between intra-individual states. It is entirely conceivable that, say, depression scores vary continuously in the population, but show discontinuous change within the individual; in fact, despite the continuous character of such scores in classical taxometric analyses (Haslam et al. 2012), intra-individual patters do seem to evidence discrete transitions (Hosenfeld et al. 2015, Wichers et al. 2016).

11.4 The conceptual analysis of mental disorders

The question of how mental disorders should be conceptually analyzed and philosophically understood is rarely addressed in substantive research, which is typically focused on the analysis of empirical data. This makes it quite hard to assess what kind of model authors have in mind when, say, assessing the effectiveness of therapy or the genetic determinants of mental disorders. However, it seems that a sizeable portion of the current mainstream work is based on a premise of (some form of) biological reductionism. Although it is hard to pinpoint exactly what this position should be taken to entail, it appears clear that many researchers minimally assume that, in order to further our understanding of mental disorders, we need to intensify our research endeavors on the functional and structural analysis of the brain in relation to mental disorders, in order to uncover their "biological basis." That is, the current paradigm regards progress in neuroscience as a necessary condition for real progress in clinical psychology and psychiatry, and some even see it essentially the only way forward (Insel and Cuthbert 2015).

This is somewhat ironic, because a sober evaluation of the literature can only lead to the conclusion that, for the common mental disorders, no convincing biological basis has been found, at least if such a biological basis is defined as a common causal condition that produces symptomatology, analogous to the way a lung tumor causes chest pain or internal bleeding causes hypovolemic shock. Surely, there are many biological correlates of mental disorders, but the correlations in question are usually weak and not specific to the disorders in question. The same appears to hold for the genetic basis of mental disorders; although some specific genetic effects do exist, these are generally weak, and the most widely accepted view now seems to be that mental disorders are polygenic to such a high degree that it is altogether unclear whether the sum total of the hundreds of thousands of genetic effects may ever lead to a cognitively comprehensible analysis of, say, the genetic basis of depression (see also Turkheimer, *in press*). Had genome-wide association studies (GWAS) uncovered major genetic effects, as they have in, say, diabetes or some variants of cancer research, one could optimistically speculate on the existence of a limited number of biological pathways that would connect the relevant genes to specific endophenotypes (typically related to brain function), which then would themselves cause specific disorders. However, in face of a bewildering multitude of statistically weak relations between a great many genes and relevant phenotypes, this seems like a very difficult research programme indeed. It thus appears that one of the major findings in the past century of research on this topic is a negative one: none of the major mental disorders allows for a *simple* analysis in terms of biological pathways, endophenotypes, and neural mechanisms, where "simple" refers to the kind of explanatory simplicity of common biological pathways that characterizes many of the great medical discoveries (e.g., the discovery of bacterial infections, tumors, or viruses as the cause of previously ill-understood symptomatology).

Now, it is important to qualify the above conclusion, as it is easily misunderstood as general skepticism with respect to neuroscience or genetics. I do not intend such a reading. Some decades ago, a respectable scientist could still venture a major gene theory of, say, schizophrenia, as for instance, a great theoretician like Paul Meehl did (Meehl 1972). Today, such a position has become untenable, as many individual genes are implicated in the etiology of the disorder, with none having a particularly large influence (Schizophrenia Working Group of the Psychiatric Genomics Consortium 2014). Findings like these are of monumental importance, precisely because they falsify theories of mental disorders. In addition, I do not deny the importance of empirical results on, say, the relevance of the dopamine system for hallucinations in psychosis (Crow and Harringon 1994). Many biological factors are involved in many of the common mental disorders, and the investigation of such factors is of great importance. The proper conclusion to draw from the current state of affairs is not that we have learned nothing from biological approaches, or should stop doing biologically inspired research, but that analyses that treat psychiatric disorders as common causes of their symptoms, which may be uncovered through intensified focus on biology, are simply not in good shape. In fact, even though some researchers appear incurably optimistic about the viability of redefining mental disorders in terms of biological conditions (Insel and Cuthbert 2015), it seems to me that the prospects for this approach are actually rather gloomy.

This has strong implications for the way we should statistically represent and analyze data. Current research almost invariably treats symptoms as reflective measures of disorders (Edwards and Bagozzi 2000, Markus and Borsboom 2013). This means that symptoms can be counted, and that the resulting counts may be taken as measures of an underlying latent quantity or quality (e.g., Reise and Waller 2009). The resulting total scores are then related to genes, biological factors, or environmental conditions. This practice makes sense under a common cause model, but not under a network model, as it entirely ignores the internal dynamics of mental disorders that will be at play if a network model is correct. Standard approaches force a homogeneity assumption on symptoms which, it seems to me, is productive only in case the symptoms are actually exchangeable in relevant ways; that is, when they are in fact caused by the same latent disorder (Borsboom and Cramer 2013). If this is not the case, then counting symptoms or adding item responses will be utterly useless if one is trying to disentangle the causal processes that lead to and maintain disorder states (although total scores may still be useful to get an overall picture of disorder states, in which case the total score functions as an index variable, similar to the way the Dow Jones is used as an overall indicator of the state of the economy).

Is there another way forward? If disorders are indeed emergent phenomena that originate in patterns of symptom–symptom causation, the answer is yes. To show why, suppose we want to understand the ecosystem of the North Sea. What is required for this is that we develop a reasonable idea of which animals eat which other animals, and at what rate; in addition, we have to understand the equilibrium of the species in the water, and the environmental parameters that impinge on them. However, we do *not* need to know the details of the digestive system of the herring in order to model its role in the ecosystem; we simply have to know how many herrings there are, what they eat, and how fast they procreate. It is an attractive idea that the same may hold for mental disorders: what we need to know, then, is primarily which symptoms cause which other symptoms. Although it is interesting, and in certain cases may be possible, to do biological research in order to understand precisely which biological mechanisms connect two symptoms, that may not always be necessary for the purpose of understanding the dynamical system that generates and sustains mental disorders.

In fact, for such understanding, entirely different pieces of information are necessary—pieces of information that we currently lack and that future research should uncover. The minimum requirements for understanding the working of a complex network are:

- knowledge of how individual symptoms arise
- insight into which symptoms affect which other symptoms
- reasonable estimates of the functional forms and effect sizes of these causal relations
- understanding of the time scale at which the relevant symptom–symptom interactions operate.

We have only a rudimentary view of the operating principles of this system, as very little research has been directed at individual symptom dynamics and causal connections between symptoms. It is a fascinating idea that our understanding of mental disorders is not caused by an inadequate understanding of gene–brain–behavior pathways, but by an inadequate conceptualization of what we are doing.

A more holistic analysis of symptom networks may offer a road forward in the understanding of mental disorders, where biological reductionism has so far failed. However, perhaps unexpectedly, the results of such approaches may also serve to improve the resolution of biologically inspired studies. That is, if we develop a good idea of the connectivity of the symptom space, then we may develop novel ways of defining and operationalizing phenotypes for genetics and neuroscientific research. As an example, suppose that network research shows that most of the symptom–symptom connections in, say, depression, are similar in magnitude across people, but that the connection between insomnia and depressive mood is particularly variable. Then that connection should be the focus of research on individual differences, as it likely produces most of the variability in the network.

This may lead to studies that disentangle a particular part of a symptom network; for instance, by measuring the strength of a specific symptom–symptom connection using experience sampling methodology. This way, a specific network parameter could be estimated for each individual (e.g., see Wichers 2014). It is possible that, when analyzing such specific parameters, a much clearer biological picture will emerge, because we will have a much more focused research topic: instead of elusive mental disorders, we can study particular causal relations between particular variables. In addition, such research may serve a very important function in controlling disorders: If a particular symptom–symptom connection is dependent on a particular biological mechanism, then this can suggest interventions that interrupt this connection (e.g., pharmaceutical treatment). Thus, if a network model adequately describes the structure of mental disorders, we should not expect breakthroughs in research that aims to uncover simple common biological pathways that lead to disorders; however, we may very well see breakthroughs in research that aims to identify and understand biological pathways that underlie symptom–symptom relations in a networks.

11.5 Discussion

Network models offer a rich theoretical perspective mental disorders and mental health. The present chapter has attempted to lay out some of the theoretical and empirical implications that follow from this perspective. I have shown how mental health and mental disorder could be conceptualized in terms of alternative attractor states in symptom networks. If such a conceptualization turns out to be consistent with the empirical evidence, this may change our conceptualization of mental disorders and, perhaps more importantly, the way we organize empirical research psychopathology.

In particular, networks are by their nature holistic structures that can only be understood by investigating the connectivity patterns of the network as a whole (Baaási 2012). In my view, this should inspire researchers to look for causes and mechanisms underlying mental disorders in a different and largely unexplored empirical corner: rather than searching for clearly delineated biological bases of mental disorders, researchers may profitably start charting the dynamics and causal dependencies that characterize individual symptoms in psychopathology; in a second step, these may be related to biological factors, and this may considerably increase the resolution and focus of research programmes in psychopathology.

Of course, many questions arise as a result of this analysis. For example, we may wonder whether, and to what extent, the given definitions of health and disorder are general. In particular, the graph depicted in Figure 11.1 extends over many different mental disorders, but is it likely that network models indeed cover the entire space of psychopathology? Or should we expect their usefulness to be limited to particular disorders, such as depression and anxiety? In particular, some disorders (e.g., autism) may seem more amenable to a biological analysis than others (e.g., depression), and this may generate the idea that a common model is more appropriate for the former.

However, it should be clear that common causes do not equate to biological causes or vice versa: there may be common causes that are outside the person (e.g., losing a spouse may be the common cause of sadness and feelings of guilt) or biological structures that behave as networks (e.g., different organs that influence each other's functioning). In the case of autism, for instance, it is conceivable that a common cause drives the relation between, say, fixated interests and social impairment. But it is equally conceivable that fixated interests and social impairment become coupled during development (e.g., a child may gather limited social experience as a result of fixated interests, which may result in a lack of communicative expertise, which may reinforce the fixated interests). Currently, it is hard to say which disorders are amenable to what type of analysis; focused research and especially theory formation is necessary to decide these issues.

Thus, the network model does not say that all symptomatology results from network connectivity: individual symptoms can be determined outside the model (e.g., by a neurological problem or genetic variant); rather, the model holds that it is in the mutualistic interplay of symptoms that the symptomatology rises to the level of disorder. The issue, then, is not whether symptoms are solely caused by other symptoms (this is probably never the case), but whether symptom activation (from whatever source) is causally effective in steering the developmental pathway of the other symptoms that we ultimately recognize as a disorder. In this sense, we might venture the hypothesis that disorders classically traced to neurological malfunction, like autism or schizophrenia, do in fact behave as networks; this is fully consistent with the assumption that some of their primary symptoms are fixed outside the network, perhaps by biological factors.

Another important question is whether disorders that are characterized by single symptoms should be considered to be covered by the definitions given here. This is indeed questionable. If a single symptom is activated structurally, without causing any other problems and without engaging in feedback relations, it would seem that a network model misses the mark. Thus, if primary insomnia occurs without any other symptom, then a network model is inappropriate: in this case, the variance of the symptom is determined outside the network, and the causes of the problem should be sought outside the network too. On the other hand, we would not consider treating single symptoms like insomnia if people did not consider them problematic, and to consider them problematic seems to imply that such problems are already engaged in a network structure, albeit a minimal one: namely, they cause distress or functional impairment, either in the person or in their environment. In contrast to medical conditions, which may exist without causing any distress, pain, impairment, or discomfort (e.g., one may have a brain tumor without having the slightest overt symptomatology), psychiatric conditions appear to have an intrinsically relational aspect, in which they minimally stand in one causal relation; namely, they should cause trouble.

References

Barabási, A.-L. (2012). The network takeover. *Nature Physics*, **8**, 14–16.

Borsboom, D. (2008). Psychometric perspectives on diagnostic systems. *Journal of Clinical Psychology*, **64**, 1089–1108.

Borsboom, D., Cramer, A.O.J., Schmittmann, V.D., et al. (2011). The small world of psychopathology. *PLoS ONE*, **6**, e27407.

Borsboom, D. and **Cramer, A.O.J.** (2013). Networks: An integrative approach to the structure of psychopathology. *Annual Review of Clinical Psychology*, **9**, 91–121.

Boschloo L., van Borkulo C.D., Rhemtulla M., et al. (2015). The network structure of symptoms of the Diagnostic and Statistical Manual of Mental Disorders. *PLoS ONE*, **10**, e0137621.

Caspi, A., Houts, R.M., Belsky, D.W., et al. (2014). The p factor: One general psychopathology factor in the structure of psychiatric disorders? *Clinical Psychological Science*, **2**, 119–137.

Cramer, A.O.J. (2013). *The Glue of (Ab)Normal Life: Networks of interacting thoughts, feelings and behaviors.* Unpublished Dissertation, University of Amsterdam, the Netherlands.

Cramer, A. O. J., and **Borsboom, D.** (2015). Problems attract problems: A network perspective on mental disorders. Emerging Trends in the Social and Behavioral Sciences: An Interdisciplinary, Searchable, and Linkable Resource.

Cramer, A.O.J., Borsboom, D., Aggen, S.H., and **Kendler, K.S.** (2012). The pathoplasticity of major depression. *Psychological Medicine*, **42**, 957–965.

Cramer, A.O.J., Waldorp, L.J., van der Maas, H., and **Borsboom, D.** (2010). Comorbidity: A network perspective. *Behavioral and Brain Sciences*, **33**, 137–150.

Crow, T.J. and **Harrington, C.A.** (1994). Etiopathogenesis and treatment of psychosis. *Annual Review of Medicine*, **45**, 219–234.

Edwards, J.R. and **Bagozzi, R.P.** (2000). On the nature and direction of relationships between constructs and measures. *Psychological Methods*, **5**, 155–174.

Hacking, I. (1999). *The Social Construction of What?* Cambridge, MA: Harvard University Press.

Hosenfeld, B., Bos, E.H., Wardenaar, K.J., et al. (2015). Major depressive disorder as a nonlinear dynamic system: bimodality in the frequency distribution of depressive symptoms over time. *BMC Psychiatry*, 15,

Epskamp, S., Maris, G., Waldorp, L.J., and **Borsboom, D.** (*in press*). Network psychometrics. In P. Irwing, D. Hughes, and T. Booth (eds.) *Handbook of Psychometrics*. New York: Wiley.

Foucault, M. (1973). *The Birth of the Clinic: An Archaeology of Medical Perception.* London: Routledge.

Fried, E.I. (2015). Problematic assumptions have slowed down depression research: why symptoms, not syndromes are the way forward. *Frontiers in Psychology*, **6**, 309.

Fried, E.I., Bockting, C., Arjadi, R., et al. (2015a). From loss to loneliness: The relationship between bereavement and depressive symptoms. *Journal of Abnormal Psychology*, **124**, 256–265.

Fried, E.I. and **Nesse, R.M.** (2015). Depression sum-scores don't add up: Why analyzing specific depression symptoms is essential. *BMC Medicine*, **13**, 72.

Fried, E.I., Boschloo, L., van Borkulo, C.D., et al. (2015a). Commentary: Consistent superiority of selective serotonin reuptake inhibitors over placebo in reducing depressed mood in patients with major depression. *Frontiers in Psychiatry*, **6**, 117.

Fried, E.I., Nesse, R.M., Guille, C., and **Sen, S.** (2015b). The differential influence of life stress on individual symptoms of depression. *Acta Psychiatrica Scandinavica*, **131**, 465–471.

Haslam, N., Holland, E., and **Kuppens, P.** (2012). Categories versus dimensions in personality and psychopathology: A quantitative review of taxometric research. *Psychological Medicine*, **42**, 903–920.

Insel, T.R. and **Cuthbert, B.N.** (2015). Brain disorders? Precisely. *Science*, **348**, 499–500.

Keller, M. C., Neale, M.C., and **Kendler, K.S.** (2007). Association of different adverse life events with distinct patterns of depressive symptoms. *American Journal of Psychiatry*, **164**, 1521–1529.

Kendler, K.S., Zachar, P., and **Craver, C.** (2011). What kinds of things are mental disorders? *Psychological Medicine*, **41**, 1143–1150.

Kessler, R.C., Merikangas, K.R., and **Wang, P.S.** (2007). Prevalence, comorbidity, and service utilization for mood disorders in the United States at the beginning of the twenty-first century. *Annual Review of Clinical Psychology*, **3**, 137–158.

Kim, N.S. and **Ahn, W.** (2002). Clinical psychologists' theory-based representations of mental disorders predict their diagnostic reasoning and memory. *Journal of Experimental Psychology: General*, **131**, 451–476.

Kindermann, R., and **Snell, J. L.** (1980). Markov random fields and their applications (Vol. 1). Providence, RI, USA: American Mathematical Society.

Kolaczyk, E.D. (2009). *Statistical Analysis of Network Data: Methods and models.* New York: Springer.

Kraepelin, E. (1907). *Clinical Psychiatry: A Text-Book for Students and Physicians.* (Abstracted and adapted from the seventh German edition of Kraepelin's *Lehrbuch der Psychiatrie* by A. Ross Diefendorf, MD). New York: Macmillan.

Krueger, R.F. (1999). The structure of common mental disorders. *Archives of General Psychiatry*, **56**, 921–926.

Lux, V. and **Kendler, K.S.** (2010). Deconstructing major depression: A validation study of the DSM-IV symptomatic criteria. *Psychological Medicine*, **40**, 1679–1690.

Markus, K. and **Borsboom, D.** (2013). *Frontiers of Validity Theory: Measurement, causation, and meaning.* New York: Routledge.

Meehl, P.E. (1962). Schizotaxia, schizotypy, schizophrenia. *American Psychologist*, **17**, 827–838.

Meehl, P. E. (1972). Specific genetic etiology, psychodynamics, and therapeutic nihilism. *International Journal of Mental Health*, **1**, 10–27.

Meehl, P.E. (1992). Factors and taxa, traits and types, difference of degree and differences in kind. *Journal of Personality*, **60**, 117–174.

Newman, M.E.J. (2010). *Networks: An introduction*. New York: Oxford University Press.

Nolen-Hoeksema S. and **Watkins, E.R.** (2011). A heuristic for developing transdiagnostic models of psychopathology. Explaining multifinality and divergent trajectories. *Perspectives on Psychological Science*, **6**, 589–609.

Pearl, J. (2000). *Causality: Models, reasoning and inference*. Cambridge, MA: MIT Press.

Raju, T.N.K. (2006). Hot brains: Manipulating body heat to save the brain. *Pediatrics*, **117**, 320–321.

Reise, S.P. and **Waller, N.G.** (2009). Item Response Theory and clinical measurement. *Annual Review of Clinical Psychology*, **5**, 27–48.

Scheffer, M., Bascompte, J., Brock, W.A., et al. (2009). Early-warning signals for critical transitions. *Nature*, **461**, 53–59.

Schizophrenia Working Group of the Psychiatric Genomics Consortium. 2014). Biological insights from 108 schizophrenia-associated genetic loci. *Nature*, **511**, 421–427.

Sturt, E. (1981). Hierarchical patterns in the distribution of psychiatric symptoms. *Psychological Medicine*, **11**, 783–794.

Turkheimer, E. (in press). The hard question in psychiatric nosology. In: Kendler, K.S., & Parnas, J. (Eds.). *Philosophical Issues in Psychiatry*, Vol. 4: Nosology. Oxford: Oxford University Press.

Van Borkulo, C.D., Borsboom, D., Epskamp, S., et al. (2014). A new method for constructing networks from binary data. *Scientific Reports*, **4**, 5918.

Van Borkulo, C.D., Boschloo, L., Borsboom, D., et al. (2015). Association of symptom network structure with the course of depression. *JAMA Psychiatry*, **72**, 1219–1226.

Van de Leemput, I.A., Wichers, M., Cramer, A.O.J., et al. (2014). Critical slowing down as early warning for the onset and termination of depression. *Proceedings of the National Academy of Sciences of the U S A*, **111**, 87–92.

Wichers, M. (2014). The dynamic nature of depression: a new micro-level perspective of mental disorder that meets current challenges. *Psychological Medicine*, **44**, 1349–60.

Wichers, M., Groot, P.C., Psychosystems, ESM Group, and **EWS Group** (2016). Critical slowing down as a personalized early warning signal for depression. *Psychotherapy and Psychosomatics*, **85**, 114–116.

World Health Organization (1948). Preamble to the Constitution of the World Health Organization as adopted by the International Health Conference, New York, 19–22 June, 1946; signed on 22 July 1946 by the representatives of 61 States (Official Records of the World Health Organization, no. 2, p. 100) and entered into force on 7 April 1948.

Woodward, J. (2003). *Making Things Happen: A theory of causal explanation*. Oxford: Oxford University Press.

Chapter 12

I bet on Borsboom

Eric Turkheimer

I will pay myself the compliment of observing that Borsboom's contribution to this volume and my own (Chapter 5) have a great deal in common. (Although, of course, Borsboom's personal contribution to the research he describes far exceeds my own negligible contribution to psychiatric nosology.) Both of us are concerned with the relations between phenotype and genotype, psychology and neurology, and the difficulty of locating psychiatry in the complex conceptual spaces that are so defined. Moreover, we are both concerned with how a scientific account of the relationship between low-level (genes, neurons) and high-level (intentions, emotions) events in humans might relate to a psychometric description of the same phenomena. What is particularly striking, however, is how the two essays end: with protests against the prevailing biologism of the contemporary scientific era. I suspect that he, like I, heard from our editor that the conclusions seemed a little abrupt, a little strident. Why are we both so concerned to press the point that a careful consideration of philosophy and psychometrics should give pause to the relentless travel downward in the hierarchy of sciences?

Borsboom regards current efforts to discover the biological basis of mental disorders to be a failure, in obvious need of some kind of course correction, and I certainly agree with him. Borsboom's tone here is so even-handed and reasonable that it is easy to forget that what he says flies in the face of almost everything that is happening in modern scientific psychopathology. The view that the future of psychopathology research is to be found in DNA or neurons is so widespread, so deeply entrenched in the established structures of the American Psychiatric Association and the National Institutes of Health that even laying down a gauntlet, as Borsboom has done here, does not elicit a response of any kind. Where is the defense of traditional latent variable models, or of biological explanation of behavioral syndromes?

Genome-wide association studies (GWAS) are occasionally celebrated (Visscher et al. 2012), but as far as I know this approach has never been defended on philosophical grounds. I, for example, recently published (Turkheimer 2016) the assertion that GWAS is "unapologetic, high-tech p-hacking," pretty much the worst insult one can throw at a social scientist these days, and it was met with utter silence. That is the question I would like to address here. Despite Borsboom's extraordinary scientific effort toward building his network theory into a viable alternative to latent variable models on the one hand and bottom-up biological explanation on the other, there exists no meaningful debate about the nature of psychopathology or the best methods to study it: there is only a monolithic scientific establishment and isolated communities of intellectual dissidents. Why? I see two major reasons.

The first is a profound difference between the camps in their attitudes toward theory, never mind philosophy. When I read, for example, the Insel and Cuthbert (2015) paper that Borsboom cites, my strongest impression is not so much that I disagree with their theoretical basis for assuming that we can or ought to pursue psychopathology on a biological level, but rather that they do not seem to recognize that the assertion *requires* a theoretical basis. It is self-evident. I would say that they pull a reductionist rabbit out of their hat, except there is no hat, and no pulling: all of a sudden the biogenetic rabbit just appears, and its very presence seems to preclude further discussion of how it got there or what we expect it to do now.

This is not, I recognize, a matter of philosophical obtuseness on their part: it is a difference in outlook. We can conduct amazing science in the human brain and genome nowadays. We can image the brain in a dozen different modalities, record the activity of individual neurons, trace the transmission and expression of DNA in glorious detail. We *can* do these things, we *do* do these things, and what possible incremental good could come from worrying about what all the resulting data might mean? For the mainstream scientific establishment, technology is what it is: astounding and vast, and if we just let the science do its thing sooner or later it will all get sorted out.

I actually spend more time thinking about the genetics of complex behavior than its neurology, and there, as I mentioned, the great technology of the day is GWAS and its various acronymic spawn, like GCTA (genome-wide complex trait analysis) and GREML (genomic-relatedness-matrix restricted maximum likelihood). In my opinion GWAS of highly complex human behavior, of which the genomic apotheosis is educational attainment (see, e.g., Mukherjee et al. 2013), is a waste of the time and effort of the most gifted geneticists and social scientists of our time. But from the point of view of the people actually doing this work, my point of view is not so much wrong as irrelevant, because by their lights, *GWAS does exactly what it was designed to do*, that is searching for single-nucleotide polymorphisms (SNPs) with small statistical associations with phenotype. Given a large enough sample, it finds them. Not even I can argue that a stunningly sophisticated scientific method, applied correctly, is a bad thing. The method, like I said, is what it is, and the results are what they are. Only then can you worry whether those results mean something important. Borsboom and I do worry, but by and large the establishment does not. The difference is almost temperamental.

The other reason the bottom-up establishment and the top-down outsiders are unable to talk to each other is an unspoken frustration with the progress of top-down scientific psychopathology. Even if Borsboom has found a much more carefully specified way to talk about it, the idea that psychopathology is psychological, to be explained using relational systems of minds, beliefs, ideas, intentions, and cultures, is hardly new. It is what Sigmund Freud thought, it is what B. F. Skinner thought, it is what Erving Goffman thought, it is what Julian Rapaport thought.

The other theme I detect when I read Insel and Cuthbert (2015) is the argument of the contemporary political partisan: whatever the shortcomings of biological science for the study of complex human characteristics, it beats the alternative. I am not someone who thinks Freud was wrong about psychopathology; Freud created a revolutionary and profound system of ideas that, despite the continual force of his genius across his entire career, failed to crystallize into a science. The great theories of psychopathology were theories first, with an IOU on the science that was never paid off. In its frustration, the modern psychopathology establishment, epitomized by the bleakly atheoretical technology of GWAS, has stood that strategy on its head: do the science now, and hope that the theory will come later. Neurologic and genomic science may or may not have anything important to say about why some people become depressed, but at least brain science is demonstrably science, satisfying on its own terms. And as noted above, one can always decide to just appreciate it as such, and leave the whining to others.

Borsboom is no whiner. He has put an alternative on the table. The purveyor of new social scientific methodology has a very high bar to clear—the psychoanalysts, behaviorists, system theorists, and community psychologists all expected that their ideas would finally show the way to real scientific behavior of human function and dysfunction, but it seems safe to say that none ever did. It was this collective failure of high-level social science that pointed us down the reductionist rabbit hole we find ourselves in today. The proof will come when someday—and it is an absolutely astounding fact that this has never once happened in the history of scientific psychopathology—some methodology establishes methods, models, and observations that make a real, concrete difference in the lives of the psychologically afflicted. Maybe the GWAS community will discover a SNP that leads to a pathway that leads to a drug that makes such a difference. I doubt it, but if it happens they will have been right, and I will have been wrong. Network theory won't discover a drug; it will prove its worth when it can predict suicide attempts. Personally, I am betting on Borsboom, or on some future version of the insight he has developed: psychopathology is the result of a complex network of interactions among mid-level *psychological* constructs.

References

Insel, T.R. and **Cuthbert, B.N.** (2015). Brain disorders? Precisely. *Science*, **348**, 499–500.

Mukherjee, S., **Montgomery, G.**, **Nyholt, D.**, et al. (2013). GWAS of 126,559 individuals identifies genetic variants associated with educational attainment. *Science*, **340**, 1467–1471.

Turkheimer, E. (2016). Weak genetic explanation 20 years later: Reply to Plomin et al. (2016). *Perspectives on Psychological Science*, **11**, 24–28.

Visscher, P.M., **Brown, M.A.**, **McCarthy, M.I.**, and **Yang, J.** (2012). Five years of GWAS discovery. *American Journal of Human Genetics*, **90**, 7–24.

Part II

Reification, epidemics, and individual symptoms

Section 5

Reification of mental illness

Chapter 13

Introduction to "On reification of mental illness: Historical and conceptual issues from Emil Kraepelin and Eugen Bleuler to DSM-5"

Josef Parnas

Dr. Hoff's chapter addresses a fundamental issue in nosology and, in fact, in the mind–body realm. The term "reification" used here means a reduction of mental phenomena to their putative biological substrates. There are other terms with similar semantics, such as objectivation, reduction, and reductionism. Reification stems from the Latin *res*, i.e. "thing", and the term is often used in ordinary parlance for converting abstractions, ideas, or concepts into concretely existing objects.

Hoff gives us a nice narrative of the naturalistic point of view of Kraepelin and the more syncretic views of Bleuler. The author tends to see the project of operational criteria in the third edition of *Diagnostic and Statistical Manual of Mental Disorders* (DSM-III) and the tenth edition of the *International Classification of Diseases* (ICD-10) as a primarily "nominalistic" undertaking which means creating a reliable diagnostic classification without a concomitant belief that these categories reflect existing natural kinds. However, it must be remembered that the concept of operational criteria and operationalism emerged in the context of massive biological research with the hope of "carving nature at its joints." Thus the creation of the DSM-III was both on a conceptual and a concrete pragmatic level associated with the activity of the so-called neo-Kraepelinians. In other words, reification of the DSM-III and its subsequent editions was unavoidable and deeply harmful to the field (Parnas and Bovet 2015). The latest project of the U.S. National Institute of Mental Health, the Research Domain Criteria (RDoC) enterprise, is not only an attempt at reification but borders on eliminativism, a claim that mental states do not exist and that all talk about the mental should be replaced by talk about the brain.

This paper touches upon the ontological status of mental and social phenomena, acknowledging the importance of biology but also of subjectivity and intersubjectivity. This unresolved status of the mental realm is today perhaps the most interesting scientific issue which occupies philosophers and scientists alike.

Reference

Parnas, J. and **Bovet, P.** (2015). Psychiatry made easy: operation(a)lism and some of its consequences. In K.S. Kendler and J. Parnas (eds.) *Philosophical Issues in Psychiatry III*, pp. 190–213. Oxford, UK: Oxford University Press.

Chapter 14

On reification of mental illness: Historical and conceptual issues from Emil Kraepelin and Eugen Bleuler to DSM-5

Paul Hoff

14.1 Introduction

"What *is* an illness?"—"How do we *define* an illness?" These two questions may at first sight look similar. However, when taking their epistemological presuppositions into account, they are distinctly different. The first question tacitly implies that there *is* something existing independently from the diagnostician or the researcher. The second question, in a way, is more modest: It concedes that it is us, the people in charge of making diagnoses and creating research plans, who *actively define* their frameworks including the borders between separate areas of study, e.g., between diagnoses or diseases. By this, however, the issue of the existence of real things, real psychiatric disease entities in our case, "behind" such definitions, is not simultaneously addressed nor, of course, answered.

In this chapter I will argue that what is meant by "mental illness" is neither a group of natural disease entities, as Emil Kraepelin believed, nor is it arbitrary or openly deceptive for undisclosed political reasons, as antipsychiatric authors like Thomas Szasz (1920–2012) postulated (Szasz 1961).[1] Any naive reification of mental illness, in other words regarding mental illnesses as once and for all *given things*, is as misleading as the opposite position that renders any medical and scientific approach to psychopathological conditions empty and unjustified. The concept of reification, operating on a highly abstract level, touches fundamental aspects of nosology—in psychiatry and in medicine in general—and leads to substantial consequences for medical practice. The idea of psychiatric reification is discussed here with regard to the influential conceptual frameworks set up by Emil Kraepelin (1856–1926) and Eugen Bleuler (1857–1939), and is then followed up to

[1] However, Szasz himself strictly repudiated being called "antipsychiatric". As he saw it, his fierce criticism was targeted at medicalization of mental illness and at coercive measures, stating that psychiatry willingly accepted the exercise of social control and hence adopting the role of a mental health police.

present-day diagnostic manuals: the fifth edition of the *Diagnostic and Statistical Manual of Mental Disorders* (DSM-5) (APA 2013) and the tenth edition of the *International Classification of Diseases* (ICD-10) (WHO 1992). Their nominalistic approach should, given its theoretical framework, clearly favor a non-reifying understanding of mental illness, although in actual clinical practice the opposite may happen quite frequently. Finally, the recent concept of Research Domain Criteria (RDoC), standing in the tradition of denosologization or deconstruction of mental illness, is taken into account regarding possible links to the notion of reification. To be clear: I am not criticizing the scientific salience of the RDoC approach. However, I will argue that an epistemologically narrow understanding of the suggested research domains and their consequences for psychiatric nosology will risk a subtle, implicit, if unintended return to a poorly reflected version of reifying mental illness.

The general epistemological background of our topic is created mainly by the tension, well-known to psychiatry, between two perspectives: Respecting subjective experiences as viable scientific topics (i.e., idiography), on the one hand, and searching for generalizable rules beyond individual cases (i.e., the nomothetic approach), on the other hand. Therefore, the chapter concludes by interrelating the theoretical notion of reification with an important practical, albeit philosophically charged element of *any* psychiatric work, interpersonality.

14.2 Reification of mental illness as philosophical realism

Epistemologically strong versions of reifying mental illness are rooted in philosophical realism. The core idea of that concept, which indeed has a long tradition in philosophy, is the assumption of an "outer world" which continuously affects us by sensory inputs, but which in itself exists independently from any human activity. If applied to psychiatric nosology, this line of thought will lead to the postulate of distinct mental illnesses that are independent of scientific concepts by which researchers might try to detect or explain them (Kendler 2016). In the history of psychiatry, such an approach often adopted a neuroscientific framework and declared that mental illnesses are brain diseases ("... and nothing else," one might add referring to the strictest variant of this position). However, reification of mental illness may also be present in a psychological or social sciences context.

14.3 The idea of reifying mental illness in Emil Kraepelin's and Eugen Bleuler's writings

14.3.1 Emil Kraepelin

As for nosological issues, Emil Kraepelin was a particularly influential figure in the history of psychiatry. He preferred pragmatic attitudes and arguments, a strategy that worked well for his central aim which was to establish psychiatry as a respected (and powerful) scientific discipline within academic medicine. However, this strategy also distinctly supported Kraepelin's tendency to underestimate the manifold theoretical presuppositions of his work. This is particularly true for his clear-cut philosophical realism: Kraepelin claimed to target scientific findings "that provide an accurate image of the world"; as a consequence, science became a "mirror of the world" (both 1904, vol. 2, p. 209). Research should "assert ... what is the case" (1920a, pp. 356–357) by "staying in close contact with reality" (1909, p. 529), and—nosologically most important—should abandon "artificial boundaries that are not known to nature" (1899, vol. 2, p. 404).

Consequently, Kraepelin's core nosological postulate was the existence and scientific accessibility of "natural disease entities" ("natürliche Krankheitseinheiten") in psychiatry, nowadays often labelled as "natural kinds" (Zachar 2000, Read et al. 2004, Kendler and Jablensky 2011). On the clinical level, he modified the details of his nosological system over and over again, whereas, on the theoretical level, the fundamental framework was characterized by a remarkable stability: Between the second and ninth editions of his textbook (i.e., from 1887 to 1927!) Kraepelin did not substantially change his postulate of a "natural" system of mental, especially psychotic, disorders. Therefore, for him, a "true" psychiatric nosology could never only be a product of the specific scientific method applied. Pathological anatomy, etiology, or clinical symptomatology including long-term course of illness (the latter being his own lifelong focus of research), all, according to Kraepelin, necessarily converge in the same "natural disease entities." These *are* natural kinds no matter what research pathway they are systematically approached from. Briefly speaking: Psychiatric disease entities, being natural kinds, are to be *detected, not constructed* by research.

As could be expected, Kraepelin's thoroughly realistic attitude towards mental illness provoked some criticism. For example, Alfred Erich Hoche (1865–1943) regarded the search for psychiatric disease entities as grossly premature. According to him, research methods and data that were available at his time (and that might be expected in the foreseeable future) were unable to justify a decision whether disease entities exist or not, far less to identify and differentiate them from each other. Alternatively, Hoche suggested focusing on the description, definition, and clinical evaluation of syndromes, at least postponing, if not abandoning, the search for disease entities (Hoche 1912).[2] Karl Birnbaum (1878–1950) focused on the difference between "pathogenetic" and "pathoplastic" factors in mental illness, being clearly more interested in the "inner structure" of psychotic states than Kraepelin had been (Birnbaum 1923). Robert Gaupp (1870–1953), often referring to the

---

[2] Some years later, in 1920, Hoche, together with Hans Binding, wrote a book with the title "Allowing the destruction of life unworthy of living" (*Die Freigabe der Vernichtung lebensunwerten Lebens*) (Binding and Hoche 1920). Hoche is not the only prominent psychiatric author of his time who delivered valuable scientific contributions to the field and also developed grossly inhuman, protofascistic ideas (Hoff 2016).

seminal case of Ernst Wagner,[3] postulated that delusions may well develop on psychological grounds only, which meant they could be open to heuristic approaches centring around the patient's biography and personality (Gaupp 1920, Hirsch and Shepherd 1974).

Kraepelin responded to these criticisms in later programmatic papers: "Ends and means of psychiatric research" ("Ziele und Wege der psychiatrischen Forschung") (1918), "Research in the manifestations of mental illness" ("Die Erforschung psychischer Krankheitsformen") (1919) and, the most relevant one in the present context, "Clinical manifestations of mental illness" ("Die Erscheinungsformen des Irreseins") (1920b). Here Kraepelin readily acknowledged the difficulties of linking clinical symptomatology to the supposed disease entities. He accepted the view of Karl Bonhoeffer (1868–1948) that psychopathological symptoms typically are nosologically unspecific (1910). Following this line of thought, in his 1920 paper he introduced the term "psychopathological registers" as a conceptual link between unspecific symptoms and specific diseases (Kraepelin 1920b). At first sight, this seems to come close to Hoche's position. However, for Kraepelin it was just a necessary concession owed to the status of psychiatric research methods at that time. It did not indicate a fundamental change of view (Hoff 2015).

To conclude, what kind of reification did Kraepelin foster? For him, the existence and scientific detectability of natural disease entities in psychiatry was beyond doubt. But he did not claim dogmatically that the clinical entities described in the various editions of his textbook exactly represent those natural kinds. On the contrary, he modified his nosological system repeatedly due to new empirical data, criticisms from contemporary authors, and emerging conceptual developments. But again, his respect for new data and ideas did not change the basic conviction that there are such things as natural entities in psychiatric nosology. This remained the scientific point of reference for Kraepelin throughout his career as a clinician and scientist.

14.3.2 Eugen Bleuler

Eugen Bleuler, another seminal author in the history of psychiatry, strove for a mediating link between the two basic psychiatric positions briefly mentioned above: First, to regard reliably measurable (quantitative) objective data as the very center of scientific psychiatry; second, to insist on the scientifically equally respectable status of subjective (qualitative) phenomena, accessible by heuristic

[3] After developing a chronic paranoid state with systematic delusions, Ernst August Wagner (1874–1938), a school teacher, killed his own family and several other people in a village close to Stuttgart (Germany) in September 1913. Gaupp discussed the link between Wagner's biography, personality traits, and stressful, especially humiliating life events on the one hand and the ongoing formation of his delusional convictions on the other hand. Ernst Kretschmer (1888–1964), Gaupp's pupil and co-worker, introduced the concept of "sensitive delusions" ("sensitiver Beziehungswahn"), addressing the same psychopathological context (Kretschmer 1918).

means, without, of course, having to deny the relevance of the biological level. In this respect Eugen Bleuler stood, as far as his basic psychiatric convictions were concerned, as it were "between" Emil Kraepelin and another influential contemporary author, Sigmund Freud (1856–1939) (Küchenhoff 2001).

Bleuler's work was characterized by his continuous attempts to approach the topic of psychotic illness on as many levels as possible, while at the same time taking normal psychological phenomena into consideration. On the one hand, he declined one-sided dogmatic assertions, such as the many variants of "brain mythologies" which regarded psychiatry as exhaustively comprehensible along strict, but poorly reflected materialistic lines. On the other hand, for Bleuler the psychotic person was *not only* ill, *not only* deviant, but also had (or kept) access to their healthy features—to resources, as we say today. The idea that many elements of mental illness were not fundamentally different from healthy mental life was appalling to Bleuler, mainly because of its predictable therapeutic exploitation. However, he did not disapprove of the neurobiological school of thought and the research strategies arising from it. On the contrary: like the vast majority of contemporary psychiatrists, he too was convinced that brain function played a significant role in the etiology and pathogenesis of mental illnesses.

But he went one significant step further: Bleuler, unlike most of his academic psychiatric contemporaries, saw no fundamental contradiction between brain research in the broadest sense and the psychoanalytical method of interpretation as suggested by Freud. This basic attitude led to significant criticisms by many of his fellow academic psychiatrists, e.g., by Kraepelin and Karl Jaspers (1886–1969).

In 1911, 3 years after mentioning the term "schizophrenia" for the first time in public (Bleuler 1908), Bleuler's lengthy chapter "Dementia praecox or the group of schizophrenias" was published in Gustav Aschaffenburg's *Handbook of Psychiatry* (Bleuler 1911). Although Bleuler deliberately chose not to speak of schizophrenia as a single entity, but of the group of schizophrenias, he was concerned with the question of what characteristics the otherwise very heterogeneous schizophrenic patients might have in common. Bleuler saw certain psychopathological phenomena, e.g., disturbances of association and affectivity, ambivalence, and autism,[4] as core elements of any schizophrenic illness; notwithstanding his strong belief in a general neurobiological basis of mental illness, he strictly avoided speculative analogies to brain function. In contrast to Kraepelin's prognostically pessimistic, if not overtly fatalistic concept of "dementia praecox," Bleuler described benign cases of schizophrenia with extensive or even complete recovery (Maatz and Hoff 2014, Maatz et al. 2015).

Bleuler's position towards reification of mental illness is significantly more complex than Kraepelin's and therefore more difficult to delineate. Although he

---

[4] It is crucial to understand Bleuler's terms in the specific context for which he coined them or in which he used them. In particular, "autism" meant something very different from our present-day usage, e.g., in child and adolescent psychiatry.

repeatedly mentioned the biological basis of psychiatric illness, this was more a general supposition than a specific claim that clearly distinguishable disease entities, "natural kinds," do exist in psychiatry. In other words, the neurobiological underpinning of human mental life, although generally approved, did not reach such an outstanding heuristic value for Bleuler as, for example, for Kraepelin. Above all, this might have been due to his interest in psychological and psychodynamic aspects which he developed into a second heuristic framework, decisively accepted as clinically and scientifically relevant. If one additionally takes Bleuler's cautious wording into account—"group of schizophrenias" instead of just "schizophrenia"—and his emphasis on the blurred borders between mental illness and health, one might speak of a specifically attenuated tendency to regard psychiatric disorders as independent things, i.e., to reify them.[5]

14.4 **On the idea of non-reification in DSM-5 and ICD-10**

Recently there has been considerable criticism that DSM-5 and ICD-10 inflate the number of categorically defined mental disorders and, by doing so, increase the risk of uncritical reification. In these circumstances the heading of this chapter may be unexpected.

However, a close look at the conceptual history of operationalized psychiatric diagnoses clearly proves their basically nominalistic, i.e., anti-realistic, orientation. From a methodological point of view, although handling diagnoses as conceptual categories that ideally do not overlap, operationalized diagnoses do not claim to state the "true" existence of objects like schizophrenia, bipolar disorder, or personality disorder. They are, in epistemological terms, not addressing ontological entities, but operating on a nominalistic level. Their algorithms provide guidelines in which clinical situation the diagnostician should *speak of*, for example, schizophrenia, and in which not.

Kurt Schneider (1887–1967), rarely credited as forerunner of the concept of operationalized diagnoses in psychiatry, managed to pack this complex matter in just one sentence of his *Clinical Psychopathology*. Referring to schizophrenia in general and to his "first-rank-symptoms" in particular, he stated:

> Where such experiences occur beyond doubt and no underlying somatic illnesses can be detected, we do in all modesty clinically *speak of* schizophrenia. (Schneider 1980, p. 135) (translation and italics by PH)

However, the existence of a neurobiological basis especially of psychotic disorders was beyond doubt for Schneider (as it was for Bleuler). On the contrary, Schneider stated that for the whole of medicine, disease was necessarily a *somatic* dysfunction.

---

[5] Later in life, Bleuler explicitly turned to a distinctly speculative version of naturalism, partly reminiscent of the older concept of vitalism; however, his publications from that period were scarcely recognized by the psychiatric community and are therefore not discussed here (Bleuler 1934, Möller 2001).

But since the somatic basis of schizophrenia, for example, was still largely unknown, he consequently called this a postulate, explicitly *not* pretending that psychoses could already be considered scientifically clearly distinguishable biological entities (*Somatosepostulat*, "postulate of somatosis") (Schneider 1980). This rather modest position is close to the conceptual basis of DSM-5 and ICD-10. Such nominalistic approaches are compatible with the theoretical notion of the existence of "natural kinds" in psychiatric nosology, but they do not necessarily favor a naturalistic type of reification. In other words: DSM-5 and ICD-10 deliver semantic procedures that ensure the reliability of psychiatric diagnoses, but do not claim to address "natural kinds."

DSM-5 and ICD-10 are based on the psychopathological method of description and avoid hermeneutic elements wherever possible. The presence of explicit criteria and algorithms for each diagnosis and the preferential treatment of quantitative over qualitative criteria divide operational psychiatric diagnosis from other concepts. The reasons for their development and success (regarding their worldwide use) are manifold, but two points are as outstanding as they are of practical relevance to clinical psychiatry and research. The first is the urgent need to increase the reliability of psychiatric diagnoses, which for decades was unacceptably low given the bulk of incompatible nosological concepts that surfaced in the history of modern psychiatry. This target, increased reliability, indeed has been achieved.

That is not quite the case for the second goal, which is to provide diagnostic procedures acceptable for different psychiatric schools, a common diagnostic denominator, so to speak. A strong motivator in this respect was the seminal joint Anglo-American study on functional psychoses, including schizophrenia (Wing 1971). This painstakingly demonstrated the poor accordance of diagnostic procedures in two otherwise largely comparable English-speaking countries. The study's key message was that without a generally accepted diagnostic language, it would be difficult or impossible to carry out international research projects in psychiatry. Finally, in 1980 (DSM-III) and 1992 (ICD-10), operationalized diagnoses became effective on a large scale, promising to pragmatically solve that problem both for clinicians and researchers.

However, looking back from today's perspective, these manuals have only partly been able to assume the ambitious role of a common diagnostic denominator. There was criticism right from the start that DSM and ICD were too strictly bound to descriptive psychopathology, underestimating or even ignoring the subjective and social domains of people with mental disorders.[6] Paris and Phillips (2013) provided a thorough critical overview of the conceptual basis of DSM-5 and the methodological and philosophical controversies attached to it.

---

[6] Such criticisms led to the development of operationalized psychodynamic diagnoses (OPD) (Schneider et al. 2008) and to the implementation of social functioning into the diagnostic process (ICF) (Linden et al. 2009). However, both were conceptualized not to replace but to supplement the descriptive DSM and ICD approach.

14.5 **Psychiatric nosology in the 21st century: A subtle return of reification?**

Since the publication of DSM-III in 1980, there have been signs of an increasing risk that mental illness might be *uncritically* reified. Indeed, there are two variants of that risk: a harmless one, stemming from a misunderstanding of the epistemological nature of operationalized psychiatric diagnoses, and a potentially hazardous one that could—intentionally or not—lead to an inadequate conceptual and methodological restriction of psychiatric practice and research.

The first and, in a way, harmless variant is due to a misunderstanding of DSM-5 and ICD-10 diagnostic categories as representing natural kinds, as, to use the Latin word, "*res*" in the above-mentioned sense. This is practically relevant for clinical work, education, and public opinion about psychiatry. The recent remarkable public interest in such a specialized topic as psychiatric diagnoses is rooted in fears of the "inflation" of psychiatric diagnoses. Such fears clearly accompanied the publication of DSM-5 in 2013 (Frances 2013). However, misunderstanding operationalized diagnoses in a reifying manner does not present any major conceptual problem: the coping strategy is to systematically clarify and teach the theoretical background of the present diagnostic manuals.

The second variant gives rise to significantly more questions. The concept of denosologization which has accompanied psychiatric thought at least since the middle of the nineteenth century has to be recognized in this context. It declared the search for clearly separable "natural disease entities" premature, if not misleading from its very beginning. Wilhelm Griesinger (1817–1868), for example, being dissatisfied with the speculative nosological systems of the first half of the nineteenth century, voted for the concept of *Einheitspsychose* ("unitary psychosis") (Griesinger 1861). From his perspective, there was no scientifically viable grouping of different psychotic disorders, but just one psychosis which showed distinguishable stages from affective disturbances via openly psychotic symptoms to catatonic states and to severe cognitive deficiences. As mentioned earlier, Alfred Erich Hoche, decades after Griesinger, had criticized Emil Kraepelin's position as premature, if not naive, and opted for clinical syndromes—and not diagnoses—as primary research targets.

Towards the end of the twentieth century, Herman van Praag brought new attention to the idea of denosologization. He suggested that we should weaken the influence of classical nosological constructs and group mental disorders according to their neurobiological correlates (e.g., disturbances of the serotonergic system) rather than their psychopathological features (e.g., anxiety, obsessive-compulsive thoughts, depressive mood) (van Praag et al. 1987). Later, the concept of "deconstruction" of psychiatric diagnoses became even more popular (van Os and Tamminga 2007, Gaebel and Zielasek 2008). This did not, however, merely address the replacement of psychopathological by neuroscientific boundaries, but supported any attempt to move beyond the classical (mostly Kraepelinian) nosological entities. Very recently, Norman Sartorius (2015) asked exactly the same questions: "Why do we need a diagnosis? Maybe a syndrome is enough?" It seems ironic, that at present—in opposition to the overall tendency for denosologization—the influence of naturalistic types of reification might increase again by focusing psychiatric research mainly on neurobiological phenomena.

This development was encouraged by the arrival of measurable, i.e., quantitative, neurobiological criteria as candidates for validating psychiatric diagnoses ("endophenotypes," "biomarkers"). Additionally, there is a steady decline in the acceptance of psychopathology as an indispensable basis of the diagnostic process, especially if it reaches beyond description, e.g., by adopting phenomenological methods. Taken together, these factors led to the question whether the psychopathological status could be gradually or even fully replaced by neurobiological criteria.

An influential voice in this context is the National Institute of Mental Health (NIMH) research group that introduced the concept of RDoC (Insel et al. 2010). The skeptical attitude towards mainly psychopathological approaches is evident in the subtitle of their recent publication "Precision medicine comes to psychiatry" (Insel and Cuthbert 2015). From the RDoC perspective, psychopathology-based diagnostic procedures create patient groups who share clinical symptoms and, of course, a diagnostic term according to DSM-5 or ICD-10. However, from a neuroscientific point of view, these groups might not be homogeneous at all. Consequently, RDoC suggests "deconstructing" the classical symptom-based categories and studying patients (e.g., those with any type of anxiety or mood disorder) "across several analytical platforms to parse current heterogeneous syndromes into homogeneous clusters" (Insel and Cuthbert 2015). These analytical platforms should include data on the polygenic risk score, brain activity, physiological (e.g., inflammatory) markers, behavioural processes and, finally, life experiences including social, cultural, and environmental factors.

In Insel and Cuthbert's view, studying large groups of patients with the clinical diagnosis of, for example, major depressive disorder, by all these methods simultaneously, will result in more stable and valid "data-driven categories," called clusters. These clusters could then function as a basis for stratified clinical trials of newly developed drugs. Ideally, a new psychopharmacological agent might then be tailored exactly to the biochemical and genetic status of the individual patient (an approach that is often, albeit not unambiguously, labelled as "personalized medicine").

The RDoC approach is the most recent step in a longstanding and thoughtful tradition of denosologization in psychiatry. However, as this tradition has proven, a new way of generating or interpreting scientific data does not implicitly answer the basic philosophical questions that necessarily accompany the psychiatric field:

- What is the relationship between brain activity, subjective experiences, and personal autonomy?
- How may the two opposite poles of psychiatric work, measuring data and understanding the patient's "inner world," be properly combined so that effective treatment options are provided?
- What are the scientific status and practical relevance of interpersonality in psychiatry?

Such considerations are not meant to be understood as a fundamental criticism, but as a caveat. In the first place, RDoC is a promising scientific tool, but not a nosological, let alone a philosophical or anthropological, theory. If the RDoC approach is to be prevented from adopting a unidimensional naturalistic attitude that may or may not include reification of its newly defined clusters, the scientific impact of psychopathology in a broader sense that stretches beyond mere symptom description has to be strengthened (Gallagher and Zahavi 2008, Hoff 2008, Fuchs 2009, Stanghellini 2009, Parnas 2011).

Finally, I want to briefly illustrate this theoretical context by a clinically essential example, interpersonality. Even if neuroscientifically oriented concepts of denosologization like RDoC refrain from a simplified reification of mental illness, the fundamentally interpersonal character of any psychiatric procedure—prevention, diagnosis, treatment—would still not be adequately dealt with. In other words, the core features of the therapeutic relationship, as powerful a tool as it is in psychiatry and psychotherapy, cannot be scientifically addressed, let alone understood, only by the collection of neuroscientific data. What we need in medicine and in psychiatry in particular is a balanced combination of knowledge (facts), skills (the ability to handle medical problems), and values (a framework that guides medical decisions and actions). All three elements have to join together in interpersonal acts that are the bottom line of both diagnostic and therapeutic procedures (see Figure 14.1). At this point, strictly quantitative, data-driven approaches are necessarily flawed, not because they are generally inapplicable to psychiatric research, but because they are inadequate or, at least, incomplete when the fields of personal autonomy and interpersonality are at stake.

Here the conceptual basis of psychiatry and psychotherapy is closely linked to a philosophical position which also placed the notion of interpersonality at its very center: I mean transcendental philosophy as introduced by Immanuel Kant (1724–1804) and developed further, not to say radically, by Johann Gottlieb Fichte (1762–1814) (Hoff 1997, Asmuth 2007, von Manz 2014, Hoff 2017, in press). During the twentieth century, Karl Jaspers (1883–1969), Martin Buber (1878–1965), and Helmuth Plessner (1892–1985) also stressed the fundamental role of interpersonality,

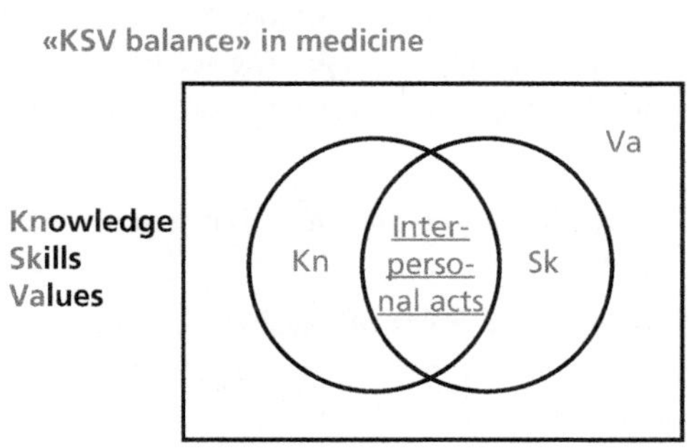

Figure 14.1 The balance of knowledge, skills, and values as prerequisite of interpersonal acts in medicine (i.e., of a stable therapeutic relationship)

albeit from theoretically different points of view (Jaspers 1946, Plessner 1975, Buber 2006). In the present context these issues of psychiatric anthropology cannot be elaborated further. However, it is probably worthwhile re-evaluating the Kantian and the Fichtean approaches since they might provide substantial inputs for psychiatry's basic issues. One of these issues, of course, is nosology.

14.6 Summary

- When using the term "mental illness," we refer to a concept, not to a given thing, i.e., not to an ontological entity. This view, however, by no means underestimates or denies the subjective and social reality of mentally ill individuals and their suffering from these conditions.
- To acknowledge subjectivity and interpersonality as indispensable elements of psychiatry, although they do not fit into strictly naturalistic frameworks, will not impede neurobiological research. On the contrary, it will strengthen it.
- The epistemological approaches of Immanuel Kant and Johann Gottlieb Fichte, along with twentieth-century authors, are rarely debated in psychiatry nowadays. They not only oppose dogmatism, but credit interpersonality with a central position. Their potential capacity to account for conceptually rich and practically relevant arguments within the ongoing debate on psychiatric diagnosis and nosology should be recognized.

References

American Psychiatric Association (2013). *Diagnostic and Statistical Manual of Mental Disorders*, 5th edn. Arlington, VA: American Psychiatric Association.

Asmuth C. (ed.) (2007). *Transzendentalphilosophie und Person*. Bielefeld: Transcript.

Binding, K. and **Hoche, A.E.** (1920). *Die Freigabe der Vernichtung lebensunwerten Lebens. Ihr Mass und ihre Form*. Leipzig: Meiner.

Birnbaum, K. (1923). *Der Aufbau der Psychose. Grundzüge der psychiatrischen Strukturanalyse*. Berlin: Springer.

Bleuler, E. (1908). Die Prognose der Dementia Praecox (Schizophreniegruppe). *Allgemeine Zeitschrift für Psychiatrie und Psychisch-Gerichtliche Medizin*, **65**, 436–464.

Bleuler, E. (1911). Dementia praecox oder Gruppe der Schizophrenien. In G. Aschaffenburg (ed.) *Handbuch der Psychiatrie*, pp. 1–420. Leipzig: Deuticke (Reprinted Nijmegen: Arts & Boeve, 2001).

Bleuler, E. (1934). Mnemismus, Psychoide. *Schweizer Archiv für Neurologie und Psychiatrie*, **33**, 177–191.

Bonhoeffer, K. (1910). *Die symptomatischen Psychosen im Gefolge von akuten Infektionen und inneren Erkrankungen*. Leipzig: Deuticke.

Buber, M. (2006). *Das dialogische Prinzip*, 11th edn. Gütersloh: Gütersloher.

Frances, A. (2013). *Saving Normal: An insider's revolt against out-of-control psychiatric diagnosis, DSM-5, big pharma, and the medicalization of ordinary life*. New York: HarperCollins.

Fuchs, T. (2009). *Das Gehirn—ein Beziehungsorgan. Eine phänomenologisch-ökologische Konzeption*, 2nd edn. Stuttgart: Kohlhammer.

Gaebel, W. and **Zielasek, J.** (2008). The DSM-V initiative deconstructing psychosis in the context of Kraepelin's concept on nosology. *European Archives of Psychiatry and Clinical Neuroscience*, **258** (suppl 2). 41–47.

Gallagher, S. and **Zahavi, D.** (2008) *The Phenomenological Mind. An introduction to philosophy of mind and cognitive science*. London: Routledge.

Gaupp, R. (1920). Der Fall Wagner. Eine Katamnese, zugleich ein Beitrag zur Lehre von der Paranoia. *Zeitschrift für die gesamte Neurologie und Psychiatrie*, **60**, 312–327.

Griesinger, W. (1861). *Die Pathologie und Therapie der psychischen Krankheiten*, 2nd edn. Stuttgart: Krabbe.

Hirsch, S.R. and Shepherd, M. (eds.) (1974) *Themes and Variations in European Psychiatry: an anthology*. Bristol: Wright.

Hoche, A.E. (1912). Die Bedeutung der Symptomenkomplexe in der Psychiatrie. *Zeitschrift für die gesamte Neurologie und Psychiatrie*, **12**, 540–551.

Hoff, P. (1997). Fichte und die psychiatrische Forschung. *Fichte-Studien*, **13**, 241–255.

Hoff, P. (2008). Do social psychiatry and neurosciences need psychopathology—and if yes, what for? *International Review of Psychiatry*, **20**, 515–520.

Hoff, P. (2015). The Kraepelinian Tradition. Dialogues in Clinical Neuroscience, **17**, 31–41.

Hoff, P. (2016). Geschichte der Psychiatrie. In H.J. Möller, G. Laux, and H.P. Kapfhammer (eds.) *Psychiatrie, Psychosomatik, Psychotherapie*, 5th edn, vol. **1**, pp. 1–27. Berlin, Heidelberg: Springer.

Hoff, P. (2017, in press) Von Kant zu Fichte: Transzendentales Denken und die Grundlegung von Psychiatrie und Psychotherapie im 21. Jahrhundert. In M. Ivaldo, H.G. von Manz, and I. Radrizzani (eds.) *Vergegenwärtigung der Transzendentalphilosophie. Das philosophische Vermächtnis Reinhard Lauths*. Würzburg: Königshausen und Neumann.

Insel, T., **Cuthbert, B.**, **Garvey, M.**, et al. (2010). Research Domain Criteria (RDoC): toward a new classification framework for research on mental disorders. *American Journal of Psychiatry*, **167**, 748–751.

Insel, T. and **Cuthbert, B.** (2015). Brain disorders? Precisely. Precision medicine comes to psychiatry. *Science*, **348**, 499–500.

Jaspers, K. (1946). *Allgemeine Psychopathologie*, 4th edn. Berlin: Springer.

Kendler, K.S. (2016). The nature of psychiatric disorders. *World Psychiatry*, **15**, 5–12.

Kendler, K.S. and **Jablensky, A.** (2011). Kraepelin's concept of psychiatric illness. *Psychological Medicine*, **41**, 1119–1126.

Kraepelin, E. (1899). *Psychiatrie. Ein Lehrbuch für Studirende und Aerzte*, 6th edn. Leipzig: Barth.

Kraepelin, E. (1904). *Psychiatrie. Ein Lehrbuch für Studierende und Ärzte*, 7th edn. Leipzig: Barth.

Kraepelin, E. (1909). *Psychiatrie. Ein Lehrbuch für Studierende und Ärzte*, 8th edn. Leipzig: Barth.

Kraepelin, E. (1918). Ziele und Wege der psychiatrischen Forschung. *Zeitschrift für die gesamte Neurologie und Psychiatrie*, **42**, 169–205.

Kraepelin, E. (1919). Die Erforschung psychischer Krankheitsformen. *Zeitschrift für die gesamte Neurologie und Psychiatrie*, **51**, 224–246.

Kraepelin, E. (1920a). Wilhelm Wundt. *Zeitschrift für die gesamte Neurologie und Psychiatrie*, **61**, 351–362.

Kraepelin, E. (1920b). Die Erscheinungsformen des Irreseins. *Zeitschrift für die gesamte Neurologie und Psychiatrie*, **62**, 1–29.

Kretschmer, E. (1918). *Der sensitive Beziehungswahn. Ein Beitrag zur Paranoiafrage und zur psychiatrischen Charakterlehre*. Berlin: Springer.

Küchenhoff, B. (2001). Die Auseinandersetzung Eugen Bleulers mit Sigmund Freud. In D. Hell, C. Scharfetter, and A. Möller (eds.) *Eugen Bleuler—Leben und Werk*, pp. 57–71. Bern: Huber.

Linden, M., **Baron, S.**, and **Muschalla, B.** (2009). *Mini-ICF-APP. Mini-ICF-Rating für Aktivitäts- und Partizipationsstörungen bei psychischen Erkrankungen*. Bern: Huber Hogrefe.

Maatz, A. and **Hoff, P.** (2014). The birth of schizophrenia or a very modern Bleuler: a close reading of Eugen Bleuler's 'Die Prognose der Dementia praecox' and a re-consideration of his contribution to psychiatry. *History of Psychiatry*, **25**, 431–440.

Maatz, A., **Hoff, P.**, and **Angst, J.** (2015). Eugen Bleuler's schizophrenia—a modern perspective. *Dialogues in Clinical Neuroscience*, **17**, 43–49.

Möller, A. (2001) Grundpositionen im Spätwerk. In: D. Hell, C. Scharfetter, and A. Möller (eds.) *Eugen Bleuler—Leben und Werk*, pp. 104–112. Bern: Huber.

Paris, J. and **Philipps, J.** (eds.) (2013). *Making the DSM-5. Concepts and controversies*. New York: Springer.

Parnas, J. (2011). A disappearing heritage: the clinical core of schizophrenia. *Schizophrenia Bulletin*, **37**, 1121–1130.

Plessner, H. (1975). *Die Stufen des Organischen und der Mensch. Einleitung in die philosophische Anthropologie*, 3rd edn. Berlin: de Gruyter.

Read, J., Mosher, L.R., Bentall, R.P. (eds.) (2004). *Models of Madness. Psychological, social and biological approaches to schizophrenia*. Hove: Brunner-Routledge.

Sartorius, N. (2015). Why do we need a diagnosis? Maybe a syndrome is enough? (Editorial). *Dialogues in Clinical Neuroscience*, **17**, 6–7.

Schneider, K. (1980). *Klinische Psychopathologie*, 12th edn. Stuttgart: Thieme.

Schneider, W., **Klauer, T.**, and **Freyberger, H.J.** (2008). Operationalized psychodynamic diagnosis in planning and evaluating the psychotherapeutic process. *European Archives of Psychiatry and Clinical Neuroscience*, **258** (suppl. 5), 86–91.

Stanghellini, G. (2009). The meanings of psychopathology. *Current Opinion in Psychiatry*, **22**, 559–564.

Szasz, T. (1961). *The Myth of Mental Illness. Foundations of a theory of personal conduct*. New York: Harper & Row.

Van Os, J. and **Tamminga, C.** (2007). Deconstructing psychosis. *Schizophrenia Bulletin*, 33, 861–862.

Van Praag, H.M., **Kahn, R.S.**, **Asnis, G.M.**, et al. (1987). Denosologization of biological psychiatry or the specificity of 5-HT disturbances in psychiatric disorders. *Journal of Affective Disorders*, **13**, 1–8.3.

Von Manz, H.G. (2014). *Interpersonalität und Ethik*. Würzburg: Königshausen & Neumann.

Wing, J.K. (1971). International comparisons in the study of the functional psychoses. *British Medical Bulletin*, **27**, 77–81.

World Health Organization (1992). *ICD-10 Classification of Mental and Behavioural Disorders (Including Disorders of Psychological Development). Clinical Descriptions And Diagnostic Guidelines*, Chapter V (F). Geneva: World Health Organization.

Zachar, P. (2000). Psychiatric disorders are not natural kinds. *Philosophy, Psychiatry, and Psychology*, 7, 167–182.

Chapter 15

Reification of mental illness: Some considerations

Dan J. Stein

In his thought-provoking chapter, Paul Hoff examines the work of Kraepelin and Bleuler, in order to address the reification of mental illness. Questions about the reification of mental illness in turn raise some of the perennial issues at the intersection of philosophy, science, and psychiatry. Thus, for example, many authors concerned with conceptual questions in the social sciences have argued about whether these disciplines should address both objective reality and subjective phenomena, and whether practitioners should emphasize more "erklären" (i.e., explanation) or "verstehen" (i.e., understanding) (Stein 2008). Analogously, authors at the intersection of philosophy and psychiatry have argued about whether mental illnesses should be conceptualized using an essentialist or a nominalist framework, and whether practitioners should emphasize more disease (i.e., biomedical explanation) or "illness" (i.e., patients' experience) (Stein 2008).

Hoff's emphasis on the history of psychiatry is clearly important when considering these debates. To quote Cicero, "*Nescire autem quid antequam natus sis acciderit, id est semper esse puerum*" (to be ignorant of what occurred before you were born is to remain always a child). That said, Hegel argued that people have never learned anything from history, or as George Bernard Shaw pithily put it, "We learn from history that we learn nothing from history." Indeed, Hoff makes an important contribution by tracing conceptual debates back through time, and by noting how cutting-edge concepts in the Research Domain Criteria (RDoC) framework partly reflect century-old approaches to mental disorder. Clinicians and researchers may well benefit from fully understanding such historical continuities, and from being able to ascertain when cutting-edge authors are merely offering old wine in new bottles.

One key issue that Hoff raises is the nature of mental illness. He emphasizes that a strong version of reification takes a naturalist and a realist approach (which he characterizes as emphasizing natural disease entities and the naturalization of mental and social phenomena). In Hoff's depiction of the perspective of the strong version, mental illness is seen as existing independently of any scientific concept. Put differently, mental illness, like other natural kinds, exists as part of objective reality, entirely separate from the particular theories or accounts that scientists or practitioners may subjectively hold about disorders. And he counters that mental illness instead refers to a concept, and not to a given thing. Certainly it is problematic when clinicians, researchers, or the public adopt an essentialist approach to mental disorders, seeing psychiatric nosology as an exercise in carving nature at her joints, and in providing the necessary and sufficient criteria that delineate the biological or psychological essences of different conditions (along the lines of establishing a periodic table for psychiatry). Given the multiple cross-level mechanisms underlying psychiatric disorders this entails a range of conceptual errors, and may help foster errors in clinical practice and in research laboratories.

I agree with Hoff that a conceptual position with roots in positivism (historically, a particular strand of analytic philosophy) may indeed strictly differentiate scientific concepts and objective reality. However, a conceptual position with roots in naturalism and realism (broader philosophical positions which aim to underpin the possibility of science and scientific progress), may nevertheless hold that scientific concepts are social constructs (Bhaskar 1978). Put differently, while scientific constructs are certainly theory-bound and in the social sciences also value-laden, at the same time science progresses by accounting for the real structures and mechanisms of the world. Similarly, I would argue that mental illness is not merely a concept; instead, our scientific constructs in psychiatry, although again theory-bound and value-laden, make progress by delineating real psychobiological structures and mechanisms (Stein 2008). Thus while I accept the point that many erroneously and egregiously view mental disorders as strong natural kinds, with necessary and sufficient features that will emerge from empirical study of the world out there, I would assert that a naturalist and realist stance does not necessitate such essentialism. Instead, a naturalist and realist stance can emphasize that categories (including the category of mental disorder) have both transitive elements (they are social constructs, they are theory-bound and value-laden) and intransitive elements (they reflect structures and mechanisms in the world) (Bhaskar 1978), with psychiatric disorders falling on the weak end of the spectrum of natural kinds (Stein 2014).

A second key issue that Hoff raises is that of subjectivity and interpersonality; he argues that these are indispensable elements of psychiatry. He argues that a focus on subjectivity and interpersonality strengthens neurobiological research rather than impedes it. And he concludes that it is important for psychiatric researchers not to take naturalistic short-cuts, reducing psychology to biology, which would amount to premature reification. Certainly it would be problematic for psychiatry and for psychiatric nosologies to neglect subjectivity or interpersonality; these cannot be ignored or elided.

I agree with Hoff that a conceptual position with roots in positivism (again, a specific position within philosophy) may well differentiate objectivity (or science) from subjectivity (or non-science). However, a conceptual position with roots in naturalism and realism (a broader set of philosophical positions) may nevertheless hold that sciences such as psychiatry necessarily involve dealing with both the objective and the subjective, and aim to provide both "erklären" (i.e., explanation) and "verstehen" (i.e., understanding) (Bhaskar 1978). Further, a focus on biological research does not necessarily entail a reduction of psychology to biology;

indeed, good biological research may well involve work that addresses emergent layers of complex phenomena, and the multiple mechanisms that operate within and between such levels. Thus while I fully accept that psychiatry involves subjectivity/interpersonality, it would seem to me that both our current psychiatric nosologies (e.g., DSM-5, ICD-11) and the RDoC framework also hold this view, and that they do not necessarily attempt to reduce subjectivity/interpersonality to biology (Cuthbert and Insel 2013). This is not to say that our current nosologies and the RDoC framework do not have important conceptual weaknesses; rather it is to assert that these lie elsewhere (Stein 2014).

In sum, my view is that Hoff's work, emphasizing the work of key historical figures in psychiatry, and warning about the hazards entailed by the reification of mental disorder, makes an important contribution to current conceptual debates at the intersection of philosophy, science, and psychiatry. However, it seems to me that his arguments about the nature of mental illness, and about subjectivity/interpersonality, primarily address an outdated conceptual approach with roots in positivism (a "classical" position). I would submit that conceptual approaches with roots in naturalism and realism can entail a more sophisticated and complex approach to mental disorder, which emphasizes that psychiatry and psychiatric nosology are both evidence-based and values-based, and which avoids the risk of reification of mental illness (an "integrative" position). That said, I suspect Hoff and I share many aspirations for nosology in particular, and psychiatry in general, including a wish to avoid essentialism and reductionism, a wish that efforts such as DSM-5 and RDoC would be more widely recognized as providing only tentative and partial windows on psychiatric conditions, and a wish to encompass the full complexity of mental disorders including both disease mechanisms and illness experiences. A recent reading of Kraepelin suggests that he too took a more integrative approach than has often been suggested (Engstrom and Kendler 2015).

References

Bhaskar, R. (1978). *A Realist Theory of Science*, 2nd edn. Brighton: Harvester Press.

Cuthbert, B.N. and **Insel, T.R.** (2013). Toward the future of psychiatric diagnosis: the seven pillars of RDoC. *BMC Medicine*, **11**, 126.

Engstrom, E.J. and **Kendler, K.S.** (2015). Emil Kraepelin: icon and reality. *American Journal of Psychiatry*, **172**, 1190–1196.

Stein, D.J. (2008). *Philosophy of Psychopharmacology*. Cambridge: Cambridge University Press.

Stein, D.J. (2014). An integrative approach to psychiatric diagnosis and research. *World Psychiatry*, **13**, 51–53.

Stein, D.J. (2014). Psychopharmacology and natural kinds: A conceptual framework. In H. Kincaid and J.A. Sullivan (eds.) *Classifying Psychopathology: Mental Kinds and Natural Kinds*, pp. 65–73. Cambridge, MA: MIT Press.

Section 6

Psychiatric epidemics

Chapter 16

Introduction to "Factors in the development of psychiatric epidemics"

Kenneth S. Kendler

In this thoughtful essay, Michael First, a psychiatric nosologist who has spent much of his career involved in work relating to the *Diagnostic and Statistical Manual of Mental Disorders* (DSM) and knows the subject deeply, tackles the tough problem of "psychiatric epidemics." Many claims, some going back centuries, have been made for changing rates of psychiatric illness in the general population. As far as I recall from my reading, the claims are, with appropriate alarm, always for increases. I cannot recall someone noting that rates of psychiatric illness are on the decline. Most typically, the suggested increases have been linked to the evils of "modernization," the faster pace of life, the greater degrees of stress. Other claims, especially those getting attention in recent decades, have been more diagnostically specific. First focuses in this essay on four disorders all of which have been the source of recent controversy regarding evidence, of varying degrees of quality, of changing incidence rates: dissociative identity disorder (aka "multiple personality disorder"), pediatric bipolar disorder, autism spectrum disorder (ASD), and attention deficit hyperactivity disorder (ADHD).

An especially helpful feature of this essay is how methodologically First takes the reader through a "differential diagnosis" of the possible causes of an "epidemic." He outlines three etiologies which in my words would be: (1) a true increase in incidence, (2) an increase in treated incidence but not true incidence, and (3) an iatrogenic epidemic due to broadening of diagnostic criteria. As First makes clear, it can be devilishly difficult to discriminate between these three (non-mutually-exclusive) explanations. This is because the gold-standard data—high-quality epidemiological surveys done at frequent enough intervals with a stable set of diagnostic criteria and interview probes—are quite hard to come by. We know, for example, that prevalence rates from different interviews, each of which claim to be operationalizing the same set of diagnostic criteria, can actually produce quite different prevalence rates. Treated prevalence data is inherently problematic. As First outlines, if special services are provided for individuals with a particular diagnosis, it is not rocket science to predict that the prevalence of that diagnosis will rise independent of what the true population prevalence may be. Changes in the structure of insurance coverage can similarly impact on treated prevalence.

Diagnostic fads within the field of psychiatry also have to be taken into account. I came of age in psychiatry at a time when it was very popular to rediagnose people with schizophrenia as having bipolar illness. We were rather disrespectful of our elders and sure that we knew better. It was claimed (although this is an exaggeration) that two long-distance phone calls on the inpatient unit were enough to get you a diagnosis of bipolar illness and a lithium trial. Years later, most of the patients were back under their original diagnosis label, because lithium treatment had failed. At a similar time, the diagnosis of "borderline personality disorder" (most commonly shortened to just "borderline") also rose in popularity. As psychiatric residents, we were apt to brag about how difficult our "borderline patient" was—manipulative, suicidal, frequently self-cutting, and so on. Having read a fair amount about the so-called epidemic of dissociative identity disorder (often with reports of early sexual abuse associated with bizarre cultic activity), the data, while still only suggestive, is most consistent with an especially malignant diagnostic fad (Hacking 1998b, McHugh 2008).

To make matters worse, there are well-demonstrated risk factors of psychiatric illness (e.g., unemployment, social dislocation related to migration, traumas related to natural or other disasters) the prevalence rates of which can change substantially and quickly in relation to historical events like economic depression, war, terrorism, and natural events like earthquakes and tidal waves. These are likely to produce real "epidemics" of psychiatric illness although the research infrastructure is rarely in place to study these in an ideal way.

There is one area that First does not discuss where true epidemics are well documented—drug abuse. New drugs or new forms of old drugs can rapidly become more accessible or cheaper due to shifts in the invention, production, and distribution of illicit substances (including the diversion of drugs from prescription to illicit use such as oxycodone in the United States). The "crack epidemic" has its own *Wikipedia* entry that begins "The American crack epidemic was a surge of crack cocaine use in major cities across the United States between 1984 and the early 1990s." Such epidemics do lead to rapid and true shifts in population incidence. Indeed, the epidemiology of illicit drug use disorders is a constantly shifting landscape.

Finally, a discussion of psychiatric epidemics would not be complete without a brief reference to Ian Hacking's intriguing if controversial book *Mad Travelers* (Hacking 1998a). This book has the intriguing subtitle "*Reflections on the reality of transient mental illnesses*." This slim book recounts an epidemic in late nineteenth-century France of what we would now call amnestic fugue. Individuals, nearly always men, would disappear and resurface months later in a distant city. As their stories were put back together, it appears they "lost their identity and memory" and in a fugue state got on a train, traveling often hundreds of miles. They would then assume a new identity, often work until either they "woke up" to their old identity and remembered their family and got in touch with them, or were found by the police or distraught relatives. Hacking, in his usual quite stimulating prose, ponders the significance of this epidemic (which lasted a decade or more and was almost entirely confined to France) for our conceptions of psychiatric illness.

As is so often the case when we ponder deeply the nature of psychiatric illness, we are struck—as we consider the nature of psychiatric epidemics—by the complex mix of biological vulnerabilities and social and cultural influences that lead to these conditions. Except that here, we also have the added factors of health care access, support services, and diagnostic fads that enter into the already quite complex mix of risk factors for psychiatric illness.

References

Hacking, I. (1998a). *Mad Travelers: Reflections on the reality of transient mental illnesses.* Charlottesville, VA: University of Virginia Press.

Hacking, I. (1998b). *Rewriting The Soul: Multiple personality and the sciences of memory,* revised edn. Princeton, NJ: Princeton University Press.

McHugh, P.R. (2008). *Try to Remember: Psychiatry's clash over meaning, memory, and mind.* New York: Dana Press.

Chapter 17

Factors in the development of psychiatric epidemics

Michael B. First

17.1 Introduction

According to the Centers for Disease Control's *Principles of Epidemiology in Public Health Practice* (Centers for Disease Control and Prevention 2012), an epidemic is defined as "the occurrence of more cases of disease than expected in a given area or among a specific group of people over a particular period of time." (p. 1-72). Although the term was originally used to refer to the rapid spread of infectious disease to a large number of people within a short period of time, it has been more broadly employed to refer to any occurrence of illness that is clearly in excess of normal expectancy.

One of the challenges in applying the term "epidemic" to psychiatric illness is that it requires one to know what the normal expectancy of occurrence is for psychiatric disorders. In the domain of infectious diseases, this concept is generally straightforward—the expected prevalence of a particular infectious disease in a population in a particular geographic area during a particular period of time is usually well known based on knowledge of historical trends. For example, the occurrence of the 2014 Ebola epidemic in Africa quickly became evident once the infectious agent was identified given that the expected base rate of Ebola virus infections in Africa in 2013 was essentially zero. Moreover, the process by which epidemics of infectious diseases develop is relatively well established and typically involves previously non-infected individuals becoming exposed to an infectious agent and subsequently manifesting signs and symptoms of the infectious disease. While some epidemics in psychiatry follow the infectious disease model of increased rates of illness after exposure to a pathogen—e.g., increased incidence and prevalence of post-tramatic stress disorder (PTSD) among residents of lower Manhattan after the 9/11 terrorist attacks (Neria et al. 2011), or increased incidence and prevalence of prescription opioid addiction related to more aggressive use of opioid analgesics on the part of physicians (Mendelson et al. 2008)—the process underlying the development of most purported epidemics of psychiatric illness is much less understood. For some psychiatric epidemics, the increased occurrence of illness primarily involves individuals who had not been previously considered to be psychiatrically ill—e.g., the increased rates of attention deficic hyperactivity disorder (ADHD) diagnoses among high school students in recent years. Other epidemics—e.g., juvenile bipolar disorder (JBD), dissociative identity disorder (DID)—have involved individuals who are already suffering from psychiatric symptoms (and thus considered likely to be psychiatrically ill) who are then "discovered" to have a particular diagnosis that appears to better explain their symptoms.

Over the past 30 years, there have been a number of articles addressing epidemics of certain psychiatric disorders with some questioning the validity of the assigned diagnoses, including DID/multiple personality disorder (McHugh 1995, Hacking 1998), ADHD (Stolzer 2007, Lanphear 2012, Frances 2014), autism (Arkowitz and Lillienfeld 2007, Liu et al. 2010), JBD (Healy and Le Noury 2007, Parry and Allison 2008, Frances 2010), internet addiction (Christakis and Moreno 2009), as well as mental disorders in general (Angell 2011). Whenever there is an apparent increase in the number of cases over a relatively short span of time, there are generally three possibilities as to how to understand what is going on. First, the increase in cases may represent a true epidemic in which the actual incidence of the disorder in the population is increasing, thus warranting careful investigation into the potential underlying causes of the increases (e.g., increased exposure to a causal environmental factor). A second possibility is that the number of true cases in the general population has not changed but that there is an increase in the number of previously undiagnosed individuals coming to clinical attention for a variety of reasons, such as increased clinician or public awareness of the disorder, improved methods of detection, increased societal acceptance of being diagnosed with the disorder, and changes in external incentives for making the diagnosis (e.g., qualifying for educational benefits, benefits bestowed by virtue of occupying the "sick role"). Finally, given that determinations of caseness rely on subjective diagnostic criteria that are subject to periodic revision, increased diagnostic rates could be a result of broadening the diagnostic definitions over time.

Arriving at a definitive explanation for increased diagnostic rates over time is typically not possible because of significant limitations in the empirical database, leading to rancorous debates regarding the significance of such increases, especially for diagnoses whose very validity has been questioned, such as pediatric bipolar disorder (Healy and Le Noury 2007). Proponents of such diagnoses invariably attribute the increased rates to improved recognition on the part of clinicians and the public, arguing that the increased rates correct a historical underdiagnosis and undertreatment of the disorders. Critics, on the other hand, generally claim either that such increases largely involve the overdiagnosis of normal individuals (as in the case of ADHD) or a mislabeling of legitimately ill individuals that is leading to the wrong treatment (as in JBD or DID).

In this chapter, we examine several of the most controversial psychiatric diagnostic epidemics in the past 30 years, exploring in more detail those factors which may have contributed to the development of the reported increased rates.

17.2 What is the method for the determination of increased rates over time?

Before we examine some of the factors that could contribute to the development of psychiatric epidemics, it is important to consider the method used to determine that, in fact, the rates of a particular diagnosis have increased over time. As is the case with epidemics of infectious diseases, in which the detection of an epidemic of cases typically necessitates an investigation into the potential infectious source of the epidemic, the discovery of an epidemic of a psychiatric disorder inevitably raises questions about what might be causing such an increase. For example, the apparent explosion in autism cases over the past 30 years has spurred the search for presumptive causal factors, leading some to arrive at the erroneous conclusion that vaccine exposure is the cause of the rise in cases (Wakefield and McCarthy 2010). If, however, it can be clearly determined that the increase in rates is due to increased clinician and public awareness or that it is entirely explained as an artifact of the assessment process (e.g., due to the broadening of case definitions over time), then there would be no need to engage in a search for a corresponding increase in a putative causal factor.

Most commonly, increases in diagnostic rates in samples of individuals who are in treatment or who are receiving benefits (e.g., extra educational services) are used to demonstrate the occurrence of an epidemic. One way of doing this is to examine trends in psychiatric diagnosis in national surveys of healthcare encounters, referred to as "treated" prevalence since it reflects the prevalence among individuals coming in for treatment of some kind. For example, Moreno and colleagues examined rates of growth between 1994–1995 and 2002–2003 in the number of outpatient visits for children and adults with a diagnosis of bipolar disorder using data from the National Ambulatory Care Survey(Moreno et al. 2007). The estimated annual number of visits in youth (0–19 years old) with a diagnosis of bipolar disorder increased from 25 per 100,000 visits in 1994–1995 to 1005 per 100,000 visits in 2002–2003, as compared to an increase in bipolar visits in adults from 905 visits per 100,000 in 1994–1995 to 1679 visits per 100,000 in 2002–2003. Similarly, Blader and Carlson (2007) analyzed records from the annual National Hospital Discharge Survey to determine trends in the rates of hospitalization for bipolar disorder in children. They found that rates of hospital discharge with a primary diagnosis of bipolar disorder increased 438.6% in children from 1996 to 2004 (from 1.3 per 10,000 children to 7.3 per 10,000 children in 2004), 296.4% in adolescents, and 56.0% in adults.

Another source of data has been surveys conducted on individuals obtained through an epidemiologically sound sampling technique, such as the national cross-sectional random-digit-dialing landline telephone surveys used to estimate the prevalence of health indicators in the general population, conducted by the Centers for Disease Control and Prevention. Such surveys are considered by epidemiologists to be closer to the true prevalence of the disorder in the general population. Visser and colleagues (2014) examined data from the 2003, 2007, and 2011 administrations of the National Survey of Children's Health and compared the estimates of the number of children reported by their parents to have ever been diagnosed with ADHD (Visser et al. 2014). They reported that the percentage of children aged 4–17 years with a parent-reported lifetime ADHD diagnosis grew from 7.8% in 2003 to 11% in 2011, representing a 42% increase.

Increased rates of autism have also been seen in social service enrollment data. For example, in the California Developmental Disabilities Service system, the number of clients served under the category of autism as a percentage of all clients rose from 4.9% to 9.4% during the 1994–2003 period (California Department of Developmental Services 1999). In U.S. special education, the total reported number of children ages 6 to 21 enrolled under the autism category among the 50 states and the District of Columbia increased from 22,445 in the 1994–1995 school year to 140,234 in the 2003–2004 school year (U.S. Department of Education 1996).

While the fact that increasing numbers of individuals are referred for clinical or special education services has both clinical and public health significance, such trends are not necessarily accurate indicators that the prevalence and incidence of a psychiatric condition in the general population is actually increasing over time. This is because increases in disorder rates in referred samples are confounded by a number of factors that are not intrinsic to the disorder itself, including among other things changes in referral patterns, availability of services, and clinician and public awareness The gap between clinical diagnosis of autism and the actual autism phenotype (i.e., the symptoms on which the diagnosis is made) was demonstrated by Lundström et al. (2015) who compared the annual prevalence of reported diagnoses of autism spectrum disorder (ASD) in the Swedish national register to the annual prevalence of the autism diagnosis assessed by a validated parental telephone interview. They found that while there was a significant monotonic increase in the prevalence of reported autism diagnoses from 1993 to 2002 in Sweden, the prevalence of the autism symptoms assessed by the parental interview was stable.

In response to the apparent alarming increase in autism cases since the condition was first formally identified by Kanner in the 1940s, a number of investigators have conducted epidemiological studies of rates of autism. Most such studies relied on a two-stage or multistage approach, with an initial screening stage which involved sending letters or brief screening scales requesting schools and health professionals to identify possible cases of autism (Fombonne 2003). The screening stages were followed by intensive assessment phases which involved administering various diagnostic instruments to the screened subjects. Although several reviews of these studies demonstrated an upward trend of rates in recent decades, these reviews concluded that these increases most likely reflect broadening of the diagnostic definitions, increased service availability, and heightened awareness of ASD in both the lay and professional public (Fombonne 2003, 2009, Chakrabarti and Fombonne 2009, Elsabbagh et al. 2012).

17.3 **Factors contributing to the dissociative identity disorder epidemic**

The marked increase in rates of reported cases of DID over the past 100 years certainly appears to qualify as an epidemic. Initially, DID and the other dissociative disorders were considered the rarest of psychological conditions, with only 76 cases reported by 1944 (Taylor and Martin 1944). In 1954, Thigpen and Cleckley described a case which became the basis of their book (and subsequent film) called *Three Faces of Eve* (Thigpen and Cleckley 1954). From that point on, and with the publication of the book *Sybil* in 1973 (Schreiber 1973), cases of DID multiplied with approximately 6000 cases having been reported by 1986 (Elzinga et al. 1998).

Lillienfeld and colleagues (1999) have argued that iatrogenic and sociocultural factors have played a substantial etiological role in DID and account largely for the dramatic upsurge in the number of reported cases. They conceptualize DID as a syndrome consisting of

> displays of multiple role enactments that have been created, legitimized, and maintained by social reinforcement. Patients with DID synthesize these role enactments by drawing on a wide variety of sources of information, including the print and broadcast media, cues provided by therapists, personal experiences, and observations of individuals who have enacted multiple identities (Lillienfeld et al. 1999, pp. 507–508).

From this perspective, the rise in DID rates can thus be explained by a combination of the wide dissemination of the features of DID throughout the culture via the media and other sources as well as by therapists' suggestions to patients that their symptoms represent the subtle actions of several alternative personalities (alters) coexisting in the patient's mental life. Those who view DID as a defensive response to severe abuse by which individuals compartmentalize their subjective experience into alters as a means of coping with the emotional pain of the trauma (Gleaves 1996), on the other hand, attribute the increased rates of DID to improved recognition of DID on the part of trained clinicians.

17.4 Factors contributing to the pediatric bipolar disorder epidemic

The epidemic of pediatric bipolar disorder began as a result of a deliberate attempt on the part of researchers to expand the bipolar disorder construct as it applies to children. Volatile aggressive behavior is the most common reason for children being brought to inpatient care (Gutterman 1998). Such presentations typically occur in combination with deficits in impulse control and affective instability, a presentation which does not clearly conform to any of the specific categories included in the *Diagnostic and Statistical Manual of Mental Disorders* (DSM). Wozniak and colleagues in a seminal 1997 paper (Wozniak et al. 1997) proposed that in the same way developmental variations in the definition of major depression had been accepted in DSM-III, DSM-III-R, and DSM-IV (e.g., irritability substituting for depressed mood as an anchor symptom), childhood-onset mania characterized by predominantly chronically irritable mood should potentially be considered a developmental variant of adult bipolar disorder. The shift in thinking among researchers in the field from viewing mania as exceedingly rare in childhood to the idea that it may be common was solidified at an National Institute of Mental Health (NIMH) Roundtable on pediatric bipolar (NIMH 2001) in which agreement was reached that bipolar disorder exists and can be diagnosed in prepubertal children, and that such children can present with both DSM-IV and non-DSM-IV phenotypes (i.e., those given a diagnosis of bipolar-NOS), These non-DSM-IV phenotypes included both a narrow phenotype, involving manic episodes that meet DSM-IV criteria symptom criteria for mania (i.e., elevated, euphoric, or irritable mood) with ultrarapid cycling, and a broad phenotype consisting of chronic manic states characterized by severe irritability, affective storms, mood lability, severe temper outbursts, poor concentration, and impulsivity with or without clear episodicity (Pavuluri et al. 2005).

This shift in thinking among academics has been accompanied by a corresponding surge in the diagnosis of pediatric bipolar disorder by clinicians. For example, during the period from 1994–1995 to 2002–2003, the diagnosis of bipolar disorder in children increased 40-fold, as compared to nearly twofold in adults (Moreno et al. 2007). According to the Centers for Disease Control, in 2004 bipolar disorder was the most common diagnosis in psychiatrically hospitalized children under age 12 (Blader and Carlson 2007). A number of factors may have contributed to this precipitous rise in diagnosis. Much of this increased diagnosis may be the result of increased awareness of the condition among both clinicians and patients. For example, a search of MEDLINE revealed only 5 publications related to pediatric bipolar disorder prior to 1980, 27 from 1980 to 1989, 50 from 1990 to 1999, and 227 from 2000 to 2005 (Moreno et al. 2007). The expansion of bipolar cases beyond the DSM-IV definition is also reflected in the treatment literature. For example, both the broad and narrow phenotypes of bipolar disorder are explicitly discussed in Kowatch and colleagues' treatment guidelines for pediatric bipolar disorder (Kowatch et al. 2005).

The proposed existence of pediatric bipolar disorder has been reflected in the popular press. A number of articles in the lay media as well as books aimed at parents have served to popularize pediatric bipolar disorder, which likely changed parents' views about the nature of their child's psychopathology and promoted treatment seeking at an earlier age. For example, *Time* magazine's cover story on August 19, 2002, "Young and bipolar," reported that "experts estimate that an additional 1 million preteens and children in the U.S. may suffer from the early stages of bipolar disorder." (Kluger and Song 2002). The book *The Bipolar Child: The definitive and reassuring guide to childhood's most misunderstood disorder* (Papolos and Papolos 2000) was the first of several books promoting childhood bipolar to the public and sold over 200,000 hardback copies. This was accompanied by a series of books written specifically for children, such as *My Bipolar Roller Coaster Feelings Book* (Hebert 2005) and *Brandon and the Bipolar Bear* (Anglada 2004) which comes with an associated coloring book, in which "Brandon's dad makes it clear that lots of kids have things wrong with their bodies, like asthma and diabetes, and that they also have to take medicine and be careful" (Healy and Le Noury 2007, p. 215). Advocacy groups, such as the Child and Adolescent Bipolar Foundation (www.bpchildren.com) and the Juvenile Bipolar Research Foundation (www.jbrf.org) have sprung up to provide parent education and online diagnostic questionnaires.

Economic factors, especially in terms of the use of the diagnosis in inpatient settings, may also play a role, involving a progressive rebranding of the same clinical phenomenon for which hospitalized children previously received different diagnoses: for example, relabeling children who would have been diagnosed with conduct disorder as bipolar disorder. The unchanged rates of conduct disorder diagnoses during the survey years covered in the Blader and Carlson analysis of inpatient diagnoses (Blader and Carlson 2007) effectively represents a decline in the rates of conduct disorder in light of the marked rise in overall population-adjusted rates of children's psychiatric diagnoses. In a process known as "upcoding," clinicians may have responded to the more stringent requirements for obtaining authorization for inpatient hospitalization by assigning a diagnosis of a major mood disorder.

Finally, Parry and Levin (2012) argue that the increase in pediatric bipolar disorder diagnoses is a function of a paradigm shift in psychiatry over recent decades from an era of "brainless psychiatry" with its emphasis on psychodynamic and family factors predominating to the exclusion of biological factors, to a current era of "mindless psychiatry" which emphasizes neurobiological explanations for emotional and behavioral problems with limited regard for contextual meaning. They point out that diagnoses of pediatric bipolar illness are often made on the basis of diagnostic checklists that "underutilize psychodynamics, family dynamics, attachment, trauma, and context." (p. 95), with the implication that many of the cases now labelled as pediatric bipolar disorder are better conceptualized as responses to difficult family situations or trauma. Echoing Perry and Levin's concerns, Carlson and Meyers (2006) noted "the diagnosis of bipolar disorder in often made by mindlessly applying criteria . . . without an understanding of developmental history and context." (p. 963).

17.5 **Factors contributing to the autism spectrum disorder epidemic**

From the 1970s onward, the reported prevalence of ASD has increased substantially. Although once considered rare, affecting fewer than 0.05% of the population (Wing et al. 1976), lifetime prevalence is now generally agreed to be at least 1% in both young people (Bard et al. 2006) and adults (Brugha et al. 2011). This significant increase in cases over a relatively short period of time has raised questions about whether there is a secular increase in the incidence of autism that may perhaps be due to exposure to as yet unidentified environmental factors. A number of possible explanations have been identified that might explain this increase including the broadening of the concept and diagnostic criteria for autism to include milder cases (Gernsbacher et al. 2005), the practice of diagnostic substitution, in which cases formerly diagnosed as learning disabled or intellectually disabled have been reclassified as ASD (Shattuck 2006), and improved detection of pervasive developmental disorders at all ages and all levels of intellectual disability (Chakrabarti and Fombonne 2009).

As pointed out by Fombonne (2003) in a review of epidemiological surveys of autism, determining whether or not there is a secular increase in the rates of autism requires differentiating prevalence (i.e., the proportion of individuals in a population suffering from a disorder) from incidence (the number of new cases in a population over a particular time period). While prevalence estimates are useful to help guide resource allocation and planning, only incidence rates are relevant for causal research. Although different epidemiological methods have been employed by researchers to try to determine whether the incidence of autism has been increasing, most have been hampered by methodological weaknesses that make the results difficult to interpret. A common method is to examine increased rates of referrals to special education services. Unfortunately, upward trends in referrals are confounded by many factors such as changes in referral patterns, availability of services, heightened public awareness, and decreased age at diagnosis, which, unless properly controlled for, make it impossible to determine whether there is a true rise of incidence. Similarly, comparing prevalence rates determined by cross-sectional epidemiological surveys done at different times is problematic given that each survey possesses unique design features which could account for between-studies variation of cases. Fombonne concluded that "the available epidemiological evidence does not strongly support the hypothesis that the incidence of autism has increased and several other reasons could easily account for an artifactual impression of an increase." (p. 376).

One factor unique to the ASD epidemic (as compared to the other epidemics discussed in this paper) is the fact that that the DSM diagnostic criteria have changed significantly during this period in terms of both the diagnostic criteria for autistic disorder as well as the inclusion of milder cases (i.e., Asperger's disorder) under the umbrella of pervasive developmental disorders. Whereas the DSM-III criteria for infantile autism required satisfying 6 mandatory criteria, the DSM-IV criteria for the corresponding category autistic disorder offers 16 possible criteria, only 8 of which need to be present to meet criteria. Furthermore, whereas the DSM-III included only three categories (i.e., infantile autism, childhood-onset pervasive developmental disorder, and atypical autism), DSM-IV offered five categories (autistic disorder, Asperger's disorder, Rett's disorder, childhood disintegrative disorder, and pervasive developmental disorder NOS), with both Asperger's disorder and pervasive developmental disorder NOS being considered milder variants of autistic disorder. According to Chakrabarti and Fombonne (2009), this diagnostic broadening can account for nearly three fourths of current ASD diagnoses.

17.6 **Factors contributing to the ADHD epidemic**

Approximately 2 million more U.S. children/adolescents aged 4 to 17 years had been diagnosed with ADHD in 2011, compared to 2003, representing an increase of 42% over a span of just 8 years (Visser et al. 2014). As with autism, DID, and JBD, whether this increase represents a secular increase, appropriate recognition and diagnosis of cases that had previously gone undiagnosed, or an overapplication of the diagnosis of ADHD remains a matter of heated debate (Newmark 2015). Economic and other incentives have likely played a particularly important role in explaining at least some of this increase. The 2011 National Survey of Children's Health reveals wide disparities from state to state (Visser et al. 2014). For instance, a child in Kentucky is three times as likely to be diagnosed with ADHD as a child in Nevada. Most of the states with the highest rates of diagnosis are in the South, with some in the Midwest; most of the states with the lowest rates are in the West or Northeast.

Hinshaw and Scheffler (2014) examined several potential factors that might explain these state-specific differences in prevalence, comparing North Carolina and California. They reported that healthcare system policies had an indirect influence over these differences in diagnostic prevalence. They found that during the late 1980s and throughout the 1990s, 30 states, including all of the Southern states, passed consequential accountability laws in which school funding became based on students' standardized math and reading test scores, rewarding schools for doing better. One way of improving test scores is to have children diagnosed with a disorder like ADHD so that these children could get extra money from the school district to help tutor them or place them into smaller classes. Some states have even allowed students diagnosed with ADHD to be taken out of the pool that was used to judge a school. The No Child Left Behind Act (NCLB), which went into effect in 2002, set national standards and established measurable goals in an effort to improve education outcomes for students, allowing Hinshaw and Sheffler to compare those 30 states to the other 20 before and after NCLB became federal law. They found that standards-based education reform has likely played a large role in the nation's increase in ADHD diagnoses (Fulton et al. 2015). Between 2003 and 2007, in those 20 states that did not get consequential accountability until NCLB was implemented, there was a 59% increase in ADHD diagnoses among children who were within 200% of the federal poverty limit. Among middle- or upper-class children in those states, there was only a 3% increase in ADHD diagnosis. But in states that had already passed the accountability laws before NCLB, rates of ADHD diagnosis only went up 20%, which matches the national average, and there was no difference between poor and middle- and upper-class children.

It has also been hypothesized that the increase in ADHD diagnoses are at least partly being driven at the individual patient level, in which parents, teachers, and late adolescent / young adult patients are pressuring clinicians to make a diagnosis of ADHD so that the patient can get medicated, under the widely accepted belief that stimulant medication will help improve the patient's academic performance, perhaps providing a crucial edge in the competitive environment of secondary education.

17.7 Conclusion and implications for the DSM

Although reports of greatly increased rates of certain psychiatric disorders in the past 30 years suggest the possibility that we are in the midst of one or more "epidemics" in psychiatry, a closer examination of each of these situations raises numerous questions about whether any of these truly represent increased incidence of the disorder in the community, which is required to conform to the definition of a true epidemic. In most of these cases, the claims for the existence of an epidemic depends on reports of increased numbers of diagnoses made by mental health providers as opposed to evidence of increased rates of the symptomatic presentation in the community. Given that psychiatric diagnoses are typically made in order to justify the initiation of treatment or to allow the individual to obtain the benefits of the designation of being in the "sick role," a multitude of factors extrinsic to the diagnoses are likely to exert a significant influence on whether or not a person is considered to have a particular diagnosis. Moreover, in virtually every one of the above scenarios, it is nearly impossible to tell how much of the increased rates of diagnoses represent appropriately increased recognition of overlooked illness versus inappropriate mislabeling of either individuals suffering from another psychiatric disorder (e.g., labelling children with conduct disorder as having PBD) or individuals whose symptoms represent a normal developmental variation (e.g., labelling children who are developmentally immature as having ADHD). Conducting epidemiological investigations across various points in time, using the same sampling and assessment methodology at each time point, is the only way to definitively establish whether an increase in rates is evidence of a true epidemic.

The large impact of non-diagnostic factors on the rise of prevalence rates suggests that the DSM definitions themselves play a relatively minor role in determining treated prevalence. For example, the rise in ADHD prevalence from 2003 to 2011 occurred during a time in which the DSM definition of ADHD was unchanged. Evidence that the broadening of the ASD concept over the last two iterations of the DSM illustrates, however, that expanding diagnostic definitions can contribute to marked increases in prevalence. The combination of increased prevalence due to psychosocial factors combined with the impact of the expansion of diagnostic boundaries underscores the need for careful construction of DSM definitions to avoid false positives (Wakefield and First 2012).

References

Angell, M. (2011). The epidemic of mental illness: Why? *New York Review of Books*, June 23, 56.

Anglada, T. (2004). *Brandon and the Bipolar Bear.* Victoria, BC: Trafford Publishing.

Arkowitz, H. and **Lillienfeld, S.O.** (2007). Is there really an autism epidemic? *Scientific American*, December, 6.

Bard, G., Simonoff E., Pickles, A., et al. (2006). Prevalence of disorders of the autism spectrum in a population cohort of children in South Thames: the Special Needs and Autism Project (SNAP). *Lancet*, **368**, 210–215.

Blader, J.C. and **Carlson, G.A.** (2007). Increased rates of bipolar disorder diagnoses among U.S. child, adolescent, and adult inpatients, 1996–2004. *Biological Psychiatry*, **62**, 107–114.

Brugha, T.S., McManus, S., et al. (2011). Epidemiology of autism spectrum disorders in adults in the community in England. *Archives of General Psychiatry*, **68**, 459–465.

California Department of Developmental Services (1999). *Changes in the populaiton of persons with autism and pervasive developmental disorders in California's developmental services system: 1987 through 1998. A report to the legislature. March 1, 1999.* Sacramento, CA: California Health and Human Services Agency.

Carlson, G.A. and **Meyers, S.E.** (2006). Phenomenology and diagnosis of bipolar disorder in children, adolescents, and adults: complexities and developmental issues. *Development and Psychopathology*, **18**, 939–969.

Centers for Disease Control and Prevention (2012). Introduction to Epidemiology. *Principles of Epidemiology in Public Health Practice Third Edition*. R. C. Dicker, F. Coronado, D. Koo and R. G. Parrish, Centers for Diseae Control and Prevention: 1–72.

Chakrabarti, S. and **Fombonne, E.** (2009). Pervasive developmental disorders in preschool children: confirmation of high prevalence. *American Journal of Psychiatry*, **162**, 1133–1141.

Christakis, D.A. and **Moreno, M.A.** (2009). Trapped in the net: will internet addiction become a 21st century epidemic? *Archives of Pediatrics and Adolescent Medicine*, **163**, 959–960.

Elsabbagh, M., Divan, G., Koh, Y.J., et al. (2012). Global prevalence of autism and other pervasive developmental disorders. *Autism Research*, **5**, 160–179.

Elzinga, B.M., van Dyck, R., and **Spinhoven, P.** (1998). Three controversies about dissociative identity disorder. *Clinical Psychology and Psychotherapy*, **5**, 15–23.

Fombonne, E. (2003). Epidemiological surveys of autism and other pervasive developmental disorders: an update. *Journal of Autsim and Developmental Disorders*, **33**, 365–382.

Fombonne, E. (2009). Epidemiology of pervasive developmental disorders. *Pediatric Research*, **65**, 591–598.

Frances, A.J. (2010). Psychiatric diagnosis gone wild: the epidemic of childhood bipolar disorder, *Psychiatric Times*, April 8.

Frances, A.J. (2014). How parents can protect kids from the ADHD "epidemic." *Huffington Post blog*, http://www.huffingtonpost.com/allen-frances/how-parents-can-protect-k_b_4767047.html

Fulton, B.D., Scheffler, R.M., Hinshaw, S.P. (2015). State variation in increased ADHD prevalence: links to NCLB school accountability and state medication laws. *Psychiatric Services*, **66**, 1074–1082.

Gernsbacher, M.A., Dawson, M., and **Goldsmith, H.H.** (2005). Three reasons not to believe in an autism epidemic. *Current Directions in Psychological Science*, **14**, 55–58.

Gleaves, D.H. (1996). The sociocognitive model of dissociative identity disorder: a reexamination of the evidence. *Psychological Bulletin*, **120**, 42–59.

Gutterman, E.M. (1998). Is diagnosis relevant in the hospitalization of potentially dangerous children and adolescents. *Journal of the American Academy of Child and Adolescent Psychiatry*, **37**, 1030–1037.

Hacking, I. (1998). *Rewriting The Soul: Multiple personality and the sciences of memory*. Princeton, NJ: Princeton University Press.

Healy, D. and **Le Noury, J.** (2007). Pediatric bipolar disorder: An object of study in the creation of an illness. *International Journal of Risk and Safety in Medicine*, **19**, 209–221.

Hebert, B. (2005). *My Bipolar Roller Coaster Feelings Book*. Victoria, BC: Trafford Publishing.

Hinshaw, S.P. and **Scheffler, R.M.** (2014). *The ADHD Explosion: Myths, medications, money, and today's push for performance*. New York: Oxford University Press.

Kluger, J. and **Song, S.** (2002). Manic depression: young and bipolar. *Time*, August 19.

Kowatch, R.A., Fristad, M., Birmaher, B., et al. (2005). Treatment guidelines for children and adolescents with bipolar disorder. *Journal of the American Academy of Child and Adolescent Psychiatry*, **44**, 215–235.

Lanphear, B.P. (2012). Attention-deficit/hyperactivity disorder a preventable Epidemic? *JAMA Pediatrics*, **166**, 1182–1184.

Lillienfeld, S.O., Lynn, S.J., Kirsch, I., et al. (1999). Dissociative identity disorder and the sociocognitive model: recalling the lessons of the past. *Psychological Bulletin*, **125**, 507–523.

Liu, K.-Y., King, M., Bearman, P.S. (2010). Social influence and the autism epidemic. *AJS*, **115**, 1387–1434.

Lundström, S., Reichenberg, A., Anckarsäter, H., et al. (2015). Autism phenotype versus registered diagnosis in Swedish children: prevalence trends over 10 years in general population samples. *BMJ*, **350**, h1961.

McHugh, P.H. (1995). Witches, multiple personalities, and other psychiatric artifacts. *Nature Medicine*, **1**, 110–114.

Mendelson, J., Flower, K., Pletcher, M.J., and **Galloway, G.P.** (2008). Addiction to prescription opioids: Characteristics of the emerging epidemic and treatment with buprenorphine. *Experimental and Clinical Psychopharmacology*, **16**, 435–441.

Moreno, C., Laje, G., Blanco, C., et al. (2007). National trends in the outpatient diagnosis and treatment of bipolar disorder in youth. *Archives of General Psychiatry*, **64**, 1032–1039.

Neria, Y., DiGrande, L., and **Adams, B.G.** (2011). Posttraumatic stress disorder following the September 11, 2001, terrorist attacks: a review of the literature among highly exposed populations. *American Psychologist*, **66**, 429–446.

Newmark, S. (2015). A true ADHD epidemic or an epidemic of overdiagnosis? *PsychiatryAdvisor.com*, July 28. http://www.psychiatryadvisor.com/adhd/a-true-adhd-epidemic-or-an-epidemic-of-overdiagnosis/article/429034/

NIMH. (2001). National Institute of Mental Health research roundtable on prepubertal bipolar disorder. *Journal of the American Academy of Child and Adolescent Psychiatry*, **40**, 871–878.

Papolos, D. and **Papolos, J.** (2000). *The Bipolar Child: The definitive and reassuming guide to childhood's most misunderstood disorder.* New York: Random House.

Parry, P. and **Allison, S.** (2008). Pre-pubertal paediatric bipolar disorder: a controversy from America. *Australian Psychiatry*, **16**, 80–84.

Parry, P.J. and **Levin, E.C.** (2012). Pediatric bipolar disorder in an era of mindless psychiatry. *Journal of Trauma and Dissociation*, **15**, 51–68.

Pavuluri, M.N., Birmaher, B., and **Naylor, M.W.** (2005). Pediatric bipolar disorder: a review of the past 10 years. *Journal of the American Academy of Child and Adolescent Psychiatry*, **44**, 846–871.

Schreiber, F. (1973). *Sybil.* Washington, DC: Henry Regnery.

Shattuck, P.T. (2006). The contribution of diagnostic substitution to the growing administrative prevalence of autism in US special education. *Pediatrics*, **117**, 1028–1038.

Stolzer, J.M. (2007). The ADHD epidemic in America. *Ethical Human Psychology and Psychiatry*, **9**, 109–116.

Taylor, W.S. and **Martin, M.F.** (1944). Multiple personality. *Journal of Abnormal and Social Psychology*, **39**, 281–330.

Thigpen, C.H. and **Cleckley, H.M.** (1954). A case of multiple personality. *Journal of Abnormal and Social Psychology*, **9**, 135–151.

U.S. Department of Education (1996). *Eighteenth Annual Report to Congress on the Implementation of the Individuals with Disabilities Act.* Washington, DC: Department of Education.

Visser, S.N., **Danielson, M.L. Bitsko, R.H.**, et al. (2014). Trends in the parent-report of health care provider-diagnosed and medicated attention-deficit/hyperactivity disorder: United States, 2003–2011. *Journal of the American Academy of Child and Adolescent Psychiatry*, 53, 34–46.

Wakefield, J.C. and **First, M.B.** (2012). Placing symptoms in context: the role of contextual criteria in reducing false positives in Diagnostic and Statistical Manual of Mental Disorders diagnoses. *Comprehensive Psychiatry*, **53**, 130–139.

Wakefield, A.J. and **McCarthy, J.F.** (2010). *Callous Disregard: Autism and Vaccines—The truth behind a tragedy.* New York: Skyhouse Publishing.

Wing, L., **Yeates, S.R.**, **Brierley, L.M.**, and **Gould, J.** (1976). The prevalence of early childhood autism: comparison of administrative and epidemiological studies. *Psychological Medicine*, **6**, 89–100.

Wozniak, J., **Biederman, J.**, **Kiely, K.** et al. (1997). Mania-like symptoms suggestive of childhood-onset bipolar disorder in clinically referred children. *Journal of the American Academy of Child and Adolescent Psychiatry*, **34**, 867–876.

Chapter 18

Diagnostic epidemics and diagnostic disarray: The issue of differential diagnosis

Josef Parnas

Michael First's chapter concludes that the reported rises in prevalence of certain diagnostic categories such as dissociative identity disorder (DID), pediatric bipolar disorder (PBD), autism spectrum disorder (ASD), and attention deficit hyperactivity disorder (ADHD) cannot be considered, given the available evidence, as true epidemics. We simply lack proper systematic epidemiological studies. Moreover, First aptly points to the fact that a reported increase in a frequency of a diagnostic category may be due to multiple factors ranging from a true rise of incidence to changes in treatment seeking behavior, availability of treatment facilities, and mislabeling. This last issue I would like to elaborate in this comment.

Seen from a European perspective, and more specifically from the Danish psychiatric register information, we have observed dramatic increases in the diagnoses of borderline personality disorder (BPD) and ADHD especially in adulthood. The borderline diagnosis is quickly replacing schizophrenia as the most common diagnosis for first admissions to psychiatric hospitals. In a previous paper in the *Philosophical Issues in Psychiatry* series (Parnas 2012), I pointed to the fact that patients with what was once called hebephrenia but without grotesquely flamboyant features are systematically misdiagnosed as suffering from BPD. Hebephrenia has basically disappeared as a diagnosis for first-admission cases with schizophrenia. It is my common clinical experience, confirmed by our systematic empirical studies, that patients diagnosed elsewhere as suffering from BPD or ADHD in fact often fulfill the criteria for schizophrenia. It is also remarkable that clinicians and scientists find no conceptual dissonance between the concept of personality disorder and chronic psychotic features (Yee et al. 2005, Slotema et al. 2012). Clearly we are dealing here with instances of mislabeling.

This mislabeling can be attributed to the problems of differential diagnosis in the current criteria-based diagnostic systems. Essentially an explicit notion of differential diagnosis has disappeared from clinical parlance and from psychiatric education in Europe. One can perhaps even say that the notion of differential diagnosis has no meaning for diagnostic systems such as the fifth edition of the *Diagnostic and Statistical Manual of Mental Disorders* (DSM-5) and the tenth edition of the *International Classification of Diseases* (ICD-10). Why is it so? The concept of differential diagnosis implies a cognitive activity on the part of the clinician, who is weighing the available evidence, consisting of historical data, context, and the gestalt that the patient presents, with an eye to the actuarial factor.

However, the diagnostic categories in the operational systems are defined by a number of so-called criteria (which means simple, lay-language symptom descriptions), some exclusion and inclusion rules, and very weak or no hierarchical considerations. The symptoms, which overlap categories, have been basically removed; thus, for example, it is a novelty for some clinicians to learn that anxiety is often a part of early schizophrenia. The symptoms are viewed as isolated autonomous entities definable in themselves and independent of each other and the larger whole or gestalt of which they form a part. A patient who has a sufficient number of those criteria—usually reported on a very superficial level—then receives this particular diagnosis. What would the notion of differential diagnosis mean in such a context?

In the clinician–patient encounter, the doctor should in principle address all inclusion and exclusion criteria for all DSM and ICD disorders which is hardly feasible. Differential diagnosis in these systems is presented as a decision tree for a structured interview each one beginning with a specific situation (First 2014). There is no theory or conceptualization of the gestalt/prototype of the illness, which normally guides further exploration. Thus, for example a young man who is sitting in the waiting room in a lotus position mumbling to himself and occasionally laughing in a silly manner will be diagnosed as depressed if he answers yes to a sufficient number of depression questions but responds negatively to structured questions about persecution, hallucinations, or influence phenomena (Parnas 2015). There is no room to consider that he might be dissimulating and no suggestion of how to interview a dissimulating patient. In other words, he may not find the structured questions relevant to his own experiences (Norgaard et al. 2013). In the absence of prototypical considerations, all clinicians invariably acquire their own prototypes simply because prototypes are an intrinsic feature of human cognition. Because these prototypes are unsupervised and not subjected to rigorous academic discussion they are very often based on single prominent features, leading to what might be called "associative diagnosis." When the patient says "I am feeling down," then the diagnosis of depression dominates the cognitive field of the clinician; if the patient says that he cuts himself, a BPD diagnosis emerges. In this diagnostic approach, there is no room for evaluating and grasping the basic organization of the patient's mental life, e.g., whether the entire picture is proximate to a psychotic decompensation.

Another way of approaching diagnosis is to incorporate prototypical considerations where each larger diagnostic group—such as the schizophrenia spectrum, affective illnesses, or organic disorders—presents its characteristic gestalt or prototype (Parnas and Bovet 2015). Prototypical considerations do not preclude a detailed symptomatic description. On the contrary, a gestalt is dynamically interacting with its parts. In clinical terms, the overall picture confers a certain diagnostic value on the single symptoms whereas the single symptoms constitute the gestalt as a clinical reality. This is a common part–whole relation prevalent in biology and essential in understanding mental life. Thus in a comprehensive semi-structured phenomenological interview the interviewer is guided by such initial gestalts which become discarded, modified, or strengthened during the course of a conversation rather than an interrogation (Jansson and Nordgaard 2016).

Seen in the light of these considerations, I disagree with First that the DSM system as such only plays a minor role in the unusual fluctuations of diagnostic frequencies. As readers may know, the original idea behind the DSM-III was to retain prototypical narrative descriptions supplemented by lists of criteria. However, only the latter survived the publication process. There seems to be a consensus that we need to improve the qualitative and descriptive aspects of psychopathology. This is a prerequisite for any successful phenotype-substrate correlation. I think that in this context phenomenology is highly needed (see Parnas and Parnas, this volume, Chapter 26).

References

First, M. (2014). *Handbook of Differential Diagnosis.* Arlington, VA: American Psychiatric Publishing.

Jansson, L. and **Nordgaard, J.** (2016). *The Psychiatric Interview for Differential Diagnosis.* New York: Springer.

Nordgaard, J., Sass, L.A., and **Parnas, J.** (2013). The psychiatric interview: validity, structure, and subjectivity, *European Archives of Psychiatry and Clinical Neuroscience*, **263**, 353–64.

Parnas, J. (2012). DSM-IV and the founding prototype of schizophrenia: are we regressing to a pre-Kraepelinian nosology? In K.S. Kendler and J. Parnas (eds.) *Philosophical Issues in Psychiatry II*, pp. 237–60. Oxford, UK: Oxford University Press,.

Parnas, J. (2015). Differential diagnosis and current polythetic classification. *World Psychiatry*, **14**, 284–87.

Parnas, J. and **Bovet, P.** (2015). Psychiatry made easy: operation(a)lism and some of its consequences. In K.S. Kendler and J. Parnas (eds.) *Philosophical Issues in Psychiatry III*, pp. 190–213. Oxford, UK: Oxford University Press.

Slotema, C.W., Daalman, K., Blom, J.D., et al. (2012). Auditory verbal hallucinations in patients with borderline personality disorder are similar to those in schizophrenia, *Psychological Medicine*, **42**, 1873–1878.

Yee, L., Korner, AJ., Meares, RA., and **Stevenson, J.** (2005). Persistent hallucinosis in borderline personality disorder. *Comprehensive Psychiatry*, **46**, 147–154.

Section 7

Culture-bound psychiatric syndromes

Chapter 19

Introduction to "Description and explanation of the culture-bound syndromes"

Kenneth S. Kendler

Dominic Murphy, who has long been an active contributor as a philosopher to issues psychiatric, tackles a central issue in our understanding of psychiatric illness that is the subject of little current active research. Indeed, its importance and its current near absence from leading psychiatric journals is itself worth a careful look, but that will have to be at another time. Simply put, the question is the degree to which cultural and social factors shape the nature of human psychopathology. I grew up in psychiatry among the first generation of biological psychiatrists in the early 1980s. If anyone bothered to raise such an issue then, the response would have been, "Of course psychiatric disorders are the same across cultures. These are neurobiological syndromes, after all." Studies sponsored by the World Health Organization (WHO) found rather similar clinical pictures for schizophrenia (World Health Organization 1973) and depression across cultures (Sartorius et al. 1983), and the incidence of schizophrenia was also fairly similar across a diverse series of international sites (Jablensky et al. 1992)—so end of story.

Now, even these hard-core reductionists would likely accept a cultural impact on the content of symptoms. I recall my early experiences with schizophrenia patients in the west of Ireland. I was confronted with a range of delusional beliefs—especially involving a variety of Catholic saints, none of whom I had ever heard of—which was distinctly different from the content I was used to seeing in my prior training. But how could it be otherwise? Anyone with eyes open would see such changes over historical time. I recall speaking with an older psychiatrist who was practicing when the first Russian satellite was launched and spoke of the profusion of "sputnik delusions" in his patients. When I first started practicing, I would never see a patient with the belief that a hard drive had been installed in their brain. In the years since, this has not been an uncommon delusional theme. The first influencing machine in the world's literature, described by Haslam in 1810 (Haslam 2013), was a loom. Now they are all computers.

But this does not get to the deeper root issue that Murphy tackles. Are there psychiatric syndromes which are—*tout court*—"culture bound" and only manifest in a particular cultural context? Or, are there a limited number of ways in which our human mind–brain system can dysfunction (not counting the "hardware" damage seen in neurological conditions) and is the nature of that dysfunction shaped by our cultural experiences? I have long been attracted to the conceptual approach to this broad issue proposed by Karl Birnbaum in a well-known article published in 1923. It is worth quoting:

> The essential clinical phenomena which occur in any illness are, first, those which refer to the actual cause of the illness, and which endow it with a specific character, its quality of being "thus and no other"; secondly, those which may be said to shape the disorder in that they give content, coloring, and contour of the individual illnesses whose basic form and character have already been biologically established. The former group of phenomena I would *call pathogenic,* and the latter *pathoplastic.* (Birnbaum 1974, p. 203)

Defined in this way, "pathoplastic" would refer to a range of factors from biographical to community, and broader social and cultural forces. I favor Birnbaum's theory but it is devilishly difficult to find a way to empirically answer the question of whether two syndromes from distinct cultures are "pathogenically" the same but "pathoplastically" different, versus different "all the way down." One method might be on the horizon. Using genome-wide genetic markers and one of several aggregating statistical methods, we can now calculate the genome-wide genetic correlation between two different syndromes. If we had a collection of cases of controls for disorder 1 in culture 1 and disorder 2 in culture 2, we could potentially figure out if they arise from closely related genetic variants. (One nasty fact that would interfere with this plan is that we would have to correct for genetic differences across the sample which, if they arise from quite different ethnic groups, could prove difficult.) But such a method would be a big advance.

I also want to advocate for another quantitative approach that is a small part of the broad problems that Murphy is struggling with in this paper—a psychometric approach to cross-cultural differences in psychiatric syndromes. This approach addresses the following question: Do diagnostic criteria for a given disorder behave in the same way across cultural groups? (While not my main interest here, a part of this is the problem of translation of DSM criteria across languages—in this case across major language groups—which is itself an issue of no small import that I will not treat here.) We have for some years been conducting a large-scale study of major depression in Chinese women (Flint et al. 2012) and often got the following criticism, largely based on the widely read work by Kleinman (1982):

> How do you know that the depression you are studying in China has anything to do with the depression that we see and treat in the US or Western Europe?

Using fairly standard psychometric techniques (e.g., confirmatory factor analysis) we can ask whether the structures of intercorrelations in the DSM criteria for major depression are similar between our sample of Chinese women and parallel samples in Western countries (North American and Western Europe) versus among the Western samples themselves (Kendler et al. 2015). This is a smaller question than the deeper one we might want to answer, but it has the important advantage that it is one we can actually answer. The empirical results were quite clear: The degree of resemblance was so great they were essentially the same. That is, for all intents and purposes, the DSM criteria in our Chinese sample are performing similarly to how they behave in parallel Western samples. So perhaps the prospects for an empirical synthesis between psychiatry and social and cultural theory are not quite as dark as Murphy concludes.

The issues addressed in the essay are so interesting in part because they illustrate the degree to which psychiatry really sits at the crossroads of the biological and human sciences. How is the dysfunction of the human mind–brain system influenced by neurobiology on the one hand and culture on the other? What could be a more intriguing question?

References

Birnbaum, K. (1974). The making of a psychosis: the principles of structural analysis in psychiatry. In S.R. Hirsch and M. Shepherd (eds.) *Themes and Variations in European Psychiatry: An anthology*, pp. 199–238. Charlottesville, VA: University of Virginia Press.

Flint, J., Chen, Y., Shi, S., and **Kendler, K.S.** (2012). Epilogue: Lessons from the CONVERGE study of major depressive disorder in China. *Journal of Affective Disorders*, **140**, 1–5.

Haslam, J. (2013). *Illustrations of Madness (Psychology Revivals)*. London: Routledge.

Jablensky, A., Sartorius, N., Ernberg, G., et al. (1992). Schizophrenia: manifestations, incidence and course in different cultures. A World Health Organization ten-country study. *Psychological Medicine Monograph Supplement*, **20**, 1–97.

Kendler, K.S., Aggen, S.H., Li, Y., et al. (2015). The similarity of the structure of DSM-IV criteria for major depression in depressed women from China, the United States and Europe. *Psychological Medicine*, **45**, 1945–1954.

Kleinman, A. (1982). Neurasthenia and depression: a study of somatization and culture in China. *Culture, Medicine and Psychiatry*, **6**, 117–190.

Sartorius, N., Davidian, H., Ernberg, G., et al. (1983). *Depressive Disorders in Different Cultures: Report on the WHO collaborative study on standardized assessment of depressive disorders*. Geneva: World Health Organization.

World Health Organization (1973). *Report of the International Pilot Study of Schizophrenia. Volume 1: Results of the initial evaluation phase*. Geneva: World Health Organization.

Chapter 20

Description and explanation of the culture-bound syndromes

Dominic Murphy

20.1 Introduction

Throughout the sciences of the mind our established findings and models rest on research into what Henrich et al. (2010) call WEIRD (Western, educated, industrial, rich, democratic) subjects. Theorists are beginning to worry about the possible shortcomings of this body of evidence. Within psychiatry, it has long been acknowledged that considerable variation across cultures in the presentation of mental illness is the order of the day, to the extent that whether or not we can even talk about the same diagnosis occurring in different cultures is itself a contested matter. Given the extent of this cultural variation, the concern is that we are mistaken in resting our theories on a small and unrepresentative sample of humanity.

The understanding of this cultural variation is a pressing matter for psychiatry, and will become more important as Western psychiatric training takes hold in more and more countries, and as psychiatrists in Western societies learn to deal with more and more diverse populations. There is a broader issue at stake too: psychiatry is a field which has generated a body of theoretical literature on the integration of explanatory models and descriptions of behavior and experience. It is an ideal science in which to develop theories that could then be exported to the wider scientific communities. There is an increasing wealth of comparative and anthropological studies that seem to offer a rich body of evidence that can tell us more about how the mind works across cultures and enable us to test existing hypotheses with a view to expanding the range of cultural variation that the human sciences may cover. Anthropologists have for a long time documented numerous variations in cultural practice but these descriptive projects have often failed to make contact with the explanatory projects of the cognitive and brain sciences (some of the exceptions will be noted later in this chapter). Psychiatry sits at the intersection of neurological and cultural forces, and offers a testing ground for synthetic models that implement theories about the relations between them. The upshot of this theory-building and theory-testing could be used to both increase our understanding and treatment of mental illness and to enhance our broader understanding of the mind. Ultimately, one would hope that the integration of descriptive and explanatory projects across the cognitive and anthropological sciences might help address normative puzzles, as we aim to decide whether cultural practices that strike Western communities as deviant should be copied, suppressed, or tolerated.

This paper aims to lay the groundwork for a philosophical understanding of cultural variation in psychiatry by setting out some of the main conceptual questions and revealing some of the terrain. It has two main themes: first, I will investigate the recent history of psychiatry since the introduction of culture-bound syndromes (CBS) in the fourth edition of the *Diagnostic and Statistical Manual of Mental Disorders* (DSM-IV; American Psychiatric Association 1994) and the move away from them in the fifth edition (DSM-5; American Psychiatric Association 2013). CBS are patterns of behavior, cognition, and emotion that are generally limited to, and bound up with, specific societies or sociocultural areas, but are regarded as forms of mental illness rather than merely cultural differences. As instances of "deviant deviance" (Hughes 1985, p. 3), CBS enable us to tackle important questions in the philosophy of psychiatry, concerning explanation, causation, and classification. As well as CBS, psychiatry also explains some conditions as instances of standard DSM diagnoses, which are universal but take different forms in different cultures. I will discuss these two strategies, which I call particularizing and unversalizing mental disorders

Second: I will look at what it means for a syndrome to be bound up with a particular culture. Some authors have proposed to expand the concept of CBS to include (controversial) behavioral syndromes described by Western psychiatry, such as multiple personality disorder (Hacking 1995), anorexia nervosa (Lee 1996), and attention-deficit disorder (Lakoff 2000). Such Western syndromes are often conceptualized as social constructions. Are non-Western CBS social constructions too? The issues here concern the viability of social constructionist models in cases where the individual minds that are altered by social forces are presumed to work in untypical ways. I will end by asking whether CBS and other culturally distant pathological behavior can be described in ways that do not beg any theoretical questions.

20.2 **Universalism and particularism**

CBS entered official Western psychiatric classification in 1994 in DSM-IV. An appendix to DSM-IV provides a working definition of CBS and a glossary of 25 examples (American Psychiatric Association 1994, pp. 897–903). The glossary was recommended by an independent group of medical anthropologists and cross-cultural psychiatrists as a way to increase the overall cultural validity and sensitivity of DSM-IV.

DSM-IV (p. xxiv) introduced the notion of CBS to express the idea that some cultures exhibited distinct forms of mental illness, but it was especially concerned with conditions that Western psychiatrists might see at home, typically among immigrants. This reflects a sensitivity to cross-cultural differences in psychopathology that was growing at the time as medical anthropology made headway in psychiatry.

DSM-5 has heavily qualified the concept of CBS. It has reformed psychiatry's approach to what it now calls cultural formulation. DSM-5 has moved to a model of "cultural concepts of distress" (p. 758) which are ways that "cultural groups experience, understand and communicate suffering, behavioral problems or troublesome thoughts and emotions." DSM-5 supplements its conceptual reform with a thorough overhaul of the "Outline for Cultural Formulation" that was introduced in DSM-IV-TR, in part in response to pleas from cross-cultural psychiatrists dissatisfied with the old ways (e.g., Canino and Alegria 2008). It reflects an unprecedented investment in applying anthropology to psychiatry by the DSM-5 Cultural Issues Subgroup, who ran field trials of the new Cultural Formulation Interview (CFI) in six sites around the world (Aggarwal 2013). The CFI calls for systematically assessing the cultural or ethnic groups to which subjects belong, and the ways in which they understand their problem and experience it.

Despite the rhetoric, it is unclear how the new appreciation for culture in psychopathology can influence the field. The treatment of these issues remains cursory (less than 20 pages out of 900) and poorly integrated with the diagnostic criteria in the main body of the manual. And if one thinks of one's own culture as just the way things are, or ought to be, then one will continue to see cultural influences as interesting only if they are non-Western.

DSM-5 follows its predecessor in coping with cross-cultural variety in two ways. It sees it as either a local version of a universal diagnosis whose paradigm is the description of that diagnosis in DSM-5, or as a culturally specific, not Western, local condition. The first, universalizing, strategy involves taking a condition such as depression or anxiety, and treating it as universal—found in every culture, despite local differences in character. The problem with this view is apparent when we ask how much variation is permissible before we must speak of a new condition, and whether some types of variation count more than others. For example, Arthur Kleinman (1988) argued that depression takes different forms around the world:

> Depression experienced entirely as low back pain and depression experienced entirely as guilt-ridden existential despair are such substantially different forms of illness behavior with different symptoms, patterns of help-seeking, course and treatment responses that though the disease in each instance may be the same, the illness rather than the disease is the determinant factor.

The Chinese experience and the experience of depression in the West are so different, Kleinman argued, that Chinese and American subjects might as well have different diagnoses. Kleinman stresses differences in experience amounting to a different disease. On the other hand, Kitanaka (2011) argues that biomedical psychiatry has transformed the Japanese understanding of depression, to see it not as a rare and very serious condition but as a complex of alienation and exhaustion tied to overwork and social pressure. An interesting point about Japan is that depression, being conceptually tied to middle-class overwork, is gendered as male, whereas in the West women are twice as likely to be diagnosed with depression (Kitanaka 2011, p. 17). Despite her stress on social causes and social meaning, Kitanaka does not argue that depression in Japan is a different condition to that in the West.

Another example is *wacinko*. It is found only among the Oglala Sioux in the northwestern United States. *Wacinko* is a state of withdrawn, mute anger, directed at someone else, which may last for years. The Oglala live in the United States, but their culture is not shared with most Americans, and neither is *wacinko. Wacinko* is often a reaction to disappointment or interpersonal problems. Some Lakota writers see it as a form of strategic behavior, aimed at manipulating another person's will. But because in extreme cases some subjects may commit suicide, this condition has been seen by Western-trained psychiatrists as a form of reactive depression (Lewis 1975)

These are examples of depression, or depression-like, conditions. They illustrate some of the questions to be answered if one adopts the unificationist route and sees different diagnoses as manifestations of the same underlying condition. What are the important features of the condition, such that it can be identified in individuals across cultures? How much difference, and what sorts of difference, should persuade us that we have distinct conditions rather than variations of the same one?

The same questions can be asked about differences within a culture, of course, since psychiatric disorders vary notoriously across sufferers. They also arise in comparing the past with the present—it has been argued that the forerunners of today's anorectics can be found among the self-harming female saints of the middle ages (Bell 1985) or the "fasting girls" of the nineteenth century (Brumberg 1988, Busby 2003).

So, how different do we allow two conditions to be before we stop considering them as manifestations of a single DSM category? DSM-IV holds that conditions the world over conform to its diagnoses, but is silent on what that amounts to. One possibility is to change the DSM diagnosis somewhat. It has been suggested that anxiety disorders, for example, should have their "worry domains" expanded because people from other cultures may worry about things that Euro-Americans do not seem to get exercised about (Lewis-Fernández et al. 2009). The assumption here is that anxiety disorders are common enough in all human cultures to merit treating as a universal, but that this can be missed if clinicians do not appreciate the different triggers, reactions, and conceptions that distinguish the anxiety disorders in different populations. Lewis-Fernández and his team (2010) argue that a majority of Latino sufferers from *ataque de nervios* would meet panic disorder criteria, for example, if the DSM amended the requirement that a panic attack lasts only a few minutes. *Ataque de nervios* was listed as a CBS in DSM-IV-TR. Its symptoms commonly include a mix of classic panic attack symptoms such as palpitations and sensations of bodily heat and loss of control, but it may involve uncontrollable shouting and threats of violence, together with other symptoms less often found in panic attacks. Lewis-Fernández is a lumper; he is at least open to the idea that *ataque de nervios* can be assimilated to existing anxiety diagnoses provided we take the variation in symptomatology more seriously. We need to recognize the greater variety of symptoms among sufferers from anxiety who live in Western cultures but do not show the typical symptoms of a Westerner.

On this view, it is not the DSM diagnosis that should be universalized, but a broader category of which the DSM privileges one instance. One way to make this case would be to prescind from symptoms and think in terms of common mechanisms. Horwitz and Wakefield (2007, p. 199) for example

> agree with Kleinman's distinction between disease as a universal underlying dysfunction and illness as the culturally shaped expression of a given dysfunction . . . [but] if there are indeed underlying common dysfunctions, then treatment presumably depends in large part on the science of identifying and intervening in such dysfunctions irrespective of their cultural presentation.

This is in part a point about labeling, since on this view the name of the diagnostic category refers to the underlying dysfunction (the "disease") rather than its manifestations (the "illness"). The larger point, for our purposes, is that idea that unity in diversity is established by identifying what it is that has gone wrong in the mind/brain. We assume that is shared across cultures, but the inputs that trigger the dysfunctional mechanism, as well as the outputs that it then produces, will be culturally labile.

The second tactic used by American psychiatry to deal with the problem of cultural diversity has been the concept of "culture-bound syndromes." Many CBS have been recognized by psychiatrists. DSM-IV-TR defined CBS as "recurrent, locality-specific patterns of aberrant behavior and troubling experience that may or may not be linked to a particular DSM-IV diagnostic category" (p. 898). The distinction between different manifestations of a diagnosis and a CBS is drawn clearly:

> Although presentations conforming to the major DSM-IV categories can be found throughout the world, the particular symptoms, course, and social response are very often influenced by local cultural factors. In contrast, culture-bound syndromes are generally limited to specific societies or culture areas and are localized, folk, diagnostic categories that frame coherent meanings for certain repetitive, patterned, and troubling sets of experiences and observations.

DSM-IV-TR treats *ataque de nervios* as a CBS and not a form of panic disorder on the grounds that it is often associated with a precipitating event. This distinguishes it from panic disorder, in which the attacks are *unexpected* surges of fear of discomfort with no clear precipitator (DSM-5, p. 209). Phobias are also marked by episodes of fear, but in phobias there are reliable links between the attacks and a specific kind of stimulus. This specific relationship is absent in *ataque. Ataque de nervios* does not conform to the diagnostic exemplar closely enough to count as panic disorder as is stands, and DSM-5 did not adopt the amendments to the panic disorder criteria that Lewis-Fernández advocated.

The assumption in mainstream psychiatry is that Western conditions are not culture-bound; they represent abnormalities in a universal human endowment. DSM-5 (pp. 243–244) for instance, treats muscle dysmorphia as a regular diagnosis, not a CBS. This is despite prevalence data for the wider condition of body dysmorphic disorder being noted only for Germany and the United States, and the characteristic behaviors being weightlifting and steroid use, which largely exist in specific Western contexts. Avoidant/restrictive food intake disorder is noted as occurring in the United States, Canada, Australia, and Europe (DSM-5, p. 336). Although these countries are not identical to each other, one would expect a wider range of cultures before it can be seen as universal. The point is that DSM-5 has main text for diagnoses that occur in the West and a special appendix for the rest of the world. It is hard not to see this as the expression of a view that Western minds are the norm. In this picture, CBS can come to be seen not as distinctive local forms of illness or distress, but as different expressions of the same underlying abnormality that Western subjects exhibit. There should be dysmorphia everywhere, but it will not always look American. It will, however, be the expression of a condition that is best understood by modeling the minds of people from NATO countries and then treating other populations as deviant. The changes introduced in DSM-5 represent some improvements over the DSM-IV treatment of CBS, but the basic problematic assumption that Western minds are the default model is still there.

Despite some hopeful signs in DSM-5, then, I do not think it has moved away from the traditional picture in psychiatry with its two approaches: the idea that cultural variation is either the distinctive cultural shaping of a universal condition or the idea that that CBS are peculiar local forms of distress with no claims to generality.

That is, the understanding of (e.g.) depression that derives from Western psychiatry is seen as the basic case, and other conditions are viewed as falling under the relevant diagnosis depending on how far they resemble the Western condition. Other conditions are local matters of no real psychiatric import, for they do not make us rethink our categories. Of course, nothing I have said so far means any of this is wrong, so now let me draw some morals via a discussion of the wider issues.

I have mentioned two ways that psychiatry deals with cultural variation: assimilation to the Western norm, or marginalization as CBS. It is interesting that these occur together, because they can be seen as defining two opposite strategies: one insists on the psychic unity of human kind, despite local noise, and the other argues that there is no sense in which psychology is shared cross-culturally. The latter strategy sees every CBS as a distinctive mental kind that cannot be understood other than in context, and cannot be assimilated to a wider condition.

Conditions like these raise the question of line-drawing in an interesting way. If these three objections are valid, i.e., if CBS and DSM disorders cannot be conceptualized as fully distinctive sets or kinds of disorders, how then are we to think of their relationship?

Four options remain:

- CBS are not disorders and only DSM disorders exist.
- CBS are disorders but they can be incorporated in DSM disorder categories or other universal categories (the universalist position).
- All mental disorders, including DSM disorders, are to be considered as CBS (the particularist position).
- The current DSM position is correct and there exist both universal DSM categories and particular CBS (though the DSM is unwilling to countenance the possibility that some of its own diagnoses may be CBS).

What it would it take to successfully defend any of these options? Empirical findings alone cannot tell us—or, more accurately, to answer the question psychiatry relies on empirical findings that need to be embedded in broader models derived from the human sciences. To see why, let's start with a claim that underpins the universalist position.

DSM-IV claimed a limited universalism, in that sense that it acknowledged the existence of CBS but also insisted that "presentations conforming to the major DSM-IV categories can be found throughout the world" (American Psychiatric Association 1994, p. 898). It is unclear what it takes for a "presentation" to "conform" to a DSM category: the natural reading is that conformity is a matter of displaying the signs and symptoms that make up the criteria for a diagnosis. But signs and symptoms always stand in need of interpretation. We need to know what makes two pieces of behavior, in different cultures, the same symptom or a different one. Even simple measures of bodily activity depend for their meaning on context—a racing pulse might indicate a panic attack, or it might mean you have just won the lottery. So here is one sort of context—signs and symptoms cannot be identified in isolation but only as categories in systems of classification. In the West, folk psychology and other culturally familiar ways of carving up human nature serve as systems of classification. They supply the concepts for many of the descriptive criteria found in DSM. Although they are certainly supplemented by technical concepts, and often operationalized in ways that are loosely attached to common sense, our familiar pictures of human nature are at the bottom of our psychiatric categories. Suppose these pictures are themselves culturally specific? If they are, we may miss the significance of a piece of behavior that does not fit into our way of thinking, but nonetheless expresses the same underlying condition.

Further, some conditions may well be found throughout the world even though they are not considered as disorders. Hearing the voices of the spirits of the dead is listed as one of the symptoms of a mental disorder, i.e., complicated bereavement, in DSM-IV, while it is a common experience in the mourning processes and rituals of some non-Western societies (Bentall 2003). So are we wrong or are they? The obvious answer, as well as the politest one, is that neither we nor they are wrong, because how a person deals with bereavement depends on their culture, and whether you have a interaction with your culture that strikes your peers as normal or abnormal might have something to do with whether your psychology is working as it should.

Adjudicating between the four options mentioned above requires a social theory that lets us state observations about human behavior in ways that are independent of particular psychiatric claims. This is not the only place where psychiatry could do with a theory that it currently lacks, but we do have some models in social theory, and in the second part of the paper I want to look in more detail at CBS, and discuss some of the epistemic problems they raise. Just as the idea of conforming to a DSM diagnosis is obscure, so too is the notion of something's being culture-bound, so in the next section I focus on this issue as a way of illustrating some of the complications that might be involved in connecting psychiatry and social theory.

20.3 Culture-bound syndromes: some epistemic problems

In theory, CBS are those folk illnesses in which alterations of behavior and experience figure prominently, relative to local norms. CBS are conceived of as limited: they exist among specific societies. Standard psychiatric diagnoses are not thought of in this way, even if they are culturally limited. Multiple personality disorder/ dissociative identity disorder (DID), for example, was widely diagnosed in the United States in the 1980s, but seldom found elsewhere. That does not lead psychiatrists to treat it as a CBS, even though it seems to fit the definition. (In fact DSM-5 has introduced the "possession form" of DID, to include experiences of possession as well as those of internal takeover of the personality by an alter.) In such cases, skepticism is likely to focus on the idea that there is a genuine condition here at all, but CBS are not seen as unreal or artifactual, just not standard.

The term "culture-bound" carries at least two different meanings. One is that of being limited to a part of the world, usually the area occupied by a particular ethnicity or culturally distinct society—what Cawte (1974, p. 107) calls "culture-specific." Some CBS are indeed endemic to specific societies or sociocultural areas, even though many are not. Secondly, the boundedness of CBS can also be interpreted as their being culture-reactive, i.e., bound up within a particular culture. In this sense, CBS are intimately connected with, and modulated by, the culture they emerge from. Both transcultural psychiatry and medical anthropology thrive on exactly this assumption, i.e., that culture matters in psychopathology (see, e.g., López and Guarnaccia 2000). The obvious complication is that all mental illness—indeed, all human behavior—is modulated by culture in this way. This is what opens the door for those who think that all mental disorders are culture-bound. Gold and Gold (2014) have discussed the emergence of what they consider to be a new form of psychopathology—the "Truman Show delusion" in which subjects imagine themselves to be the protagonist of a reality TV show (like the hero of the movie after which the disorder was named). The existence of the show is known to the people around the subject, who are leagued in a conspiracy about it. Gold and Gold (p. 213) argue that the cultural space for this condition has been opened up by the rise of new forms of media and an attendant loss of privacy.

The Truman Show delusion might seem to be a candidate CBS, but at the same time it illustrates the difficulties attending the notion of "culture-bound"; the initial subjects were New Yorkers, but reality TV has befouled the airwaves all over the world. If, as the Golds think, the condition is due to interactions between new cultural forms and existing aspects of human psychology, then it seems as though it might be a candidate universal—a form of paranoia.

So, it seems as though the two meanings of culture-bound I mentioned above are in conflict, since something can be modulated by culture in a way that is specific to a location, yet in principle able to spread across the world if the modulation taps into universal mechanisms. Only British people could have been driven to madness by soccer in the 1860s, but now it could happen anywhere.

It would be helpful to have some more precise questions to ask if we are to understand what it means to be bound by a culture. First, what exactly does it mean for a culture to bind a particular syndrome or set of symptoms? Second, at which level(s) of explanation do we explain the binding? There are diverse possibilties: aetiology, epidemiology, neurophysiology, diagnosis, therapy, symptom-formation, and so forth.

A move that appeals to a lot of scholars is to redefine "being (culturally) bound" as "being (socially) constructed." This is especially appealing in cases like *malgri* (Cawte 1974), from the Wellesley Islands in the Gulf of Carpentaria (northern Australia), in which symptoms seem bound up with local beliefs in a very direct way. *Malgri* chiefly involves abdominal pain and distension, perhaps accompanied by leg or head pain; it is explained locally as due to entering the sea after eating terrestrial food without first washing one's hands in fresh water, or eating food from the sea and going ashore without washing in salt water. Washing prevents the local totemic spirit from entering your body, but that will only happen if you stray outside the territorial range associated with your group (p. 110) and enter a zone where the local spirit does not know you. The degree of specific cultural impingement in *malgri* seems a lot deeper than the degree involved with the Truman Show delusion—almost any society could be influenced by reality TV, but the necessary contingencies for *malgri* are bound up with a way of life and a religious practice. The syndrome also seems functional, since observation of the totemic rules peacefully perpetuates territorial borders. In a case like this, the load-bearing parts of the explanation seem to cry out for anthropology or social theory rather than psychology or psychiatry—it looks a lot more like a ritual than a disease.

But to legitimize the redefinition we would have to show that "being culture-bound" and "being socially constructed" refer to the same phenomena. Now, there do exist striking similarities between some non-Western CBS and mental illnesses that have been seen as Western social constructions. The hysterical fugues of late nineteenth-century France (Hacking 1998), for example, are remarkably similar to epidemics of *grisi siknis*—a CBS found among the Miskito people in Nicaragua and Honduras (Dennis 1981: I owe this example to Pieter Adriaens). Of course, however, one can argue that there are also fundamental similarities across syndromes in both cultures: they can be considered as transient mental illnesses, in Hacking's sense of existing only at a certain time and place (Hacking 1999).

Thinking of CBS as social constructions brings in a wide variety of concepts, arguments and theories that are actively being debated in philosophy, providing us with a template of asking and unravelling difficult questions (Hacking 1999, Mallon 2007, Haslanger 2012). However, we also want to know how cultural forces might act on the mind. Henrich et al. (2010) survey a number of experimental results that suggest that people of European descent are not representative of human beings generally. This does not just include performance on high-level cognitive tasks. It also involves systematic differences at lower levels. The Muller–Lyer illusion, for example, is not an illusion at all as far as the San foragers of the Kalahari are concerned.

Results like this are significant for psychiatry because they suggest that cultural differences can run very deep within our psychology. Some experimental differences in cross-cultural cognitive psychology, such as those detected by Richard Nisbet (2003) between people of European and East Asian descent, implicate high-level processing systems. The Muller–Lyer results may show the effects of culture on very low-level visual processing. The mechanism that the original experimenters (Segall et al. 1966) suggested to explain the results is that the visual system in Western subjects adapts early in life to an environment full of "carpentered corners." People from Western countries grow up in a world of right angles and this biases their visual system to make specific inferences about distance from the edges and contours in the visual field. But this early environment is not the norm in human history, so it may be that WEIRD people are the exception to the human rule. Conversely, Segall et al.'s results suggest that children experience the Muller–Lyer illusion more than their elders, including African children. That may suggest that Africans grow up among buildings with rounded edges, to which they adapt. Perhaps Africans are exceptions to the normal pattern of development in which the visual system is set up to expect a world of edges (edge detection is a very important part of early vision and visual development). Or perhaps there is no default system and nobody is an exception, and the visual system is just highly malleable. We do not know, though the issue seems amenable to empirical proof. The point is that we have no grounds for thinking either that very early, low-level processes are exempt from culture, nor that Westerners have minds that are the human norm. Even basic aspects of the mind can be cross-culturally distinguished. Geurts (2003) argues that the senses are culturally constructed: so that her subjects, the Anlo-Ewe in Ghana, have a different folk model of the sensorium, which privileges balance and reception of sound as the most important senses, rather than sight as in the Western "five-sense" model. She argues that this has significant implications for moral development and conceptions of health and disease. But, in fact, the idea that there are more than five senses has been recently canvassed among Western philosophers, and actually enumerating the senses turns out to be very difficult; the debate kicked off by Keeley (2002) turns out to be hard to resolve, especially once we widen its focus to include non-human animals. Is your sense of balance a distinct, sixth sense? Keeley proposed a materialist program that individuates senses in terms of specific organs linked to the physical transduction of energy. This is very different from an approach like that of Geurts, which essentially says the senses are whatever the local culture takes them to be. This tension between the scientific approach and local ways of knowing gets to the heart of the issues under discussion, for the natural way of following a universalist program is to look for, and privilege, the neuropsychology of a presumed universal diagnosis. The skeptical response is that even basic neuropsychology can be shaped by culture.

Putting things as I have done in this section leads to natural synthesis: CBS should be seen as representing the effects of specific cultural traditions and contexts on mental machinery that may itself be built differently in different places. Here the obvious mechanism to appeal to is that of a mental representation, understood as a physical phenomenon realized in brain tissue that represents social properties and also causes behavior. This lets us consider material mechanisms for the transmission of cultural forces (Sperber 1996) and also opens the possibility of integrating syndromes (collections of symptoms) with underlying brain systems (where the representations are realized). A synthesis of these two approaches lets us see social construction as the effect of culturally transmitted symbols on brain systems, where the mental machinery houses the representations that enable behavior, and CBS are constituted by the output of that representational structure in that context. It is a natural extension of this line of thought to suppose that all mental illnesses, including those in the main body of the DSM, are really CBS. It would equally apply to the universalizing strategy as to the particularizing one, since universal conditions would reflect a greater degree of sharing -either of minds or of culture (or both) and purer CBS would reflect a lesser degree.

The strategy is widely applicable because the basic structure of the synthesis—culture embodied in representation leading to behavior—applies to almost every behavior ever enacted by anyone. Now, the fact that it is so widely applicable might seem to show that the synthesis is too crude, and maybe too trite, but the details can be worked out in productive and interesting ways, and the commitment to variation in cognitive structures around the world is a substantial empirical bet. The problem with the synthesis is not that it is too trite. The problem is that it makes everyone come out looking normal. That is, we are treating candidate mental illnesses as if they can be explained by the same dynamics that we would use to describe non-pathological social roles.

This pretty obviously begs the question, since in treating CBS like any socially constructed phenomena we are taking sides with those who do not see them as pathologies at all. If psychopathology is explicable by the same dynamic as socially constructed phenomena in general it is not a problem, perhaps, but they might not be so explicable. Here is an analogy. Suppose you are an adaptationist who thinks that everything in biology should be approached in the light of evolution via natural selection. Whatever the merits of this as a general attitude, it would lead you astray if you asked about the adaptive function of every form of illness or disease, since the theory is, very crudely, designed to explain the normal range of function. People get sick for reasons unrelated to natural selection. Though it may be that some phenomena, like morning sickness or menopause, are adaptive despite being seen as pathologies, it is not generally true that forms of illness should be explained as adaptive phenomena; blocked arteries have no adaptive function, even if arteries do.

Similarly, a theory designed to explain socially constructed phenomena as the interplay of representational and cultural structures will go badly wrong if CBS are in fact mental illnesses that have quite another cause. For example, nobody would call obedience to food taboos or religious dietary regulations a form of psychopathology. They are clearly cultural forms transmitted over time, and potentially explicable using the blend of social theory and cognitive theory I gestured at just now. Suppose we use those same intellectual tools to explain *malgri* as a form of social control based around foodways. This might provide a satisfactory explanation but it is pretty obviously question-begging, because it leaves no room for any explanation that uses clinical psychiatric concepts. The concern is that explanations which appeal to cultural transmission assume a normal mind, which rules out psychiatric explanations in advance. We could explain the reproduction of psychotic symptoms across generations in the West as instances of cultural transmission, given that subjects may very well acquire from the wider culture some hints as to what stereotypical psychotic symptoms look like. On the other hand, we should resist the idea that, once we have appealed to the mechanisms of social construction and cultural transmission, there is nothing left to explain. Existing models of social construction need to be supplemented by explanations that appeal to neuropsychological abnormalities.

Explaining CBS as social constructions, then, biases inquiry against seeing them as mental disorders. But the behavioral items comprising the syndromes only make sense against a background of interpretation supplied by local norms. This raises the problem of how we are to describe their constituent signs and symptoms in the first place: the difficulty of seeing whether a pattern of behavior is pathological or not is sharpened when the behavior is displayed in a culture that is not one's own. In a familiar culture certain behaviors might strike an observer as plainly aberrant and in need of psychiatric explanation. But that perspective is not open to somebody observing another culture. I noted above that symptoms, like other items of behavior, need interpretation. Even to count a piece of behavior as a symptom it needs to be brought under a concept—a state of mind classed as deluded or anxious, or a bodily movement seen as compulsive rather than informed by ritual.

Treating CBS as social constructions transmitted across the generations via standard mechanisms or learning and imitation sidesteps this issue—it represents behaviors as falling under conceptual structures that make sense relative to an interpretation supplied by the local context. But, as noted, it does so at the cost of adopting models that take normal human psychology for granted. The challenge of explaining CBS is to incorporate psychological abnormality into the models, so that behaviors can be seen as evidence of psychopathology, but this needs to be done without pre-judging the question whether they are in fact pathological—we need a neutral descriptive language. Getting the description right involves a series of judgements about the correct representation of what is there, which takes the usual difficulties in both psychiatry and anthropology and adds them together. It is really unclear how we are to set out CBS as explananda without taking sides on whether they are local, culturally bound pathologies, whether they are particular forms of universal pathologies, or whether they are pathologies at all.

20.4 **Conclusion**

I have suggested that psychiatry is undecided between seeing culture-bound phenomena as (1) purely socially constructed, (2) as local forms of universal pathological conditions, or (3) as local pathological conditions. There are real conceptual problems involved in trying to build models that can distinguish between these options, and since the extent to which human psychology varies across cultures is unknown, the correct conceptual framework for describing symptoms is unclear, and most existing models of cultural transmission and/or social construction are designed to explain non-pathological phenomena. Some sort of synthesis between psychiatry and social theory is clearly necessary and inevitable, but the current prospect is very dark.

Acknowledgements

I am very grateful to Ken Kendler and Joe Parnas for the invitation to present some of these ideas to the Fourth Copenhagen Conference on Philosophy and Psychiatry. Ken also provided helpful comments on an early draft. Some of the material in part one is revised from an earlier effort (Murphy 2015) and I thank Steeves Demazeux and Patrick Singy for their help with that piece. I owe a special debt to Pieter Adriaens for sharing his thoughts (and unpublished writings) on culture-boundedness and social construction, which were very helpful.

References

Aggarwal, N.K. (2013). Cultural psychiatry, medical anthropology and the DSM field trials. *Medical Anthropology*, **32**, 393–398.

American Psychiatric Association (1994). *Diagnostic and Statistical Manual of Mental Disorders*, 4th edn. Washington, DC: American Psychiatric Press.

American Psychiatric Association (2013). *Diagnostic and Statistical Manual of Mental Disorders*, 5th edn. Washington: American Psychiatric Press.

Bell, R.M. (1985). *Holy Anorexia*. Chicago: University of Chicago Press.

Bentall, R.P. (2003). *Madness Explained: Psychosis and human nature*. London: Penguin.

Brumberg, J.J. (1988). *Fasting Girls: The history of anorexia nervosa*. Cambridge, MA: Harvard University Press.

Busby, S. (2003). *A Wonderful Little Girl: The true story of Sarah Jacob, the Welsh fasting girl*. London: Short Books.

Canino, G. and **Alegria, M.** (2008). Psychiatric diagnosis—is it universal or relative to culture? *Journal of Child Psychology and Psychiatry*, **49**, 237–250.

Cawte, J. (1974). Malgri: a culture-bound syndrome. In J. Cawte (ed.) *Medicine is the law: Studies in psychiatric anthropology of Australian tribal societies*, pp. 106–119. Honolulu: University Press of Hawaii.

Dennis, PA. (1981). Part three: Grisi Siknis among the Miskito. *Medical Anthropology*, **5**, 445–505.

Geurts, K.L. (2003). *Culture and the Senses: Bodily ways of knowing in an African community*. Berkeley, CA: University of California Press.

Gold, J. and **Gold, I** (2014). *Suspicious Minds: How culture shapes madness*. New York: Free Press.

Hacking, I. (1998). *Mad Travelers: Reflections on the reality of transient mental illnesses*. London: Free Association Books.

Hacking, I. (1999). *The Social Construction of What?* Cambridge, MA: Harvard University Press.

Haslanger, S. (2012). *Resisting Reality: Social Construction and social critique.* Oxford: Oxford University Press.

Henrich, J., Heine, S. J., and **Morenzayan, A.** (2010). The weirdest people in the world. *Behavioral and Brain Sciences*, **33**, 61–83.

Hughes, C.C. (1985). Culture-bound or construct-bound? The syndromes and DSM-III. In R. Simons and C. Hughes (eds.) *The Culture-Bound Syndromes*, pp. 3–24. Dordrecht: Reidel.

Keeley, B.L. (2002). Making sense of the senses: individuating modalities in humans and other animals. *Journal of Philosophy*, **99**, 5–28.

Kitanaka, J. (2011). *Depression in Japan: Psychiatric cures for a society in distress.* Princeton, NJ: Princeton University Press.

Kleinman, A. (1988). *Rethinking Psychiatry: From cultural category to personal experience.* New York: Free Press.

Lee, S. (1996). Reconsidering the status of anorexia nervosa as a Western culture-bound syndrome. *Social Science and Medicine*, **42**, 21–34.

Lewis, T.H. (1975). A syndrome of depression and mutism in the Oglala Sioux. *American Journal of Psychiatry*, **132**, 753–755.

Lewis-Fernández, R., Guarnaccia, P.J., and **Ruiz, P.** (2009). Culture-bound syndromes. In B. Sadock, V. Sadock, and P. Ruiz (eds.) *Comprehensive Textbook of Psychiatry*, 9th edn, Volume II, pp. 2519–2538. New York: Wolters Kluwer/Lippincott Williams & Wilkins.

López, S.R., Guarnaccia, P.J. (2000). Cultural psychopathology: uncovering the social world of mental illness. *Annual Review of Psychology*, **51**, 571–598. Erratum in *Annual Review of Psychology*, 2003;54:vii.

Mallon, R. (2007). A field guide to social construction. *Philosophy Compass*, **2**, 93–108.

Murphy, D. (2015). Deviant deviance: cultural diversity in DSM-5. In S. Demazeux and P. Singy (eds.) *The DSM-5 in Perspective: Philosophical reflections on the psychiatric Babel*, pp. 97–110. New York: Springer.

Sperber D. (1996). *Explaining Culture.* Oxford: Blackwell.

Segall, M.H., Campbell, D.T., and **Herskovits, M.J** (1966). *The Influence of Culture on Visual Perception.* New York: Bobbs-Merrill.

Chapter 21

Reflections on culture-bound syndromes

Paul S. Appelbaum

After graduating from medical school in Boston and before beginning a psychiatric residency there, I spent a year doing a medical internship in Israel. The hospital where I worked was in Beersheva, in the south of the country, often referred as the "capital" of the Negev desert region. Although it has since grown enormously, in the mid-1970s Beersheva was a dusty city of perhaps 80,000 people, almost all of them born somewhere else in the world. I treated people from Morocco and other North African countries, Russia, Denmark, Georgia, Romania, Iraq, Hungary, and elsewhere, along with a small number of native Israelis. As the regional medical center for the southern part of the country, my hospital also had responsibility for the treatment of the Bedouin population living in the Negev.

As may be evident, most diagnosis and treatment was conducted with the help of an interpreter, but it quickly became apparent that I was dealing with very different patients, complaints of illness, and social situations than I had come to know in Boston. One of the most striking complaints I heard soon after entering the wards was common to the Bedouin patients and to Jewish immigrants from the Maghreb. "Raglayim ko'ave li," they would say in Hebrew or in its Arabic equivalent: "My legs are hurting me." My first impulse was to examine their legs to determine the nature of the problem. Thrombophlebitis? Intermittent claudication? Osteoarthritis? Lymphangitis?

As experienced local doctors already knew, however, these complaints almost never corresponded to identifiable pathology in the lower limbs. Rather, they seemed to be a way of communicating generalized distress, whether physical (e.g., "I don't feel well") or mental (e.g., "I'm upset about something"). Indeed, the patients' overall presentations often seemed to include symptoms related to depression, including a dysphoric affect, psychomotor agitation, and anxiety. It struck me that in similar circumstances in the United States, patients would complain about abdominal discomfort (e.g., "My stomach hurts"). Indeed, even young American children often use abdominal complaints as a generalized expression of unhappiness (e.g., "I can't go to school today—my tummy hurts."). I wondered if I were seeing a culturally determined variant of the presentation of non-specific distress, of which depression was just one precipitant.

The phenomenon stuck in my mind, and when I returned to Boston to begin residency at the conclusion of my internship year, I tracked down a copy of Robert Burton's classic seventeenth-century description of depression, *Anatomy of Melancholy* (1638), to see what kind of somatic symptoms were reported. Interestingly, Burton noted that people with melancholy frequently complained of abdominal discomfort, a category that he referred to as "windy Hypochondriacal Melancholy" (at 2633). Since depression is often associated with constipation (Garvey et al. 1990), presumably on the basis of reduced intestinal motility, one could point to a physiologic basis for their perception that something was awry in their abdominal cavities—and for the apparent continuity of presentation from seventeenth-century England to the United States today. But if it were strictly a matter of people with depression reporting their interpretations of altered peristaltic activity, the Bedouin and Maghrebi Jews for whom I cared should also have localized their somatic distress associated with depression to their digestive systems rather than to their legs. It appeared that something more complicated was going on here that could not be attributed in a simple way to pathophysiologic changes in bodily function.

Does my experience in Beersheva have any implications for our broader understanding of culture-bound syndromes? Some obvious words of caution are in order. I did not survey representative samples of distressed and/or depressed patients in either Boston or Beersheva. My impressions may be distorted by the patients I happened to see and may be limited by the language and cultural barriers that stood between us. Moreover, I was a young and inexperienced physician who may have erred in either his observations or interpretations of the situation. However, for the sake of this exercise, let's grant the validity of my impressions and ask where they may lead.

These observations suggested to me that the symptomatic manifestations of disease—physical or mental—can be shaped by cultural preconceptions, including what part of the body we think should hurt when we are not feeling well. It appears that in parts of the Middle East the answer to that question is "the legs," whereas in the United States and perhaps in Europe as well, "the abdomen" is the more common response, and has been for several centuries. According to Kleinman (1987), in China it may be more likely that the locus is the lower back, even—when distress is due to depression—to the exclusion of the symptoms associated with dysphoria that define depression in the West. Presumably, drawing on the typology offered in Dominic Murphy's elegant exploration of culture-bound syndromes (this volume, Chapter 20), that puts me on the side of the "unificationists," i.e., I appear to be endorsing the view that common underlying mechanisms may result in very different symptomatic presentations in different cultures—but nonetheless remain manifestations of the same disorder.

However, I am not sure that the answer is quite that simple. Indeed, a one-size-fits-all model—whether what Murphy calls the "universalist" or "particularist" approaches—may not be enough to explain cultural variation in psychiatric symptomatology. I suspect that across disorders there is a gradient of the extent to which symptoms are determined by common biological processes—e.g., presence of thought disorder and negative symptoms in schizophrenia (World Health Organization 1975)—versus environmental/cultural factors—e.g., the content of delusions in schizophrenia (Jay 2003). At the extremes, culture may play little role in the manifestation of a disorder—e.g., Alzheimer's disease—or may play so dominant a role as to determine whether a disorder exists in the first place—e.g., classical hysteria, which since Freud's time appears largely to have disappeared from the Western world (Shorter 1992).[1] This is not quite the same as Murphy's suggestion that "all mental illnesses, including those in the main body of the DSM, are really [culture-bound syndromes]," but it acknowledges that in fact many of them may be.

If the notion of a gradient of cultural responsiveness (which seems more congenial than speaking deterministically of syndromes as "culture-bound") has something to be said for it, then a comprehensive diagnostic framework would need to locate approximately where on the spectrum a given disorder sits, and to alert clinicians to the culturally responsive variants that have been reported. That would get us out of a conceptual problem identified by Murphy, i.e., the relativistic notion that Western presentations of mental disorders faithfully reflect the underlying illnesses, whereas presentations in other cultures are distorted by sociocultural influences. Given the absence of cross-cultural studies of many mental disorders, locating disorders on a spectrum of culture responsivity may not be a task that can be accomplished today or in the near future, but perhaps it suggests a useful research agenda for cross-cultural psychiatrists and medical anthropologists.

Of course, such an approach would not address many of the other issues that Murphy correctly points to as associated with the current category of culture-bound syndromes. We would still need to explain what culture is and how it acts to affect symptomatic presentations, and to struggle with the enduring line-drawing dilemmas of the field: where do we locate the boundary between normality and illness, and when do we define disorders as distinct rather than as variants of a common underlying condition? And we should not be surprised if the *Diagnostic and Statistical Manual of Mental Disorders* (DSM), as a product of American psychiatry, no matter the extent to which it has proven useful in other parts of the world, continues to privilege those syndromes and their variants that are more likely to be seen by North American psychiatrists, in either native-born or immigrant populations.

But asking, "How much is this disorder affected by cultural influences and in what ways?" may turn the discussion of culture-bound syndromes in a more

[1] Note that this conclusion—although congruent with most psychiatrists' impressions—is controversial in two ways. Some commentators contend that changes in psychiatric nosology rather than in the manifestations of patients' presentations are responsible for the "disappearance" of hysteria (Micale 1993); others suggest that conversion symptoms can still be found, not in the psychiatric clinic, but across the hall in neurology (Stone et al. 2008).

useful direction than looking to dichotomize disorders into those that are culturally influenced and those that are not.

References

Burton, R. (1638). *The Anatomy of Melancholy.* Project Gutenberg edition: http://www.gutenberg.org/files/10800/10800.txt.

Garvey, M., Noyes, R., and **Yates, W.** (1990). Frequency of constipation in major depression: relationship to other clinical variables. *Psychosomatics*, **31**, 204–206.

Jay, M. (2003). *The Air Loom Gang.* New York: Four Walls Eight Windows.

Kleinman, A. (1987). *Social Origins of Distress and Disease: Depression, neurasthenia, and pain in modern China.* New Haven, CT: Yale University Press.

Micale, M.S. (1993). Disappearance of hysteria: a study in the clinical deconstruction of a diagnosis. *Isis*, **84**, 496–526.

Shorter, E. (1992). *From Paralysis to Fatigue.* New York: Free Press.

Stone, J., Hewett, R., Carson, A., Warlow, C., and **Sharpe, M.** (2008). The disappearance of hysteria: historical mystery or illusion? *Journal of the Royal Society of Medicine*, **101**, 12–18.

World Health Organization. (1975). *Schizophrenia: A Multinational Study. A summary of the initial evaluation period of the International Pilot Study of Schizophrenia.* Geneva: World Health Organization. http://apps.who.int/iris/handle/10665/37767.

Section 8

The coming and going of Asperger's syndrome

Chapter 22

Introduction to "On the appearance and disappearance of Asperger's syndrome"

Kenneth S. Kendler

Miriam Solomon is a distinguished philosopher of science and medicine who is relatively new to the field of psychiatry. She has chosen to comment on the fascinating story of the appearance and then disappearance of Asperger's syndrome in the *Diagnostic and Statistical Manual of Mental Disorders* (DSM). It was first added to DSM-IV as a member of the category of "Pervasive Developmental Disorders." By DSM-5, it was gone, a causality of the creation of the new diagnostic category of autism spectrum disorders. What is relatively unique about Solomon's perspective is that it emphasizes the viewpoint of the "consumers" of the DSM—those themselves affected with Asperger's syndrome and their close relatives. She poignantly quotes from several consumers who described the positive sense of having a diagnosis that applied to them—that provided "an explanation of what I'd endured my entire life."

The focus in Solomon's paper is concern about the consequences of diagnostic changes on consumers and the degree to which they should be considered in the decision-making apparatus for future DSM changes. She argues with some force that a reasonable number of people diagnosed with Asperger's syndrome were upset when their disorder was dropped from DSM-5. This seems to be because, unlike most other psychiatric disorders, affected individuals had developed a positive identification with the syndrome and support groups had been built around this category. They therefore felt, with some justification, that the legitimacy of their efforts had been undercut by the DSM-5 decision to expel their diagnosis from the manual.

Through much of her essay Solomon expresses considerable empathy with these individuals, but in the latter part of the paper she adds a further nuance. In many cases, she argues, the "Asperger" identity was founded on being "better than" the low-functioning autistic cases. This understandably decreases her sympathy for their plight.

Reading this essay again has prompted me to try to recall when, in the thousands of hours of DSM meetings I have attended since the early 1980s, I have been in discussions where issues like this were raised. It is with some embarrassment that I can only clearly recall one such discussion. It was during the development of DSM-IV when I was a member of the Schizophrenia and Other Psychotic Disorders Work Group. The discussion was brief and it involved the perennial issue—often raised over the last few decades in nosologic discussions—of whether we should eliminate the term "schizophrenia" and substitute it with another, more benign label (Lieberman and First 2007, George and Klijn 2013). The argument started with the typical observation that schizophrenia has a very negative connotation and carries a lot of stigma so that receiving such a diagnosis could have quite a negative effect on individuals. The rejoinder was that the term has a long historical tradition of research and a change in names would be disruptive. Then, it was pointed out that we have other disorders that are often seen as or even more pejorative (e.g., antisocial personality disorder, narcissistic personality disorder, and alcohol dependence) and there are no plans afoot to change them—so why schizophrenia? The topic was then dropped but, as noted, has since recurred in the psychiatric literature, in part driven by the decision in Japan to change the name of schizophrenia to "integration disorder" (Lieberman and First 2007, George and Klijn 2013).

This is no place to try to offer any definitive "DSM response" to the points raised by Solomon. Instead, I try to summarize some impressions. DSM leadership has indeed traditionally seen itself as having two major audiences—researchers and clinicians. Patients are not normally on that list. As we think about changing, adding, or (much more rarely) deleting criteria, patient's concerns barely get a mention. We are however, constantly concerned about ways of improving diagnoses so as to facilitate better care for our patients.

How common are the concerns raised by Solomon in the Asperger's story? I think not very common. DSM does not retire psychiatric disorders very often and the chances that one of those chosen in the future would, like Asperger's, have a strong positive identification among patients and diagnosis-specific support groups seems rather remote. But we do change criteria sometimes. For example, those for schizophrenia were modestly narrowed from DSM-IV to DSM-5, shifting a small percentage of the patients previously diagnosed with schizophrenia into other categories. Regardless of how rarely such issues arise, the theoretical issues posed are important ones.

What is the responsibility of the DSM process to be concerned about these questions—that patients will be harmed by diagnostic changes impacting on their self-identity and/or self-understanding? Do other branches of medicine consider this issue when they add or delete diagnoses? Should psychiatry differ in this regard because of the nature of our conditions?

This is an awkward question for me, given my long-term focus on improving the scientific rigor of the DSM process, as these issues fall a long way from the problems of validity and reliability. Solomon specifically advocates for the addition of such questions to our "circle of concern." I certainly do not feel that this reflects a major problem with the nosologic process such that patient representatives are needed on every future DSM work group to guard against changes that have major adverse outcomes on our patients. But I would subscribe to some "consciousness raising"—that the changes we make can sometimes impact in important ways on people's lived lives. I would argue that we should, at a minimum, be aware of this as a concern. I am not convinced that we need to change guidelines and build this formally into our processes, given the likely rarity of these self-identify concerns. Others might argue to the contrary and this would deserve its own deliberative process. But a broad commitment to a humanistic agenda for DSM does need to complement our scientific focus and provide some way for such concerns, when appropriate, to enter into our deliberations.

References

George, B. and **Klijn, A.** (2013). A modern name for schizophrenia (PSS) would diminish self-stigma. *Psychological Medicine*, **43**, 1555–1557.

Lieberman, J.A. and **First, M.B.** (2007). Renaming schizophrenia. *BMJ*, **334**, 7585.

Chapter 23

On the appearance and disappearance of Asperger's syndrome

Miriam Solomon

Nature never draws a line without smudging it.

Lorna Wing

23.1 Introduction

Asperger's syndrome was added to the psychiatric disease classifications in the fourth edition of the *Diagnostic and Statistical Manual of Mental Disorders*, DSM-IV (1994), and removed from the fifth edition, DSM-5 (2013), almost 20 years later. This is a short life for a psychiatric syndrome. My goal in this chapter is to examine this case in depth in order to see what can be learned from it about appropriate criteria for making changes in the DSM nosology.

The DSM is a document that aims to balance the needs for psychiatric disease classification of clinicians, research scientists, educators, and sometimes other interested parties such as patient groups and the legal profession. Just how this balance is (and should be) accomplished is a matter of debate. For example, while Robert Michels has said that the DSM has little to do with science (Michels 2015), Ken Kendler has devoted much professional energy to strengthening the scientific standards of the DSM, most recently chairing the DSM-5 Scientific Review Committee (SRC) that reviewed the recommendations of work groups (Kendler 2013).

23.2 History of Asperger's syndrome

Hans Asperger was an Austrian pediatrician who in 1944 described a case series of four boys with what we now recognize as "Asperger" characteristics: "a lack of empathy, little ability to form friendships, one-sided conversations, intense absorption in a special interest, and clumsy movements." He described them as autistic (although they were much more functional, and especially more verbal, than some of Kanner's classic cases of autism), and as "little professors." At the same time as the Nazi's Final Solution, he argued for the importance of human diversity:

> Not everything that steps out of line, and thus "abnormal," must necessarily be "inferior" (Asperger 1938)

The British psychiatrist Lorna Wing revived the category in 1981, distinguishing it from Kanner's autism, and calling it "Asperger's syndrome."

It was championed by influential psychiatrists as well as by people with the disorder. Over the next 20 years, there were around 900 published papers on Asperger's syndrome. The first diagnostic criteria appeared in 1989, World Health Organization criteria in 1993, and in 1994 it was introduced in DSM-IV. Asperger's was classified with other autistic disorders in a group called "Pervasive Developmental Disorders."

Reception of the new Asperger's diagnosis was also enthusiastic among people who identified with the diagnosis. A typical reaction was that from Katherine Annear:

> I grew up without a label and after having many thrown at me in my late teens, finding Asperger's was like finding a glove that fit.[1]

The diagnostic category helped people to understand themselves, or their affected family members, for the first time. A similar reaction from Michael John Carley:

> I was finally presented with an explanation of what I'd endured my entire life. I don't have the words to describe the biblical weight being lifted off me.[2]

The Asperger's identity (some refer to it as "Aspie," but the term is controversial) has become quite successful, even termed the "defining psychiatric malady" of the Millennial generation.[3] There are questions about overdiagnosis and also a debate about whether what is being diagnosed is a disability or merely a difference (conceptualized as "neurodiversity"), as Asperger himself suggested.

23.3 New classification of autistic disorders in DSM-5

DSM-5, published in 2013, removed the Asperger's diagnosis. The most commonly given reason for this is that the category is not sufficiently distinguished from other autism spectrum disorders (ASDs) for the diagnosis to be reliably distinguished from other diagnoses in the DSM-IV such as high-functioning autism and pervasive developmental disorder—not otherwise specified (PDD-NOS). Proposed special criteria, such as limiting the Asperger's diagnosis to those with no language delays, or those without cognitive impairment, have not in practice adequately demarcated those who are thought to have the disorder. This is because in practice, clinicians have found that rigid application of such criteria does not meet their prognostic and treatment needs. These difficulties with the reliability of criteria for diagnosis led to doubts about the scientific validity of Asperger's syndrome.

---

[1] Katharine Annear, 2013, http://www.abc.net.au/rampup/articles/2013/05/24/3766915.htm

[2] http://www.education.com/magazine/article/Understanding_Aspergers_Syndrome/

[3] See Benjamin Wallace's piece in the *New York Magazine* at http://nymag.com/news/features/autism-spectrum-2012-11/

The DSM-5 proposes a classification for autistic disorders that is in some respects simpler than the one in DSM-IV. Instead of assessments of three areas—language, social skills, and repetitive and restricted interests and behavior (RRIBs)—it considers language and social skills together as one area, and RRIBs as a second area. When language and social skills are combined, those formerly diagnosed with Asperger's do less well on the combined measure and are less distinguishable from others with autistic disorders. The given justification for combining language and social skills is that the areas of functioning are not separate; especially, the pragmatics of language requires social skills. Studies using factor analyses and cluster analyses show that language and social skills covary more closely than either do with RRIBs (Mandy et al. 2012). ASD is now a large and diverse category that includes those individuals formerly diagnosed with classic autism, pervasive developmental disorders (except for one type of case to be discussed below), and Asperger's syndrome. The ASD diagnosis is given together with assessments of the degree of severity in the two areas of impaired functioning. Those formerly diagnosed with Asperger's syndrome are generally less severely affected than those formerly diagnosed with autism or with many cases of PDD.

There is one type of case (formerly in the PDD-NOS category) that does not fit into the new ASD category: cases in which individuals have communicative and social disorders but do not have RRIBs. Rather than making them an apparently arbitrary exception to the general rule of requiring both social/communication delays and repetitive behaviors, they have been classified under a new category: social (pragmatic) communication disorder, S(P)CD. This keeps the criteria for ASDs clear, categorical, and consistent.

Since this new system of classification is only beginning to be implemented, we do not know how reliable or valid it will turn out to be. Although we expect that it removes some difficulties with the previous system, we do not yet know whether it introduces other difficulties: scientific, clinical, or public health. This is the case for *any* proposed changes in classification (unless we revert to prior classifications for which we have data, or unless there are field trials using the proposed classification). A study by Young Shin Kim et al. (2014) suggests that the new system will work well, but this study may not generalize to typical clinical contexts.

23.4 The process of producing DSM-5

DSM-5 is the product of expert consensus. More precisely, it is the product of several expert consensuses. Thirteen work groups, which were assigned tasks in their areas of diagnostic expertise, made recommendations for change that were reviewed by the SRC, the Clinical and Public Health Committee (CPHC), the DSM-5 Task Force (an expert consensus group including the chairs of the work groups) and finally by the American Psychiatric Association (APA) Board of Trustees. The charge of the SRC was to provide independent scientific review. The charge of the CPHC was to consider the implications for clinical practice and public health. The idea is that the two main constituencies served by the DSM—researchers and clinicians—have formal advisory roles, and serve as checks on the work groups. Asperger's disorder, along with other autistic disorders, was discussed by the Work Group on Neurodevelopmental Disorders.

Ken Kendler (2013) has argued that work groups have a bias in favor of making changes to DSM categories, since they want to see that their discussions make an impact. If no changes are made, no impact is visible, however wise the decisions may have been and however much new data may have been incorporated into the decision. The review committees serve as a check on this bias, asking whether the proposed changes have scientific support and whether they make clinical sense. The APA Board of Trustees makes the final decisions, taking into account the work of the work groups, both review committees, and the DSM-5 Task Force. Only the final report is published, so disagreements between the committees are not publicized.

I have written elsewhere about the importance of expert consensus for establishing medical authority and for communicating best practice (Solomon 2015). Expert disagreement, on the other hand, tends to decrease medical authority and create opportunities for other interests to shape outcomes. It is best kept behind closed doors (Solomon 2015).

23.5 **Assessing the validity of a diagnosis**

Ken Kendler has set out an influential conceptual framework for validators of psychiatric diagnoses: see Kendler (2009), which was modified from Kendler (1980). The framework comprises antecedent validators (such as family histories of a disorder), concurrent validators (such as biological markers, patterns of comorbidity, and other correlates), and predictive validators (diagnostic stability, prognosis, responsiveness to treatment). This is a wide range of possible validators, some of which are relevant to an understanding of disease etiology, and some of which are more relevant to clinical practice.

For ASDs, whether classified under DSM-IV or DSM-5 criteria, we have validators of typical strength for psychiatric disorders (i.e., not very strong). Family history plays a role, but the genetics is complex with "a mix of strong-effect genetic lesions coupled with weak-effect common polymorphisms" (Talkowski et al. 2014) in a way that does not yet let us identify consistently contributing genetic factors. There are no known biological markers. Patterns of comorbidity (which can be measured with neuropsychological tests) provide much evidence for the nature of the disorder, but these patterns are not perfectly tidy (as the DSM-IV category of PDD-NOS and the DSM-5 category of S(P)CD show). The diagnosis of ASDs does show stability over time, in that some patterns of comorbidity persist and others go through expected changes correlated with age or developmental stage. There is not much in the way of successful treatment for ASDs, and such treatments as there are (behavioral therapies and treatments for commonly associated anxiety and depression) are not specific to ASDs, but used for a variety of psychiatric conditions with the same symptoms. So the main validators of ASDs amount to patterns of comorbidity. (This situation is common for psychiatric disorders, and responsible for the DSM's focus on clusters of symptoms.)

23.6 **Assessing the DSM-5 classification of autistic disorders**

As I said earlier, we do not yet know how reliable or valid the DSM-5 classification of autistic disorders will be. We will need to gather data on new diagnoses, and see whether the combination of ASD (with degree of severity) and S(P)CD provides a clearer, more reliable, perhaps simpler classification than the one in DSM-IV.

The DSM-5 classification of autistic disorders was proposed not as a random hypothesis, but as a result of both scientific judgment and clinical experience. It is not possible to have much data on a newly proposed classification (we can only have data on classification systems we have used). The main reasons at present justifying the changes are scientific judgment and clinical experience.

Of course, I do not know anything about the discussions of classifications of autistic disorders that took place in the relevant work group, or in the SRC, or in the CPHC. Such deliberations are not made public. All I have access to are the written reports of the two oversight committees, which state in general terms the kind of criteria that they regarded as relevant and as irrelevant.

The SRC emphasizes the importance of *evidence* that justifies changes in disease classification. What is *evidence*? The answer to this question has been complicated at least since the development of evidence-based medicine in the 1990s, because the so-called "hierarchy of evidence" has (rightly) made us more critical about what counts as good evidence. At the top of the standard hierarchy of evidence are well designed and executed clinical trials, whereas "clinical experience," "expert consensus," and "pathophysiological reasoning" are at the bottom of the hierarchy. What kind of evidence does the SRC count? The report of the SRC does not make an explicit statement about this. This is an omission, not least because the standard evidence hierarchy is a poor metric for the range of evidence that the SRC considered. It is not clear where to put the genetic and imaging studies that are counted as high-quality evidence, but they are not randomized controlled trials; at best they are observational evidence. Certainly, considerations lower in the standard medical evidence hierarchy, such as observational evidence, clinical experience, and expert consensus, played an important role in suggesting the DSM-5 diagnostic criteria for ASD. In particular, they supported some widely accepted hypotheses about ASD. In this way, the hypotheses are not random unsupported assumptions, but reasonable (although fallible) supported claims.[4]

One important hypothesis guiding the creation of the DSM-5 diagnostic criteria for ASD is that the combination of social/communicative delays and RRIBs is constitutive of the disorder. This is not in the DSM-IV criteria, which in practice provided a PDD-NOS category for those without RRIBs. What *evidence* supports (or undermines) this hypothesis? The presence of individuals who have social and communicative delays but do not have RRIBs is not taken to undermine this

---

[4] To be precise, I would say that the assumptions/hypotheses are not evidence, but that there is evidence for them.

hypothesis[5]; it is used to argue for another pathological category. The assumption is a theoretical hypothesis, whose plausibility is supported by the clinical experience that social/communicative delays and RRIBs often co-occur, although they are apparently independent traits. The idea is that the hypothesis will be tested by seeing whether the new criteria will be validated (by any of the antecedent, concurrent, or predictive validators discussed above).

Another hypothesis that goes into the DSM-5 classification of ASD is that differences in degrees of severity do *not* reflect differences in underlying pathology. This is a reasonable assumption on grounds of parsimony, but not one that is supported by a set of clinical trials.

Yet another hypothesis is that language skills and social skills are best combined into a single measure of social/communicative disorders. This is based on the clinical experience that it is difficult to distinguish the two sets of skills (at least, for the pragmatic aspects of language), and on studies using factor analysis and cluster analysis to see whether the social and the communicative covary (Mandy et al. 2012). The studies are limited, and it would be misleading to claim that we have strong evidence that language and social skills are best combined into a single measure. This is a matter of scientific judgment, about which experts disagree.

A related hypothesis that is used in DSM-IV but dropped in DSM-5 is that the absence of language delays in many individuals with Asperger's signifies a significant difference from other ASDs, one worth marking in disease classification criteria, and which may stem from an important difference in underlying pathology. More recent clinical experience has shown that many of those diagnosed with Asperger's in fact have significant language delays, removing the motivation for the hypothesis (Mayes et al. 2001, Macintosh and Dissanayake 2004).

In summary, there is scientific reasoning going into the DSM-5 categorization, and the reasoning comes from assumptions that may be supported by some evidence, but that evidence is not always high-quality evidence from clinical trials or even evidence from genetic and neuroscientific studies. The DSM-5 categorization of autistic disorders is a reasonable hypothesis about nosology, which will be tested further in future clinical trials and clinical experience. *I recommend that, in future editions of DSM, whichever body does the work of the SRC should refine the criteria to include statements about the nature and strength of the evidence that goes into constructing new hypotheses.*

I now move on to the work of the CPHC. This committee was set up to consider the impact of diagnostic changes on clinical practice and public health, considering both professional and public constituencies. The typical questions that the committee asked were: Does the proposed new diagnostic category result in loss of clinical or educational services for some individuals who need them? (e.g., by falling into a "mild" category or the " social communication disorder" category)

---

5 At this time; I wonder whether, in clinical and/or scientific practice, it will prove more important to classify those with S(P)CD under ASD than to be fastidious about the new definition of ASD.

Does the proposed new diagnostic category result in overdiagnosis, such that the normal range of behavior becomes pathologized? Does the proposed new diagnostic category lead to any inappropriate treatments? I expect that all of these were discussed for the case of Asperger's, and will continue to be evaluated as DSM-5 is put to use.

I focus here on an additional consideration of the CPHC that seems to have special resonance for the case of Asperger's syndrome and ASDs. The committee report says:

> We considered that diagnoses are occasionally put to unintended purposes. Some individuals use their diagnostic labels to find personal meaning and distinctiveness, a version of "identity politics." And some patients, families, and advocates preferentially claim and adhere to certain diagnoses (eschewing others that may be more accurate) to secure and maintain social and economic benefits (Yager and Mcintyre 2014).

The CPHC does not explicitly say what should be done about such "unintended purposes." To my ear, the implication is that such unintended purposes are regrettable but need to be acknowledged. The implication is that patients, families, and advocates sometimes resist proposed changes in diagnostic categories because of their other interests. There is no statement about how patient interests should be weighed when making recommendations for changing diagnostic categories. This consideration is particularly relevant to the case of Asperger's syndrome, which has been used to justify the Asperger's identity that many patients and their families have found meaningful.

The disappearance of the Asperger's diagnosis may be what Miranda Fricker (2007) calls a "hermeneutical injustice" to people with Asperger's. What Fricker means by "hermeneutical injustice" is a lacuna in social self-understanding in an oppressed group caused by the decisions of a privileged group.[6] With the disappearance of the Asperger's diagnosis, the authors of the DSM are removing their professional support for the Asperger's identity. ASD (even with degrees of severity) does not "fit like a glove" for those with Asperger's; indeed it does not fit like a glove for anyone with ASD, because of the broadness of the spectrum of disorders covered by the category.[7] Loss of the Asperger's diagnosis may mean the loss of understanding of one's disorder (or difference). Certainly, some have experienced it as a harm. For example, John Elder Robison wrote (*New York Magazine*, July 12, 2013):

> Just like that, Asperger's was gone. You can do things like that when you publish the rules. Like corrupt referees at a rigged college football game, the APA removed Asperger's from the field of play and banished the term to the locker room of psychiatric oblivion. Their new and improved DSM went on sale two months ago, and shrinks everywhere lined up to buy it. Meanwhile, my 2007 memoir about living with Asperger's is now deemed diagnostically obsolete.

---

[6] One of her examples is the situation for sexually harassed women before the development of the concept of "sexual harassment."

[7] A familiar saying in the autism community is "If you've met one person with autism, you've met one person with autism."

My sympathy for such harm has been to some degree tempered by the knowledge that it is commonly part of the meaning of the Asperger's identity that the person is in a different—*and better*—diagnostic category than lower-functioning persons with autism. Parent and writer Lucy Berrington wrote that a benefit of the Asperger's diagnosis was that it helped parents to accept their children's developmental delays:

> The Asperger's label has helped many who don't fit the classic autism model or stereotype to get a diagnosis and accept their autism. We don't need data to tell us that Asperger's is a less unnerving diagnosis than autism for those who haven't come to terms with their own or their children's special needs . . . the Asperger's/autism dichotomy penalizes and stigmatizes classic autism.

It was a less scary diagnosis, but at the expense of reinforcing the negative attitudes toward autism. I call this the dark side of the Asperger's diagnosis. One blogger, Brigianna Spencer, puts this plainly:

> Because Asperger's becomes stereotyped as the "good," "mild," "high-functioning" autism, that leaves classic autism with the stigma of "the bad kind of autism" simply by the existence of the contrast.[8]

The Asperger's diagnosis was correlated with socioeconomic status. Those lower on the socioeconomic scale were likelier to be diagnosed with PDD-NOS or with high-functioning classic autism than those higher on the socioeconomic scale (Kauffman 2012).

A brave blogger, Michael Scott Monje Jr., unequivocally states what he thinks is going on:

> The term "Aspie" has come to be a way for those of us who want to talk about our experiences to separate ourselves from "those" Autistics. It allows us an identity that has been sanitized for our allistic audience—a way of performing eccentricity instead of disability, of showing we are "like them" but "still employable". This is disgusting.[9]

What is going on here is a phenomenon that Hilde Lindemann (in Nelson 2001) calls "hostage taking." The Asperger's identity is made positive by putting down another oppressed group, those with classic autism. (Lindemann's example is anti-gay rhetoric in Black rapper communities.) A positive identity, as Lindemann characterizes it, is a narrative that fosters the humanity and frees the agency of the members of the group. The Asperger's identity celebrates the abilities of those with Asperger Syndrome by explicitly or implicitly contrasting them with the disabilities of those with classic autism and framing them as "neurodiversities." This positive Asperger's identity comes at the cost of damaging the identity of another oppressed group.

---

[8] Quoted in Lucy Berrington's 2012 article ("What we'll miss when we miss Asperger's syndrome"); https://www.psychologytoday.com/blog/aspergers-alive/201212/what-we-ll-miss-when-we-miss-asperger-syndrome)

[9] http://wearelikeyourchild.blogspot.com/2014/01/dont-aspie-me.html

There is some truth to the claim that people with Asperger's have suffered a hermeneutical injustice because of the disappearance of the diagnostic category. And I think that this truth deserves consideration at the level of the CPHC. That is, patients, families, and their social and economic circumstances should have a voice in making revisions to the DSM. The "scientific considerations" are not so compelling that other considerations can be ignored, nor so clear that we can dismiss experiential and hermeneutic claims as unscientific.

That said, because the Asperger's identity is not innocent in the hands of many who have used it, keeping the identity is a potential injustice to those harmed by it: those with more classic autism. Hanna Rosin, who has written thoughtfully about her son's receiving and losing the Asperger's diagnosis within a period of a few months, describes the DSM-5 criteria as "democratic"[10] in that they makes no important distinctions between people on the autism spectrum. I think this is an important insight, and one that argues for the DSM-5 criteria on ethical grounds. Did it play a role at the level of the CPHC? If it did not, I think that it should, going forward, with whatever body takes the place of the CPHC in future editions of the DSM.

Hanna Rosin also writes, like others, about the transformative experience of receiving the Asperger's diagnosis. She wrote:

> almost the minute we got the diagnosis, my resistance to labeling melted, and so did my husband's. We walked willingly into another world, with its own language, rituals, and worldview.

Six months after this diagnosis, DSM-5 was published. Rosin acknowledged:

> DSM-5 no longer grants the special status that the Asperger's label once supplied to a high functioning cohort . . .

Interestingly, however, any harm she may have experienced as a result of the removal of the diagnostic category was short-lived. Over a year of reading and thinking, she came to embrace the category of ASD, interpreting it as implying "an unbroken continuum among minds that extends from autism all the way into the realm of the normal" and describing the category as in this way "democratic." This may not be an interpretation officially sanctioned by the CPHC or the authors of DSM-5. But it may become an ethically important aspect of the ASD diagnosis, and deserves to be recognized in any future discussions. It also shows that identities can usefully change over time—even as underlying causes and symptoms may not change--and sometimes mark different stages in the acceptance of a disorder.

23.7 **Conclusion**

Through considering the case of Asperger's, I have argued for the inclusion of a broader set of criteria in revising psychiatric diagnostic categories. In particular, I have argued for clarifying the scientific criteria by being more explicit about the

[10] http://www.theatlantic.com/magazine/archive/2014/03/letting-go-of-aspergers/357563/

nature of the evidence (especially from genetic and neuroimaging studies) and by recognizing the role of scientific reasoning (which is traditionally put on the bottom level of the evidence hierarchy). And I have argued for broadening the clinical and public health considerations—currently, the work of the CPHC—to include the impact on patient self-understanding and identity. This is probably best done with patient/advocacy input to, or participation in, the work of the CPHC.

Broadening the set of criteria for revising psychiatric diagnostic categories probably will not make decisions easier. But the decisions were already complex because of the variety of evidence as well as clinical and public health considerations. To those who say that broadening the criteria will make things too complex, I would argue that they are already too complex. In such situations, it is best to have all the considerations on the table.

The work of the CPHC is framed as "extrascientific." I think that this is misleading because we cannot tell a priori which considerations may prove scientifically relevant in the future. It is possible, for example, that the self-understanding of those with ASD/Asperger's will prove an important key to our future understanding of the disorder. A related point is that "scientific" considerations alone are not sufficient for doing science. As Helen Longino (1990) and others have argued, values are part of science.

The process of producing DSM-5—in particular the roles of the SRC and the CPHC—is also being reconsidered. Their work is valuable, indeed essential, but it might be achieved for future DSMs in different ways, such as by a single review committee, and/or a separate committee of patients and patient advocates. The Guidelines for Making Changes to DSM-V (10/21/09)[11] say that the most important clinical criterion is "*the magnitude of adverse effects on our patients that would arise from the deletion of the syndrome*" (italics in the original). Considering patient perspectives on diagnostic categories should be part of this assessment.

Acknowledgments

Many thanks to Ken Kendler and Sam Fellowes who commented on a previous draft of this paper.

References

Fricker, M. (2007). *Epistemic Injustice: Power and the ethics of knowing.* Oxford, UK: Oxford University Press.

Kaufmann, W.E. (2012). DSM-5: The new diagnostic criteria for autism spectrum disorders. Research Symposium—Autism Consortium, Boston, MA. http://www.autism-consortium.org/symposium-files/WalterKaufmannAC2012Symposium.pdf.

Kendler, K.S. (1980). The nosologic validity of paranoia (simple delusional disorder): a review. *Archives of General Psychiatry*, 37, 699–706.

[11] Available online as a supplementary appendix to Kendler (2013).

Kendler, K.S. (2013). A history of the DSM-5 Scientific Review Committee. *Psychological Medicine*, **43**, 1793–1800.

Kendler, K., **Kupfer, D.**, **Narrow, W.**, **Phillips, K.**, and **Fawcett, J.** (2009). *Guidelines for making changes to DSM-V*, revised 10/21/09. Washington, DC: American Psychiatric Association.

Kim, Y.S., **Fombonne, E.**, **Koh, Y.**, et al. (2014). A comparison of DSM-IV pervasive developmental disorder and DSM-5 autism spectrum disorder prevalence in an epidemiological sample. *Journal of the American Academy of Child and Adolescent Psychiatry*, 53, 500–508.

Longino, H. (1980). *Science as Social Knowledge*. Princeton, NJ: Princeton University Press.

Macintosh, K.E. and **Dissanayake, C.** (2004). Annotation: The similarities and differences between autistic disorder and Asperger's disorder: a review of the empirical evidence. *Journal of Child Psychology and Psychiatry*, 45, 421–434.

Mandy, W.P., **Charman, T.**, and **Skuse, D.H.** (2012)., Testing the construct validity of proposed criteria for DSM-5 autism spectrum disorder. *Journal of the American Academy of Child and Adolescent Psychiatry*, **51**, 41–50.

Mayes, S.D., **Calhoun, S.L.**, and **Crites, D.L.** (2001). Does DSM-IV Asperger's disorder exist? *Journal of Abnormal Child Psychology*, 29, 263–271.

Michels, R. (2015). The construction of a diagnosis is not a scientific issue. In. K.S. Kendler and J. Parnas (eds.) *Philosophical Issues in Psychiatry III: The nature and sources of historical change*, pp. 371–372. Oxford, UK: Oxford University Press.

Nelson, H.L. (2001). *Damaged Identities, Narrative Repair*. Ithaca, NY: Cornell University Press.

Solomon, M. (2015). *Making Medical Knowledge*. Oxford: Oxford University Press.

Talkowski, M.E., **Minikel, E.V.**, and **Gusella, J.F.** (2014). Autism spectrum disorder genetics: diverse genes with diverse clinical outcomes. *Harvard Review of Psychiatry*, 22, 65–75.

Yager, J. and **McIntyre, J.S.** (2014). DSM-5 Clinical and Public Health Committee: challenges and considerations. *American Journal of Psychiatry*, 171, 142–144.

Chapter 24

Impact of "severity decategorization" in DSM-5

Michael B. First

A key aspiration of the revision process for the fifth edition of the *Diagnostic and Statistical Manual of Mental Disorders* (DSM-5) was a push towards increasing its dimensionality. Before the formal start of the DSM-5 revision process in 2006, an initial research planning process was initiated in 1999 which culminated with the publication in 2002 of *A Research Agenda For DSM-V* (Kupfer et al. 2002a), one goal of which was "to transcend the limitations of the current DSM paradigm and to encourage a research agenda that goes beyond our current ways of thinking" (Kupfer et al. 2002b, p. xix). Accordingly, in the "Basic nomenclature issues for DSM-V" chapter (Rounsaville et al. 2002), the authors issued a call to consider "the advantages and disadvantages of basing part or all of DSM-IV on dimensions rather than categories." (p. 12). This was followed by the convening of 13 international research planning conferences, one of which was devoted entirely to dimensional approaches to diagnostic classification. The accompanying monograph (Helzer et al. 2008a) included nine chapters focusing on various potential implementations of dimensionality in DSM-5, e.g., "Dimensional options for DSM-V: the way forward," (Helzer et al. 2008b). Two of the five major sections of the 2011 monograph "The conceptual evolution of DSM-5" (Regier et al. 2011), which summarized the proceedings of the 2009 American Psychopathological Association Annual Meeting, concentrated on dimensional aspects of classification. Part I, "Diagnostic spectra: assessing the validity of disorder groupings" included a chapter entitled "Integration of dimensional spectra for depression and anxiety into categorical diagnoses for general medical practice" (Goldberg et al. 2011) and Part II, "Integrating dimensional concepts into a categorical system," included three chapters about dimensional implementations: "A proposal for including clinically relevant dimensions into DSM-5" (Helzer 2011), "Empirically-derived personality disorder prototypes: bridging dimensions and categories in DSM-5" (Krueger et al. 2011), "Options and dilemmas of dimensional measures for DSM-5: Which types of measures fare best in predicting course and outcome?" (Wittchen et al. 2011). Indeed, according to Regier and colleagues in one of the few papers published by the DSM-5 leadership during the revision process (Regier et al. 2009), "we have decided that one, if not the major, difference between DSM-IV and DSM-V will be the more prominent use of dimensional measures in DSM-V" (p. 649).

Ultimately, when DSM-5 was published in 2013, most of the proposed dimensional constructs ended up in Section III of DSM-5, a part of the manual intended for DSM-5 components for which it was determined that "the scientific evidence is not yet available to support widespread clinical use." (American Psychiatric Association 2013, p. 24). These included the illness severity scales, WHO-DAS-II (a scale for measuring disability) and the cross-cutting symptom measures adapted from the NIMH PROMIS project, all of which were placed in this section as a result of a vote by the American Psychiatric Association Assembly in May 2012 (American Psychiatric Association Assembly 2012) that expressed serious concerns about their clinical utility. Also included in Section III was the hybrid dimensional/categorical approach to personality disorder classification after being rejected for inclusion in the main section of the DSM-5 by the American Psychiatric Association Board of Trustees (Zachar et al. 2016).

With the exception of severity scales for intellectual disability and autism spectrum disorder (ASD), the only dimensional proposals to make it into Section II (the section containing diagnostic criteria approved for routine clinical use) were the proposals to create dimensional spectra for substance use disorder (SUD) and ASD in which a single broad category is defined with subgroupings based entirely on severity. The creation of these dimensional spectra amounts to a *decategorization based on severity* of existing DSM-IV categorical constructs in which categorical diagnoses are eliminated in favor of a broader dimensional construct. In the case of SUD, the DSM-IV categories of substance dependence and substance abuse were eliminated from DSM-5 and replaced with a single SUD category with specifiers available to indicate three levels of severity based on the number of symptoms of the broad Substance Use category that are present: "mild" if 2–3 out of the 11 symptoms have been present, "moderate" if 4–5 symptoms have been present, and "severe" if 6 or more symptoms are been present. The broadly defined DSM-5 category of ASD replaces the DSM-IV categories of autistic disorder, Asperger's disorder, childhood disintegrative disorder, and pervasive developmental disorder—not otherwise specified (PDD-NOS), with specifiers available to indicate three levels of severity based on the level of support that is needed in both the social communication and restricted, repetitive behaviors domains.

There are two main advantages to this decategorization strategy. First, it reflects the reality of the absence of sharp boundaries between categorical diagnostic subgroupings that differ largely based on severity and thus avoids misleading researchers and clinicians into thinking that the subgroupings represent distinct diagnostic entities. Furthermore, by favoring a "lumping" strategy over the more typical "splitting" strategy which has historically guided most DSM decisions, it has the effect of reducing the number of DSM categorical overall, which conforms with clinicians' preferences for fewer categories in a diagnostic classification system (Reed et al. 2011). There are, however, a number of disadvantages of decategorization in favor of diagnostic spectra. First of all, it ignores the fact that the existing DSM diagnostic categories were originally established because of the clinical value of having distinct categories for lower-severity forms of a disorder. These lower-severity categories typically involve different management strategies and have different long-term prognoses. Moreover, given the omnipresence of stigma associated with virtually all mental disorders, lower-severity categories are typically viewed by patients, families, and the public at large as less stigmatizing and more acceptable (Ben-Zeev et al. 2010).

Let us consider the cases of SUD and ASD in turn. Starting with DSM-III, SUDs have been covered by two diagnostic entities: substance dependence, a generally more severe condition which was defined in terms of the individual's impaired control over their use of a substance, and the less severe substance abuse category, which reflected problematic use. Although the original plan for DSM-III-R was to eliminate the DSM-III Abuse category because of problems which were identified with using social and occupational consequences to define abuse (Rounsaville et al. 1986), pragmatic concerns about having a diagnostic label for anyone needing help with substance use overrode validity concerns (Wakefield 2015) and the category was retained in both DSM-III-R and DSM-IV. The DSM-5 work group chose to replace the DSM-IV substance dependence and substance abuse categories with a single SUD category for two main reasons (Hasin et al. 2013). First, both factor analyses and item response theory analyses of the DSM-IV dependence and abuse items found a single unidimensional construct for all of the DSM-IV items (except for substance-related legal problems), which supported having a single broad category rather than two categories. Second, a number of problems had been identified with the DSM-IV abuse category, including lower reliability and validity compared to dependence and the fact that although abuse was assumed to be of lesser severity than dependence, some abuse items (e.g., failure to fulfill major role obligations) indicated clinically severe cases. It should be noted that an alternative solution to the abuse category problems could have been to retain the category and fix the diagnostic criteria to address the reliability and validity problems. From a conceptual standpoint, substance dependence and abuse are clearly separable with dependence being comparable to the concept of addiction in which the person has impaired control over substance use whereas abuse reflects the negative consequences of excessive substance use. There is clinical utility to the concept that individuals can develop destructive substance-related behaviors without having gotten to the point that they are unable to control their use, a distinction which is lost by having a single unidimensional construct. Moreover, the claim that the dependence and abuse items are unidimensional is weakened by the observation that this finding may in fact be an artifact of poor wording of the existing diagnostic criteria that fail to draw a clear distinction between the dependence/abuse concepts (Wakefield 2015).

The severity-based decategorization of the DSM-IV categories of autistic disorder, Asperger's disorder, childhood disintegrative disorder, and PDD-NOS appears largely motivated by problems that the DSM-5 Neurodevelopmental Work Group identified with the Asperger's disorder criteria set according to the Rationale section of the Asperger's disorder page on the DSM-5 web site (DSM-5 Neurodevelopmental Work Group 2010a). First of all, the requirement in Asperger's disorder of no significant general delay in early language development can be difficult to determine in retrospect, especially for adolescents and adults.

Moreover, the requirement that other specific pervasive developmental disorders (e.g., autistic disorder) trump the diagnosis of Asperger's disorder means that most Asperger's cases should actually be diagnosed as autistic disorder since language delay is not a required feature of autistic disorder (i.e., most cases of Asperger's disorder would meet the autistic disorder criterion B(2), "marked impairment in the ability to initiate or sustain a conversation with others"). Finally, research suggests that the requirement for lack of early language impairment does not demarcate a meaningful subgroup of autism cases in terms of course/outcome, etiology, neurocognitive profile, and treatment needs, thus supporting the perspective that Asperger's disorder is not substantially different from other forms of high-functioning autism and should be eliminated as a distinct category separate from autistic disorder.

Other researchers, however, claim that Asperger's is distinct from other subgroups within the autism spectrum (Matson and Wilkins 2008) and that the lack of differentiating findings reflects different samples being identified as Asperger's in such studies (Klin et al. 2005). Rather than supporting the elimination of Asperger's disorder, these researchers suggested modifying the Asperger's criteria to reflect the need for a more stringent diagnostic approach with a more nuanced view of onset patterns and early language.

Furthermore, a potentially significant downside of eliminating the Asperger's disorder diagnosis is the risk of increasing the stigma of those with the condition (Ben-Zeev et al. 2010). Applying the ASD label to those who have the Asperger's disorder label has the potential to increase stigma because they will be seen as the same as those with autism, despite having milder symptoms. Indeed, a study by Kite and colleagues (Kite et al. 2013) which surveyed 547 health and educational professionals about the proposed change in labeling revealed that about half of the survey participants objected to the change, with 15% citing higher stigma as the key reason. Similarly, parents of adolescents with Asperger's as well as adults with Asperger's had expressed concerns about belonging to more broadly defined autism group rather than to a milder and presumably less stigmatized Asperger's group (Calzada et al. 2012, Giles 2014). On the other hand, a 2015 internet-based study in which adults in the United States (obtained from MTurk, a site which recruits participants to take surveys) were asked to review a vignette of a child with Asperger's disorder that was accompanied by a label of ASD Asperger's, or no label at all, and to rate it in terms of stigma attitudes, found no relationship between stigma rating and whether the case was labeled with the ASD or the Asperger's label or lacked a label entirely (Ohan et al. 2015). In any case, given the potential effect on stigma of eliminating the Asperger's category, the DSM-5 work group clearly prioritized making their decision on scientific grounds (i.e., the purportedly increased validity of the ASD category despite the lack of consensus in the field regarding the supporting evidence) rather than considering the social impacts of the change.

In conclusion, the trend in DSM-5 towards decategorization based on severity, which appears to be motivated by the push in DSM-5 towards dimensionality, has significant practical downsides in terms of eliminating clinically useful distinctions and potentially increasing stigma. It is also notable that the decategorization of SUD and ASD is inconsistent with the strategy used elsewhere in DSM-5 of continuing to keep separate less versus more severe versions of a condition based on symptoms and/or prognosis, such as maintaining the distinction between schizophrenia and schizophreniform disorder, two conditions that have essentially the same symptoms but differ based on their persistence. Notably, in contrast to the Substance and Neurodevelopmental Work Groups, the Neurocognitive Work Group adopted the exact opposite strategy by adding to DSM-5 a new category, mild neurocogitive disorder, that differs from its more severe counterpart, major neurocognitive disorder, based entirely on severity and functional impairment. Although the stated rationale for adding this category to DSM-5 was to "recognize the substantial clinical needs of individuals who have mild cognitive deficits . . . but can function independently" (DSM-5 Neurocognitive Disorder Work Group 2010b), the decision to include it as a separate disorder rather than creating a single neurocognitive disorder category with specifiers for "mild," "moderate," and "severe" has not been documented. Most likely it was to avoid the stigmatization that would likely have occurred by including this condition as part of the same category that includes dementia.

References

American Psychiatric Assocation Assembly (2012). APA Assembly Notes http://alabama-psych.org/wp-content/uploads/2012/02/apa_assembly_notes_may_2012.pdf Accessed December 29, 2015.

American Psychiatric Association (2013). Use of the Manual. In *Diagnostic and Statistical Manual of Mental Disorders*, 5th edn, pp. 19–24. Arlington, VA: American Psychiatric Association.

Ben-Zeev, D., **Young, M.A.**, and **Corrigan, P.W.** (2010). DSM-V and the stigma of mental illness. *Journal of Mental Health*, **19**, 318–327.

Calzada, L.R., **Pistrang, N.**, and **Mandy, W.P.** (2012). High-functioning autism and Asperger's disorder: utility and meaning for families. *Journal of Autism and Developmental Disorders*, **42**, 230–243.

DSM-5 Neurodevelopmental Work Group. (2010a). Asperger's Disorder—Rationale section from archived version (March 19, 2010) of DSM-5 web page (https://web.archive.org/web/20100314185048/http://www.dsm5.org/ProposedRevisions/Pages/proposedrevision.aspx?rid=97#). Retrieved December 31, 2015.

DSM-5 Neurocognitive Disorder Work Group. (2010b). Minor Neurocognitive Disorder—Rationale tab from archived March 19, 2010 DSM-5 web page https://web.archive.org/web/20100312130342/http://www.dsm5.org/ProposedRevisions/Pages/proposedrevision.aspx?rid=420# Retrieved December 31, 2015.

Giles, D.C. (2014). "DSM-V Is taking away our identity": the reaction of the online community to the proposed changes in the diagnosis of Asperger's disorder. *Health*, **18**, 179–195.

Goldberg, D., **Simms, L.J.**, **Gater, R.**, and **Krueger, R.F.** (2011). Integration of dimensional spectra for depression and anxiety into categorical diagnoses for general medical practice. In D.A. Regier, W.E. Narrow, E.A. Kuhl, and D.J. Kupfer (eds.) *The Conceptual Evoluation of DSM-5*, pp. 19–36. Arlington, VA: American Psychiatric Association.

Hasin, D.S., O'Brien, C.P., Auriacombe, M., et al. (2013). DSM-5 criteria for substance use disorders: recommendations and rationale. *American Journal of Psychiatry*, **170**, 834–851.

Helzer, J.E. (2011). A Proposal for incorporating clinically relevant dimensions into DSM-5. In D.A. Regier, W.E. Narrow, E.A. Kuhl, and D.J. Kupfer (eds.) *The Conceptual Evolution of DSM-5*, pp. 81–96. Arlington, VA: American Psychiatric Association.

Helzer, J., Kraemer H., Krueger, R.F., et al. (eds.) (2008a). *Dimensional Approaches in Diagnostic Classification: Refining the research agenda for DSM-V.* Arlington, VA, American Psychiatric Association.

Helzer, J.E., Wittchen, H., Krueger, R.F., and **Kraemer, H.C.** (2008b). Dimensional options for DSM-V: The way forward. In J.E. Helzer, H.C. Kraemer, R.F. Krueger, et al. (eds.) *Dimensional Approaches in Diagnostic Classification*, pp. 115–127. Arlington, VA: American Psychiatric Association:.

Kite, D.M., J. Gullifer, and **Tyson, G.A.** (2013). Views on the diagnostic labels of autism and Asperger's disorder and the proposed changes in the DSM. *Journal of Autism and Developmental Disorders*, **43**, 1692–1700.

Klin, A., Pauls, D., Schultz, R., and **Volkmar, F.** (2005). Three diagnostic approaches to Asperger syndrome: Implications for research. *Journal of Autism and Developmental Disorders*, **35**, 221–234.

Krueger, R.F., Eaton, N.R., South, S.C., et al. (2011). Empirically-derived personality disorder prototypes: bridging dimensions and categories in DSM-5. In D.A. Regier, W.E. Narrow, E.A. Kuhl, and D.J. Kupfer (eds.) *The Conceptual Evolution of DSM-5*, pp. 97–118. Arlington, VA: American Psychiatric Association:

Kupfer, D., First, M.B., and Regier, D., Eds. (2002a). *A Research Agenda for DSM-V.* Washington, DC: American Psychiatric Publishing.

Kupfer, D., First, M.B., and **Regier, D** (2002b). Introduction. In D. Kupfer, M. First and D. Regier (eds.) *A Research Agenda for DSM-V*, pp. xv–xxiii. Washington, DC: American Psychiatric Association.

Matson, J.L. and **Wilkins, J.** (2008). Nosology and diagnosis of Asperger's syndrome. *Research in Autism Spectrum Disorders*, **2**, 288–300.

Ohan, J.L., Ellefson, S.E., and **Corrigan, P.W.** (2015). Brief report: the impact of changing from DSM-IV's "Asperger's" to DSM-5's "autistic spectrum disorder" diagnostic labels on stigma and treatment attitudes *Journal of Autism and Developmental Disorders*, **45**, 3384–3389.

Reed, G.M., Correia, J.M., Esparza, P., et al. (2011). The WPA-WHO global survey of psychiatrists' attitudes towards mental disorders classification. *World Psychiatry*, **10**, 118–131.

Regier, D., Narrow, W., Kuhl E.A., and **Kupfer, D.J.** (2009). The conceptual development of DSM-V. *American Journal of Psychiatry*, **166**, 645–650.

Regier, D.A., Narrow W.E., Kuhl E.A., and **Kupfer, D.J.** (ed.) (2011). *The Conceptual Evolution of DSM-5.* Arlington, VA: American Psychiatric Association.

Rounsaville, B., Alarcon, R., Andrews, G., et al. (2002). Basic nomenclature issues for DSM-V. In D. Kupfer, M. First, and D. Regier (eds.) *Research Agenda for DSM-V*, pp. 1–30. Washington, DC: American Psychiatric Association.

Rounsaville, B.J., Spitzer, R.L., and **Williams, J.B.** (1986). Proposed changes in DSM-III substance use disorders: description and rationale. *American Journal of Psychiatry*, **143**, 463–468.

Wakefield, J.C. (2015). DSM-5 substance use disorder: how conceptual missteps weakened the foundations of the addictive disorders field. *Acta Psychiatrica Scandinavica*, **132**, 327–334.

Wittchen, H., Hofler, M., Gloster, A.T., et al. (2011). Options and dilemmas of dimensional measures for DSM-5: Which types of measures fare best in predicting course and outcome? In D.A. Regier, W.E. Narrow, E.A. Kuhl, and D.J. Kupfer (eds.) *The Conceptual Evolution of DSM-5*, pp. 119–147. Arlington, VA: American Psychiatric Association.

Zachar, P., Krueger, R.F., and **Kendler, K.S.** (2016). Personality disorder in DSM-5: an oral history. *Psychological Medicine*, **46**, 1–10.

Section 9

Auditory verbal hallucinations

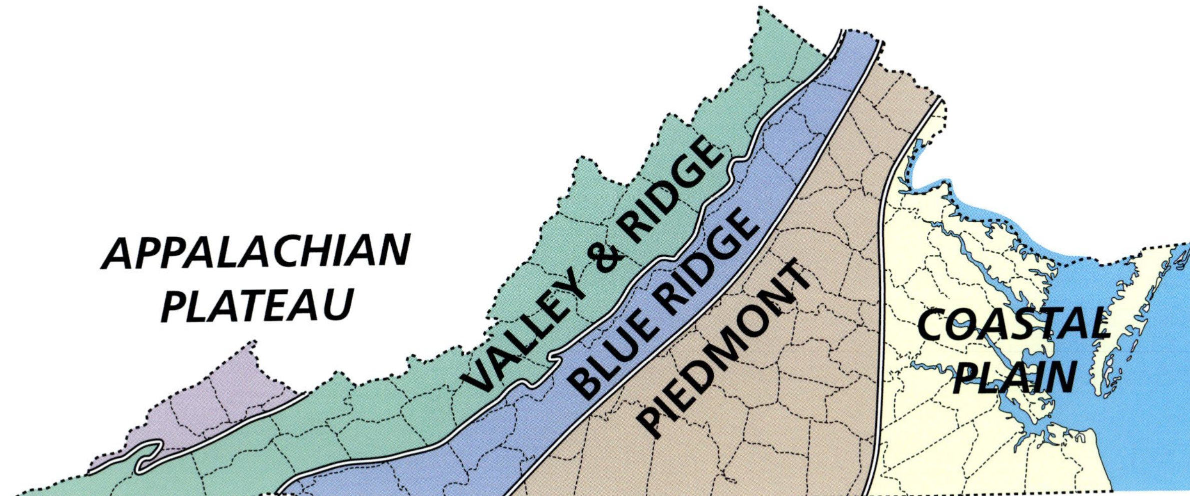

Figure 5.1 A map of Virginia, divided into meaningful but arbitrary (MBA) regions.

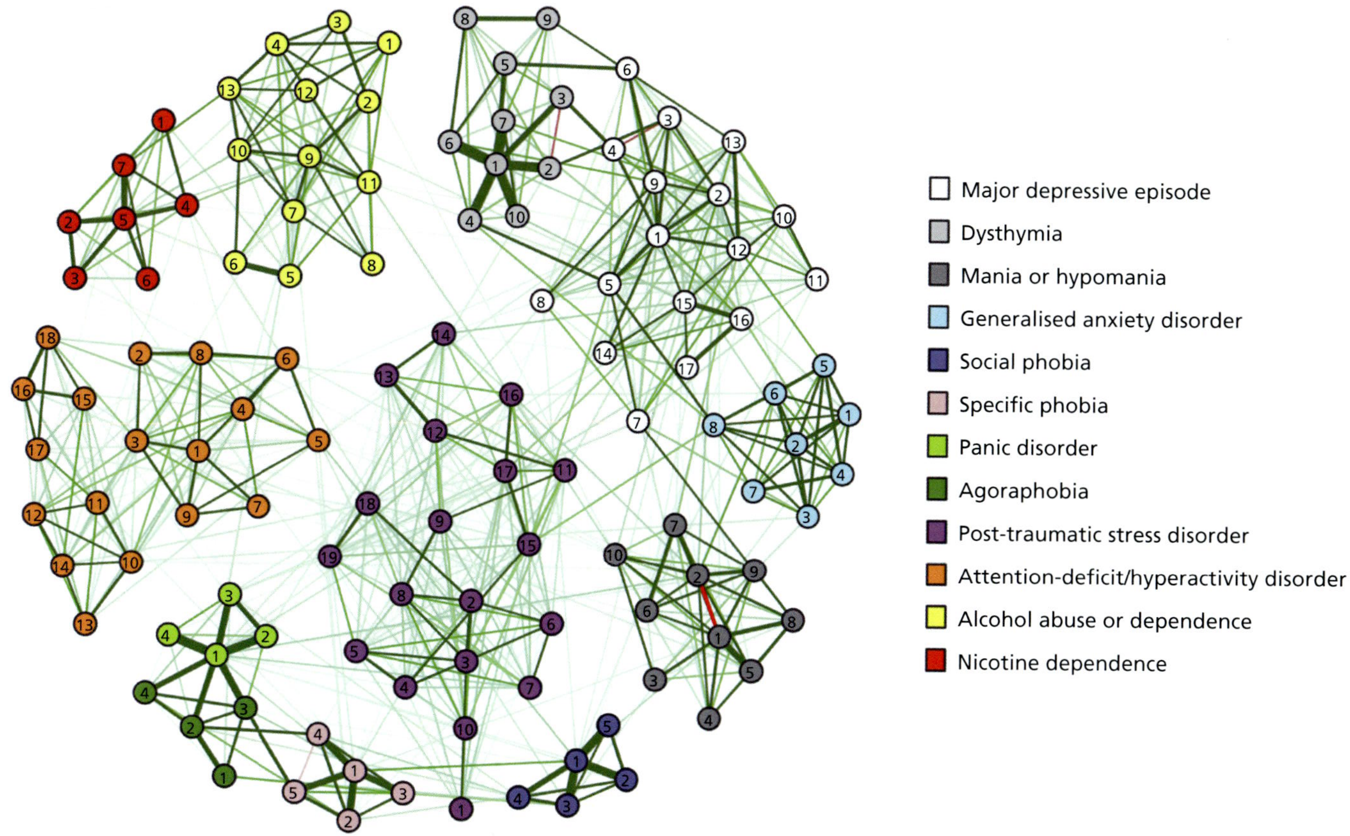

Figure 11.1 Network structure as fitted DSM-IV symptom data from a large community sample (Boschloo et al. 2015), using the R-software package IsingFit (Van Borkulo et al. 2014). Individual symptoms are represented as nodes. The strength of connections between symptoms is estimated using a penalized regression model. In the figure, stronger positive (negative) connections are represented by thicker green (red) edges. Disorders emerge out of the analysis as sets of tightly connected symptoms that tend to synchronize through the connectivity structure. Comorbidity arises as a result of edges that connect symptoms from distinct disorders ('bridge symptoms').

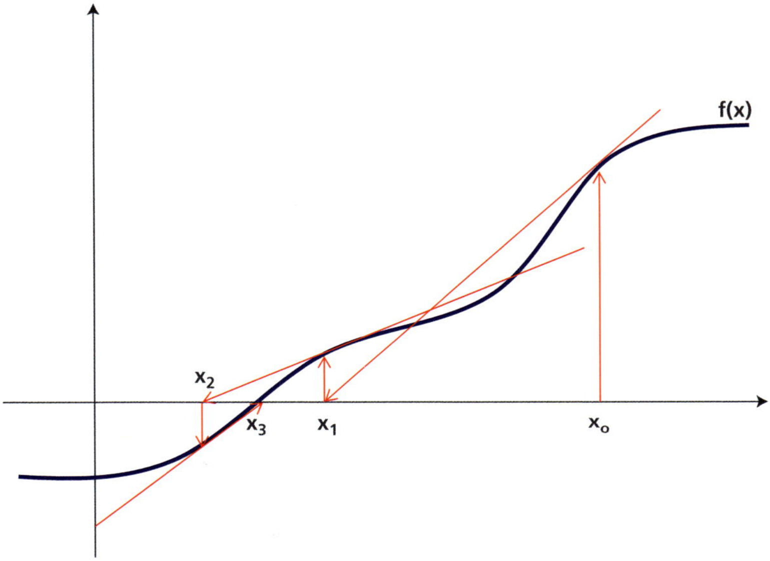

Figure 29.1 Newton's method as an example of mathematical iteration.

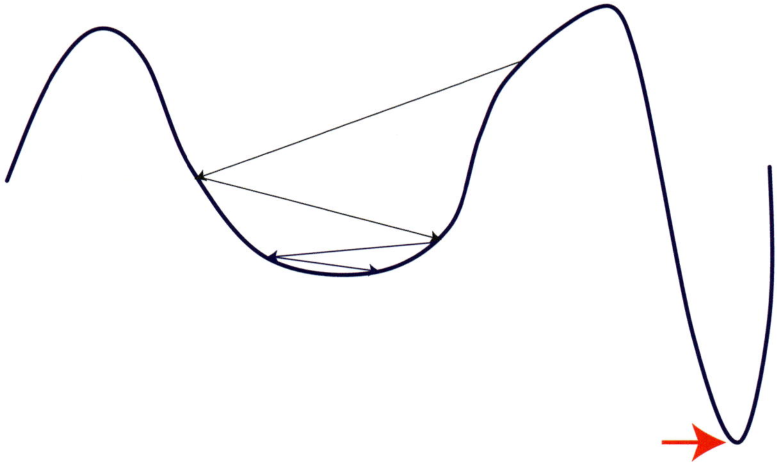

Figure 29.2 Illustration of the local minimum problem.

Chapter 25

Introduction to "The ontology and epistemology of symptoms: The case of auditory verbal hallucinations in schizophrenia"

Kenneth S. Kendler

Josef Parnas has spent his career spanning the worlds of mainstream psychiatric research and phenomenological psychiatry—a discipline based in a European philosophical tradition unfamiliar to many U.S. and British mental health professionals. He presents us with a "deep critique" of the *Diagnostic and Statistical Manual of Mental Disorders* (DSM) enterprise and, indeed, the entire diagnostic movement within psychiatry based on the operationalization of psychiatric symptoms and signs. He is not worried about problems of reliability or those of comparing different validators such as outcome or drug responsiveness. His critique is deeper and the example he chooses to illustrate his concerns is the assessment of and meaning of auditory verbal hallucinations (AVH).

One way to frame what Dr. Parnas and Dr. Urfer-Parnas (hereafter Parnas and Parnas) are driving at is whether, in psychiatry, we can assume that symptoms are things people have (like a sore throat, tennis elbow, or shortness of breath), or do they instead reflect either how people "are" or "how they experience themselves and their world." This is not a black or white distinction but a gray scale of relative objectivity and subjectivity. If the symptom is something a person "has," then it is often possible to assess it relatively well with straightforward questions. For example, for urinary tract infections we ask, "Does it burn when you urinate?" In evaluating the risk for myocardial infarction, we ask, "Do you feel pressure or pain in your chest on exertion?" There is inevitably a subjective sense to these feelings and there might be embarrassment in talking about certain human functions (e.g., urination). One can question what it means to "burn" or what exactly is meant by feeling "pressure" on my chest. But in the pragmatic world of medicine, we have for decades assumed such questions are "good enough" for regular patient care, assuming the clinician and the respondent understand one another's language and vocabulary.

Does psychiatry have symptoms like this? I think so, although this is not a topic that Parnas and Parnas discuss. Examples might include "loss of weight," "insomnia," and "phobic avoidance." I think these symptoms can, to a first approximation, be treated like the questions about burning sensations while urinating, or chest pain. Questions such as, "Have you lost weight in the last 2 weeks?", "Are you having more trouble getting to sleep at night than is usual for you?" or "Do you feel comfortable going into a crowded theater?", while subject to a range of potential problems, are generally "good enough" for regular use in clinical psychiatry with no extra fuss.

But Parnas and Parnas argue this approach is unlikely to work well with AVHs. In an ideal world, I agree. That is, questions like, "Do you hear voices that other people cannot hear?" is, in some important ways, not like asking about burning sensations or difficulty sleeping. Why not? I think at least two sets of factors are involved. First, such questions are subject to a much greater level of contextual factors than our simple questions, which can result in frequent false positives and false negatives. Indeed, with colleagues, we have shown that such a question about "voices" yields very high false-positive rates when asked in general population samples by non-clinicians (Kendler et al. 1996). For example, a respondent who is mentally healthy, but who has the experience of God communicating with him when deep in prayer, could answer "yes." Or she may think the question meant the "voice of conscience," which she experiences when she is thinking about doing something "bad." This is why I am quite skeptical about the meaning of the large literature assessing, by checklist, psychotic symptoms in the general population (van Os et al. 2009).

Second, and this is the main focus of the following essay, it might be wrong to assume that one "has" AVH in the same way as one might "have" burning urination or insomnia. The symptom strikes deeper into the sense of experienced selfhood that is poorly, and indeed inaccurately, tapped by the term "voices." Shifting to a different symptom that for me even better illustrates this problem, some individuals with severe depression experience a deep derealization (Hornstein 2009, Ratcliffe 2015). The world around them is no longer the world they lived in. It is foreboding and dark. The joy, beauty, and love they used to experience are gone. It is no longer their world. This can be clinically very important, but it is difficult or impossible to ask usefully about such experiences with the typical short question. While the query, "Does the world around you feel different?" might get the discussion going, it is hardly adequate as a definitive probe. This symptom is not something such patients "have." Rather it is something they "are." It cannot be accurately assessed by an item in a structured interview but rather as part of a longer and deeper conversation with a skilled and experienced clinician.

Given the validity of these concerns, I do not share the sense of Parnas and Parnas that this reflects a deep crisis with the DSM diagnostic system. To explain why not in this brief essay, I need to explain why there are many times when this operationalized approach to psychiatric diagnosis deserves to be called "OK but not great." That is, we need to balance pragmatic needs with practical aims. Most obviously, if I am working in a busy emergency room and I need to get a quick diagnostic view of a quite psychotic patient, I will ask, among other things, "Do you hear voices?" It is not the best, but I don't have time for the in-depth assessment. Despite its crudity it will most typically get me some important information.

Then there is the problem of research. Imagine I have $1 million to spend to do the field work for a large-scale molecular genetic study of schizophrenia and my goal is to have enough power to detect risk loci. If I have an experienced psychiatrist spend 8 hours reviewing every hospital record and talking in detail with the patient in an assessment which could tap the subtle symptoms that Parnas and Parnas are describing, that would likely cost $3000 per patient. So I would spend all my grant money to evaluate 333 patients. However, if I develop a 1 page assessment that required a quick look at hospital records and then a 20 minute interview assessing only key symptoms and signs with simple questions, that might cost $200 per patient so I could study 5000 patients. While I do not doubt the 8 hour evaluation will be of higher quality, would the error with the second method in diagnosing schizophrenia be so substantial that it would produce weaker genetic signals than the much smaller study with better assessment? I doubt it. Indeed, evidence from the major genome-wide association of schizophrenia published in *Nature* in 2014 (Schizophrenia Working Group of the Psychiatric Genomics Consortium 2014) shows this is not the case. The molecular genetic profile of cases diagnosed using such "light" phenotyping do not differ substantially from those assessed using quite intense methods.

So, I do not agree with the dire message of this essay by Parnas and Parnas. However, I want to conclude on a different note where we are in much deeper agreement. There are a variety of pressures on psychiatry today which have the aggregate effect of loosening our links to our psychopathologic heritage. It is one thing to know how to do a quick diagnostic assessment in the emergency room or for a large-scale research study, and it is another to think that is the only proper way to do a psychiatric evaluation. Especially in the non-urgent clinical work we do, which gives us the time and space for careful efforts to understand the lived experience of our patients, this remains a vital skill that should be fostered in all mental health professionals. But that is not happening in U.S. training programs where, in too many instances, a clinical assessment becomes reduced to an evaluation of the relevant DSM criteria. That is tragic. What the following lovely essay shows is the depth of subtle aspects of the assessment of "voices" and how much an exploration of these issues can improve our understanding of the experiences of our patients. Such explorations result in better clinical care and well recompense the time and effort involved in deepening our understanding of the lived experiences of those whose care is in our hands.

References

Hornstein, G. (2009). *Agnes's Jacket: A psychologist's search for the meanings of madness.* Emmaus, PA: Rodale Books.

Kendler, K.S., Gallagher, T.J., Abelson, J.M., and **Kessler, R.C.** (1996). Lifetime prevalence, demographic risk factors, and diagnostic validity of nonaffective psychosis as assessed in a US community sample. The National Comorbidity Survey. *Archives of General Psychiatry*, 53, 1022–1031.

Ratcliffe, M. (2015). *Experiences of Depression: A study in phenomenology.* Oxford: Oxford University Press.

Schizophrenia Working Group of the Psychiatric Genomics Consortium. (2014). Biological insights from 108 schizophrenia-associated genetic loci. *Nature*, **511**, 421–427.

van Os, J., **Linscott, R.J.**, **Myin-Germeys, I.**, **Delespaul, P.**, and **Krabbendam, L.** (2009). A systematic review and meta-analysis of the psychosis continuum: evidence for a psychosis proneness-persistence-impairment model of psychotic disorder. *Psychological Medicine*, **39**, 179–195.

Chapter 26

The ontology and epistemology of symptoms: The case of auditory verbal hallucinations in schizophrenia

Josef Parnas and Annick Urfer-Parnas

26.1 Basic nosological tenets

Addressing and discussing the critical theoretical issues in psychiatric nosology during the era after the fifth edition of the *Diagnostic and Statistical Manual of Mental Disorders* (DSM-5) must include a thorough consideration of symptoms and signs. It is generally accepted that symptoms and signs are the most basic elements or terms of psychiatric description and classification. The notion of "symptoms" designates the patient's subjective complaints (e.g., a feeling of pain), whereas "signs" describe the "objective," publically observable, "external," or "third-person" features.

It is remarkable that psychiatry is largely mute on the nature of these phenomena with few, typically ignored exceptions (Stanghellini et al. 2012). It seems that the very possibility of such a discussion appears as potentially subverting a widespread, tacit acceptance of the behaviorist epistemology of current psychiatry.

A systematic reflection on the nature of symptoms and signs and the methods of their exploration, description, and analysis was undertaken by Karl Jaspers in the successive editions of his *General Psychopathology* (7th edition 1963). Unfortunately, Jaspers left no visible or enduring impact on contemporary psychopathology. During the "operational revolution" leading to the creation of the DSM-III, these epistemological issues were seen, if noticed at all, as largely unproblematic and treated in a behaviorist spirit that has persisted to this day (for a detailed account, see Parnas and Bovet 2015).

Thus, the prevalent and largely implicit approach can be articulated as a following series of interdependent assumptions:

- Addressing mental phenomena such as psychiatric symptoms and signs does not require any conceptualization of the nature of phenomenal (experiential) consciousness.
- Symptoms and signs have no pathogenetically relevant meaning, apart from causing distress and dysfunction.

- Rather, the symptoms and signs are purely epiphenomenal, with a referential function, i.e., they are indicative of and reducible to the malfunctioning neural circuits.
- They are envisaged as well-demarcated, mutually independent, thing-like entities, amenable to unproblematic demonstration by a structured interview (performed by a layperson) or a checklist-based identification and quantification (Nordgaard et al. 2013, Parnas and Bovet 2015).
- Finally, symptoms and signs are definable "operationally," i.e. in brief, commonsensical, lay-language statements (Parnas and Bovet 2015).

In the following section, we address and describe the clinical–phenomenological manifestations of auditory verbal hallucinations (AVH) in schizophrenia. We have chosen AVH as a paradigmatic case of a symptom because it is a central feature of schizophrenia and happens to be one of our current research interests. We will then assess to what extent the contemporary theoretical assumptions listed above cohere with what we can learn about the phenomenology of AVH. However, we first briefly introduce the reader to the historical vicissitudes of this concept, up to the most recent Research Domain Criteria (RDoC) research program (Ford et al. 2014).

26.2 Historical background

26.2.1 Nineteenth century and early twentieth century

During the nineteenth century, there seems to have occurred a certain division of psychopathological labor between French and German psychiatry: the issue of delusion was a central topic of German psychiatry whereas the French focused on hallucinations.

The first medical definition of hallucination is commonly attributed to J. E. D. Esquirol, the author of the first modern textbook of psychiatry, *Des maladies mentales considérées sous leur rapport médical, hygiénique et médico-légal* [Mental illness as considered in medical, hygienic, and medico-legal reports] (1838). Esquirol proposed a descriptive definition of hallucination as a "perception without object." In a pathogenetic sense, however, he considered hallucination as a "psychic" (i.e., psychological) abnormality that was unrelated to a sensory disturbance. In his view, a crucial aspect of hallucination was the patient's "intimate conviction" about the truth of the experience. Thus, Esquirol considered the nature of hallucinations as being close to that of delusion.

It is noteworthy that Esquirol's descriptive definition of hallucination survived until our time basically unchanged, although partly misunderstood by reifying the descriptive connotations of the term "perception." Hallucination became viewed as a sensory event with roots in a disorder of perception: for example, the general definition of schizophrenia in recent editions of the *International Classification of Diseases* (ICD-8 and ICD-10) contains a reference to "disorders of perception," i.e. hallucinations.

The French alienists of the mid nineteenth century debated the topic of hallucination at a famous series of meetings of the Société médico-psychologique in Paris from 1855 to 1856. Some of the issues addressed there still resonate in our times (Lanteri Laura 1991, Berrios 1996):

- Do hallucinations occur in mentally healthy individuals?
- Are hallucinations a product of a cognitive or a perceptual disorder?
- Are hallucinations caused by a disorder of the brain or the peripheral sensory apparatus or both?

J. Baillarger (1846) distinguished two types of hallucinations: the psychosensory, with sensory qualities, and the "psychic" hallucinations. He described the latter as a kind of "language of thought." Another important figure, J. P. Falret, regarded hallucination as an exclusive "disorder of reason" and not a passive, sensory phenomenon (Ey 1973, p. 81). The discussion of compatibility of hallucination with the sane or healthy reason was never completely resolved. Some authors did not see this question as a conceptual challenge but simply settled by the "testimony of the notables" (philosophers, members of the medical academy, etc.). The notables, by describing their own hallucinations, provided an empirical "proof" of coexistence of hallucination and an absence of mental disorder.

The anatomo-clinical model (i.e., medical model) was extremely successful in medicine and neurology in the nineteenth century, resulting in identification and classification of illnesses according to their clinical manifestations and their underlying etiology. The alienists tried to adopt the same epistemological approach to the study of mental illnesses. The hallucination lost its "psychic" (psychological) character; potential causal links between hallucinating subjects and their hallucinations became dissolved in favor of the search for biological substrate. Hallucinations surreptitiously regained their sensory character. The previous distinction between "psychic" and psychosensory hallucination was reduced to a question of intensity of causally relevant stimuli in the sensory apparatus. Inspired by the phrenological program of neurology (strongly supported by the discovery of the functional brain areas), the alienists developed an atomistic model of the pathophysiology: an autonomous and automatic excitation of certain zones of the brain linearly produced hallucinations. Thus, F. Leuret, a famous French psychiatrist (1797–1851), wondered how was it possible that a subject could hear several voices conversing, when the brain only had two hemispheres. The mechanistic approach culminated with A. Tamburini's theory, the"irritative doctrine" he proposed in 1880: hallucination was a product of an excitation of the centers of images, "a sensorial epilepsy" (Ey 1973, p. 91,5).

According to Ey (1973, p. 960), the "mechanistic dogma" of hallucination contained three essential components: (1) organic causation; (2) hallucination is a primary phenomenon, i.e., unrelated to delusion and unassociated with the psychological life of the subject; and (3) hallucination is issued from a simple neurosensory excitation (an elementary basic process).

At the beginning of the twentieth century, G. de Clérambault (1925/1992) developed a pure mechanical/organic conception of the causes of hallucinations, which were thereby separated from delusions. He described an autonomous, "anideic" (void of any psychological content) process, which he called the "petit syndrome d'Automatisme Mental" or syndrome of passivity. This was a group of symptoms that had an initial role in the formation of psychosis.[1] They included the "echo of thoughts," the "enunciation of acts," coenesthesias (abnormal bodily sensations), thought block and thought interference, hallucinations without sensorial qualities (close to "thoughts aloud") (De Clérambault, 1925/1992, p. 35). The "automatisme mental," considered as a purely organic etiology, led to a disaggregation or splitting of the self, which was a nuclear aspect of the incipient psychosis. The content of the psychotic symptoms of "grand automatisme" was a result of an "explicative construction" (De Clérambault, p. 34), depending on the sociocultural ideas of the historical period. Psychosensory hallucinations and primary delusions (which Clérambault equated) could subsequently develop. Finally, with the progression of the disease, other, secondary psychotic phenomena could emerge.

26.2.2 Current research

It is difficult to select a start date for contemporary research in AVH. One important line of research, in neurosurgery, demonstrated that stimulation of various sensory brain areas produce perception-like experiences; notably, a stimulation of superior temporal gyrus provoked auditory hallucinations (Penfield and Perot 1963). In all subsequent research into AVH, the AVH are considered as a well-demarcated empirical object in the world. The phenotype is explored by comparing hallucinated with non-hallucinated patients and, most frequently, by correlating duration and/or severity of hallucinations with a broad range of potentially disturbed neural substrates. These studies include structural brain imaging, beginning with PEG, followed by CT scans, fMRI, and evoked potentials (McCarthy-Jones 2013). The initial focus on cortical changes was progressively expanded to changes in the white matter. There are several reports of significant correlations (Plaze et al. 2011, van Tol 2013). However, no robust pathogenic finding has been established, except the functional role of auditory cortex. One interesting hypothesis, in part phenomenologically inspired, was advanced by Frith (1996) who proposed a lack of fronto-temporal inhibitory activity, leading to amplification of the inner speech and thus leading the patient to misattribute his own "inner voice" to others. The possibility for this misattribution or misidentification was hypothesized to be grounded in a reduced or disordered connectivity between different brain areas (e.g., in the primary and secondary auditory cortex and language processing areas). Other authors (Allen et al. 2008) suggested an alteration in the balance between top-down and bottom-up processing as a core deficit in AVH. Higher brain functions are unable to focus on important objects and the "noise" attracts undeserved significance. The disturbances in the bottom-up processes lead to spontaneous activity in the auditory cortex, flooding the higher brain areas and increasing the risk for misinterpretation (Upthegrove et al. 2016).

---

[1] The "petit automatisme" of Clerambault are nearly identical to the so-called "basic symptoms," a concept developed by Gross et al. (1992). The similarity in question is both descriptive and conceptual.

In the recent National Institute of Mental Health (NIMH) research program, RDoC, the AVH is defined in the following way: "a conscious sensory experience that occurs in the absence of corresponding external stimulation of the relevant sense organ and has sufficient sense of reality to resemble a veridical perception" (Ford et al. 2014). These authors advocate the measurement of the phenotype of hallucination with a reliable rating scale, in which hallucination is treated as an empirical acoustic object and rated for pitch, duration, severity, etc. "[...] traditional notions of symptom are supplanted by an emphasis on quantification and relationship to neural system" (Ford et al. 2014, p. 295). In the RDoC multilevel approach, the neural level considered to be of relevance for the AVH begins with cochlear neurons and continues all the way up to the superior temporal gyrus. On the neurocognitive level, the RDoC suggests studying a so-called "Perception Construct," which includes several unimodal and multimodal perceptual/sensory tasks. Thus, it appears that there is unbroken conceptual and physiological continuity from the time of the alienists to the RDoC: "modern neuroscience ... sets investigators off to hunt for genes and pathophysiology to explain overlapping and heterogeneous clusters of symptoms" (Ford et al. 2014, p. 295). Nothing in the RDoC conceptual framework goes beyond what the alienists had already envisaged. The RDoC does not manifest interest in the phenomenology of AVH.

26.3 Phenomenology of AVH

We now present phenomenological features of AVH as they are typically described in the literature and encountered in our own clinical experience and in ongoing data collection in a new research project. The term "phenomenology" in this paper does not refer to the commonsense (DSM-style) description as it is understood in the anglophone literature, but refers to a phenomenological exploration of the patient's experience, which is not only concerned with the content of the experience (e.g., that a patient is persecuted by a male or female voice with a low or high pitch), but the structure of experience as well, such as its mode of arising and articulation (giveness), space, time, etc. Given that DSM-V and the RDoC consider hallucination as a perception-like experience resembling veridical perception, our phenomenological exposition will address this assumption in detail.

26.3.1 The nature of voices and their hearing

The literature is full of the adjectives "auditive" and "acoustic," which are used interchangeably, but mean something slightly different but complementary. The term *auditive* refers to the process of listening to and hearing, in other words to the receptive aspect of the experience, whereby the term *acoustic* refers to the sound which is being emitted and heard.

The term "voices" comes from folk psychology (Berrios 1996) and it is one of the terms that a psychiatric patient invariably learns very quickly. It is important to realize that patients often use the term as a metaphor for experiences that do not have much in common with auditory perception; in other words, it is necessary to explore their complaints in more detail. As an example, a patient designates his episodes of thought insertion as "hearing voices," even though there is nothing acoustic and no actual hearing is involved (no audition). In the majority of cases patients report experiencing linguistic fragments, interpellations, comments, or commands: it is exceptional for the patient to be exposed to an articulate, complex discourse. As a rule, these linguistic fragments have a self-referential content. The patient's actions are typically commented on and his person denigrated: "he's smoking now," "now he's walking to the door," "he's worthless," and so on. Sometimes the voices speak a language the patient does not know: one of our patients heard voices in an Inuit language, which she did not know. However, she claimed to understand single phrases.

The most characteristic feature of the voices is the *phenomenological poverty*. The voice may be of a specific gender or be indeterminate, is sometimes described as being robotic or mechanic, and is typically without a qualitative richness of perceptual detail. Typically, the patient describes the "voices" as being unlike real voices and only rarely confuses his hallucinations with normal perceptions. The perceptual poverty may be so extreme that the voices are *without voice*, without any loudness or sound, in sum without acoustic or auditory features (Eugen Bleuler "soundless voices"). Rather, the patient experiences flashes of meaning, which articulate themselves in an unmediated, direct manner in his mind. It is important to note that sometimes, when the psychiatrist presses the patient for more detail about the AVH, the patient becomes stuck and is unable to provide a more detailed description. Such situations may suggest that the psychiatrist tacitly operates with a perceptual model of hallucination, whereas the patient has an experience of a direct articulation of meaning without mediation of sensible qualities.

It is noteworthy that we can often observe transitions to what is called "influence or passivity phenomena." Thus, the patient may describe the voices as "signals" or "energy pulses" that impact his mind. The voices may "work" on the patient, they "torture" him, are emitted in order to control his movements. One of our patients, when cycling through the city, "heard voices" from the electric cables directing his path. Finally, the voices may become personified and the patient may claim that another person has invaded him.

26.3.2 Hallucinatory space

For our purposes, we distinguish between external space, space of the body, a so-called "lived space," and our interiority or internal space. Perception is a phenomenon *par excellence* that is deployed in the external space; it is one of the sources of "natural attitude," in which the world is given as real and mind-independent. Thus, external space is characterized by objectivity or accessibility from a third-person perspective. It contains places/things/objects in three-dimensional topographical relations to each other. The object is in a certain location and is experienced as real, existing independently of our mind. The perceptual object is always experienced partially or incompletely, i.e., from a specific (and therefore limited) perspective, and, so to say, "invites" a further exploration.

Importantly, a perceptual object appears in space as "public," accessible to others. It is crucial to understand that "publicness" is not something *inferred* about the object but is an intrinsic dimension of perceptual experience, an aspect of the object's appearance. We see an object as public and potentially exposed to other perspectives.

The objective external space becomes domesticated and modified by subjectivity and this felt, pragmatic space of human experience, action, and interaction is called a "lived space." The lived space overlaps with our "inner space" and bodily space.

The inner or internal space (immanence) is only a space in a metaphorical sense. It does not have an autonomous prior existence as a sort of a container that may become filled with mental contents. Rather, it is the stream of consciousness (thinking, imaging, . . .), as a self-presence that constitutes it as a private interiority, inaccessible to others. Normally, in our engaged involvement with the world (e.g., playing tennis), we are not explicitly aware of our interiority, except when we start thinking, imaging, self-reflecting, etc. The bodily space may be considered as a mixture or interface of externality and immanence (internal space). In one sense, it is a part of our interiority and lived space when "I am my body." On the other hand, the body also exists as an object of external space, akin to other material objects in the world (e.g., when I inspect my hands). A normal bodily experience consists of a seamless constant oscillation between the subjective-immanent and objectified dimensions. Bodily experience in schizophrenia is very often dominated by spatialization and objectivation (e.g., a patient claims that he is able to have his muscles detach themselves from each other, or that his thinking processes are localized in the posterior part of the brain). The patient often considers his body as an object that somehow does not fit his mind.

AVH are described by the patients as being in "the head," in the external space, or originating in the body. They may be experienced auditively, through the ears or "heard" by the mind. It is characteristic of all types of hallucinations (or their combination) that the patient considers them as *privately experienced* phenomena and he does not expect the psychiatrist to hear his voices. Some patients even say that the voices are in "another dimension." Even a patient with clearly externalized objectified hallucinatory voices never succeeds in inscribing them into the fabric of our shared social world. In contrast, an acute organic delirious patient perceives his visual hallucinatory object as an integral part of the visual space: he tries to convince others of the phenomenon and the hallucinatory scene is filled with potential actions. In schizophrenia, however, hallucinations "are not of this world," but rather in front of it (Merleau-Ponty 1962).

From a phenomenological perspective, there is no difference in kind but a difference of the process of externalization (self-objectification, see below). It is important to note that despite the possible externality of the voices, they are felt as being radically dissimilar from normal acoustic perceptual phenomena. Very often, they lack spatial features: they seem to exist diffusely or everywhere, they do not come from any particular direction and may violate the physical laws of space. In so-called "extracampine" hallucinations, the patients may hear voices in his workplace when he is sitting at home or hear voices that come from other cities or countries. Voices experienced only internally were previously called "psychic hallucinations" or "pseudohallucinations" (Baillarger 1846). The concept of pseudohallucination in particular has a very tortuous history and unclear meaning: e.g., Jaspers (1963) had his own definition, as an inner experience, phenomenologically midway between perception and imagery (Rasmussen and Parnas 2015).

26.3.3 The mode of givenness

Hallucinations are given (present themselves to the subject) in an abrupt, immediate fashion as the meanings that they carry. In contrast to perception, there is no temporal contour to the hallucination and no possibility for a reflective delay on the part of the subject; the meaning is given all at once, as a revelation, deprived of any perspectival incompleteness, and there is nothing more for the subject to explore. One of our patients was amazed by how much "talking" he could grasp in an instant and by the fact that he could distinguish the content of six different voices speaking simultaneously. Such an experience has no analogy in normal perception.

In this sense, the hallucination is an "aprioric" phenomenon because the articulation of its meaning bypasses the mediation by perception and cognition. The givenness of hallucination cannot be described as a relation between the subject and hallucination as an intentional object, but has a character as a disclosure and revelation within the subject (Naudin 1997, Charbonneau et al. 2001). Naturally, the process of externalization and delusional elaboration makes the well-articulated hallucination close to an intentional object. The process of self-objectivation or alienation of the parts of the self is known in phenomenology as "alterization." The patient does not *have a hallucination*, but *is hallucinated*. The subject is in a condition of complete passivity and exposure. The hallucination articulates itself in his most private sphere. He can no longer extricate himself from the hallucinatory experience (hyperproximity): he can only distract himself by listening to music or other activities.

26.3.4 "Thoughts aloud" (*Gedankenlautwerden*) and destructuration of consciousness

In the majority of patients with AVH, the hallucinations emerge upon a background of a phenomenon called *Gedankenlaufwerden* ("thoughts aloud") considered by Schneider (1950/1959) as being pathognomonic for the diagnosis of schizophrenia. This phenomenon has many variants; here we describe the most frequent one. Some patients have experienced thoughts aloud since childhood or adolescence and many such patients assume that everyone tends to hear their own thoughts aloud.

Thoughts aloud reflect a basic alteration in the structure of subjectivity. Normal thinking articulates itself as a series of meanings or associations that may be supported by fragments of imagery or inner speech with its flashes of linguistic formations. Yet the thoughts are not iconic; they are not given through phenomenal signs; we do not hear or see (read) them. There is no experiential distance between the thinking subject, his thinking act, and the thought-meaning (except for certain self-reflecting acts). The predicament of "hearing one's own thoughts aloud" reflects a distance or fissure within the subject himself. He listens to his own thoughts, which acquire spatialized and object-like character. "That which I think becomes an object detached from me. What I say becomes what one tells me" (Ey 1973, p. 420). Thoughts aloud therefore illustrates the process of alterization (becoming other) of the self, a process at the core of psychotic experience in schizophrenia:

> It is the sensible coefficient of the subjective-objective relation that becomes affected in the psychotic experience, and which we designate, in its generality, as the experience of alterity (otherness) (*l'expérience d'altérité*). It is a feeling that what is me or mine becomes modified. It is a feeling of oneself (*se sentir soi-même*) becoming other, depersonalized, modified in the psychosomatic unity of one's person, or to experience that which is a part of the subject, that which is him or his, as becoming other, i.e., being or belonging to an other (Ey 1973, p. 417).

The phenomenon of alterization is at the core of the psychotic experience (i.e., primary delusion, AVH). The psychotic experience is primarily an *intra-subjective event* having a character of revelation (epiphany, apophany; Conrad 1959). It is an emergence of *another presence, a co-presence within the intimacy of the self.* A revelation has no subject–object intentional structure. Such structure as mentioned above arises only through the processes of externalization and objectivation, i.e., through the formation of explanatory (secondary) delusions and hallucinatory elaborations. These cognitive-affective processes may be considered as a "psychotic work ("*travail psychotique*") (Ey 1973). The nature of psychotic experience has been aptly summarized by Gennart (2011):

> 1) the meaning of apophantic (revelatory) experience ... articulates itself through its very manifestation; the meaning is not grasped by the subject's efforts of interpretation or inference; rather the meaning is simply revealed to the subject by the experiences themselves. 2) the revelation of meaning imposes itself on the subject, short-cutting his liberty or his initiative of understanding (Gennart 2011, p. 324; our translation).

26.3.5 **The status of reality**

As we have mentioned above, the patient is aware that the hallucination is his private experience and not a publicly shared phenomenon (Aggernæs 1972). Thus, the patient does not ascribe an ordinary reality status to his experience.

For this reason, the definition of hallucination in the DSM-5 and RDoC is incorrect. The hallucinatory experience has an indisputable first-personal reality for the patient. This has to be understood in the following way: the patient has an experience in his first-person perspective, an affection that is undeniable and therefore, trivially, *real as an experience* (e.g., like having a toothache) and happening in the midst of his most intimate, private sphere. Moreover, the experience is associated with a manifestation of or a breakthrough to an alien presence, a reality of "another kind," a privately accessible ontological dimension, which is hidden from others. For these reasons, the experience of AVH often inscribes itself as a transformative existential event (Ey 1973). Schneider described this experience in the following way: "The significance [of the experience] is of a special kind;

it always carries a great import, is urgent and personal, *a sign or message from another world*" (Schneider 1959, p. 104). One of our patients gave the following account of this other ontological realm:

> There are two worlds. There is the unreal world, which is the world I am in and we are in. And then, there is the real world. The only thing that is real in the unreal world is my own self. Everything else—buildings, trees, houses—is unreal. All other humans are extras. My body is part of the charade. There is a real world somewhere and from there someone or something is trying to control me by putting thoughts into my head or by creating (. . .) screaming voices inside my head.

This brings us to the relation between delusion and hallucination. Hallucination is always a pathological phenomenon, "otherwise it is not a hallucination" (Ey 1973). As we have tried to explain, hallucinations emerge on the condition of alterization of the self, where parts of the self become felt as alien, as a co-presence of another reality or ontological realm. Thus, hallucinations reflect a complex alteration of the structure of subjectivity. The patient becomes dislocated from the shared social world. It is in this sense that the very experience of AVH is a psychotic phenomenon, with an origin not dissimilar from that of primary or ontological delusion (Bovet and Parnas 1993, Parnas 2004, 2015). However, it is important to remember that the hallucinated patient often develops various secondary delusions, reflecting his cognitive effort to account for hallucinations. In many clinical situations, it is simply impossible to make sharp distinctions between hallucinations, delusions, and phenomena of influence (Tatossian 1997).

26.3.6 **Double book-keeping**

The phenomenon of double book-keeping is central to grasping the nature of the experience and attitudes of patients with AVH. Bleuler (1911/1950) observers that the majority of patients with schizophrenia display two different existential attitudes: on the one hand, they may seem to be "cured" and adapted to the social world, yet at the same time exhibit psychotic phenomena. Bleuler called this crucial aspect "double book-keeping," sometimes also called double orientation. As an example, Bleuler mentions a "cured" university professor, who gave as a present to his mistress, his recently published monograph, signed "Lord of the Universe." A patient of ours, who claims that the hospital is surrounded by spies and agents waiting to kill him, nevertheless goes unconcerned for a walk in a nearby forest. Jaspers designated such behaviors as "inconsequential attitudes." Possibly the most lucid first-person description of double book-keeping is offered by Professor Saks:

> It was at this point, I think, that my life truly began to operate as though it were being lived on two trains, their tracks side by side. On one track, the train held the things of the 'real world'—my academic schedule and responsibilities, my books, my connection to my family (. . .) On the other track: the increasingly confusing and even frightening inner workings of my mind. The struggle was to keep the trains parallel on their tracks, and not have them suddenly and violently collide with each other (Saks 2007, p. 64).

In our view (Henriksen and Parnas 2014), double book-keeping does not simply reflect a coexistence of rationality and irrationality (commonly harbored by all of us) but suggests a more fundamental fact: that the patient *lives simultaneously* in two different and incommensurable ontological frameworks, which the patient seems to experience largely (but not invariably) as not conflicting. It is important to emphasize that the condition of double book-keeping does not entail a phenomenal disunity of consciousness. It is also crucial to realize that the felt contact to "another world" is not primarily an outcome of logical inference, accounting for hallucinatory or other psychotic phenomena. Rather, the access to another ontological dimension is an aspect of the alterization (self-alienation, converting a part of self into another) of self-awareness, and may precede the outbreak of overt psychosis by many years. The psychotic onset may be seen as a culmination, in which the psychotic symptoms and the experiential access to another ontological realm are interdependent aspects.

26.3.7 **Disorder of the self and AVH**

A psychotic culmination of self-alienation in schizophrenia is to be likely sought in the disorders of the so-called "core" or "minimal" self (Damasio 1999, Gallagher and Zahavi 2008), which is a basic, prereflectively operating structure of consciousness. It is an unproblematic sense of "I–me–myself" imbuing all experiencing and a sense of self-coincidence that is normally only rarely interrupted. The minimal self assures the subjectivity of experience, making it always someone's experience. Phenomenologically oriented empirical studies (Parnas and Henriksen 2014) demonstrate that in the schizophrenia spectrum disorders, the patients complain of a sense of incompleteness ("I am only half"), a failing sense of self-presence and of automatic self-identity, hyper-reflexivity, and various other forms of self-alienation and lack of immersion in the social world. These complaints frequently date to schooldays and early adolescence. The self-disorders weaken the structure of subjectivity and facilitate the process of alterization, allowing normally silent, tacit regions of the self to gain an alien prominence.

Thus, many patients report feeling fundamentally (ontologically) different from other people since childhood and adolescence. This feeling of difference is difficult for the patient to specify in terms of mundane characteristics. It is a sense of difference that is prior to the awareness of "what" is different. Description and comparison of characteristics presuppose a shared dimension on which the compared characteristics may be placed. The *Anderssein*-difference lies in the structure of subjectivity and the associated ontological framework. The patient may say that he feels "as if he came from another planet," as if he was an "extraterrestrial" or that he does not feel like a true human being or that "I feel as if the stork dropped me on the wrong planet." The most frequent formulation is to feel "wrong," a vague sense of fundamental difference for which the patient cannot find appropriate predicates (Kimura 1992).

26.4 Discussion and conclusions

26.4.1 Defining the AVH

The classical definition of AVH, as a perception without an object, has persisted into the DSM-5, ICD-10, and RDoC. From a perspective of phenomenological investigation, it is evident that AVH *are not perceptions*, in either a physiological or a descriptive sense. A perceptual experience is always deployed in the intersubjectively shared, external space with an essentially incomplete and perspectival manifestation of the object and is endowed with a temporal thickness or contour. AVH violate all these basic features of perception. Another, crucially problematic aspect of the DSM-5/RDoC definition concerns the reality status of AVH. The definitions claim that AVH "has sufficient sense of reality to resemble a veridical perception" (RDoC). Since the AVH are not perceptions but have entirely different qualities, the patient is able to distinguish his mundane (veridical) perceptions from AVH, which reveal themselves in the patient's private space. In sum, AVH is not an empirical object of this world, given to the patient through the perceptual channels. Rather, the AVH are best regarded as alienated and intrusive fragments of the patient's own subjectivity, and which tend to insert themselves and inhabit his privacy, resembling the phenomenon of haunting. A similar phenomenology-based criticism can be articulated with respect to the notions of delusion and bizarre delusion (Bovet and Parnas 1993, Sass 1994, Parnas 2004). In fact, it strikes us as amazing that the concept of AVH, so central to the psychopathology of schizophrenia, has been empirically and conceptually neglected for decades: research projects, publications, and textbooks operate with the term "hallucination" as if it was a well-understood phenomenon.

Such definition-related problems are all the more significant for the diagnostic systems (DSM-IV, DSM-5, ICD-10) that are epistemologically *founded* on the operationally defined components (Parnas 2015, Parnas and Bovet 2015). Obviously, this criticism has important consequences for clinical work, treatment, and research.

26.4.2 The epistemology of mental symptoms

The discussion of definition is, of course, part of a more general philosophical conceptualization of psychopathological phenomena. Since the medicalization of madness in the early nineteenth century, the concept of symptom (and sign) has been adopted by psychiatry from somatic medicine and considered as a well-delimited indicator of the underlying pathology. This view became dramatically and dogmatically reinforced during the "operational revolution" of the DSM-III. The symptom is considered as a self-sufficient, thing-like object, deprived of subjective meaning and significance; i.e., just an indicator of organic pathology, a little piece of the world's furniture. The symptom is believed to be definable through short statements in a way that does not require any reference to its psychopathological and broader personal context and its relation to other symptoms, larger wholes, or gestalts.

What, then, is a phenomenological response to the questions on the nature of the symptom? The answer will of course vary for different symptoms but a general response may be articulated in the following way: the symptom is not a well-demarcated entity endowed with spatial solidity and the permanence of the third-person realm (Nordgaard et al 2013). Rather, the ontology of the symptom (the nature of its being) is that of an emergent gestalt-prototype (Minkowski 1933, Parnas and Gallagher 2015), articulated, or constituted by an interaction between the structures of subjectivity, particular (cognitive and affective) experiences and mental contents and processes, personal and interpersonal factors, and the patient's environment. This implies a complex ontology that crucially also involves first- and second-person ontological dimensions. Of course, not all psychiatric symptoms exhibit such degrees of complexity, but that does not sanction a psychopathological ignorance on the part of psychiatrists. A patient complaining of deep fatigue may suffer from a cancer-related anemia (of which the symptom is an indicator). However, his complaints of fatigue may also refer to a mental exhaustion in the early stages of schizophrenia, due to a constant need for reflection in order to understand the meaning of everyday events (lack of common sense) (Blankenburg 1971).

There are several consequences flowing from this view, which pertain to the issues of definition and description, detection (psychiatric interview), classification, treatment, and, importantly, articulating phenotypes for psychiatric research.

As a way forward, we would advocate the adoption of the original idea behind the DSM-III (unfortunately unrealized), which was to base the classification on diagnostic categories illustrated by rich prototypical narrative description and discussions of differential diagnoses. These descriptions should be supplemented by symptom lists to assure systematicity of description (Parnas and Bovet 2015).

In our view, it is naive and harmful to continue to hold that symptoms are a bunch of phenomenal primitives that quasi-randomly combine to form diagnostic classes and can be defined in themselves, acontextually and "atheoretically," in isolation from more encompassing wholes and without any need for background knowledge. For example, to detect a delusion, the psychiatrist needs not only to know the propositional content of the patient's statements but also their context, the patient's way of arguing, his experiences and a lot of other (e.g., historical) information. Moreover, the psychiatrist must master a host of other relevant concepts in order to classify the patient as being delusional (e.g., reality, psychosis, overvalued idea, hallucination). As the exposition of the AVH illustrates, a faithful psychopathological description demands a significant clinical knowledge and conceptual sophistication.

The whole of the gestalt colors the single components in a certain way, conferring on them a diagnostic specificity. The single components constitute the gestalt as a clinical reality. A skillful clinical assessment reflects this part–whole dynamism of the gestalt. It is important to note that the concept of a gestalt-prototype does not indicate something ephemeral or atmospheric. The epistemology of this approach is consistent with contemporary cognitive research (Parnas and Bovet 2015). The "objectivity" of gestalt is assured by the intersubjective agreement.

As we and others have demonstrated, phenomenologically oriented studies may achieve quite impressive reliability levels (Vollmer-Larsen and Parnas 2007, Nordgaard et al. 2014).

For all the reasons addressed above, psychopathology is a scholarly discipline, demanding a phenomenological conceptual framework. As Jaspers noted, a psychiatrist needs "to know what people experience and how they experience it."

References

Aggernæs. A. (1972). The experienced reality of hallucinations and other psychological phenomena, an empirical analysis. *Acta Psychiatrica Scandinavica*, **48**, 220–238.

Allen, P. Larøi, F., McGuire P.K., and **Aleman A.** (2008). The hallucinating brain: a review of structural and functional neuroimaging studies of hallucinations. *Neuroscience and Biobehavioral Reviews*, **32**, 175–191.

Baillarger, J. (1846). *De l'influence de l'état intermédiaire à la veille et au sommeil sur la production et la marche des hallucinations. Mémoires de l'Académie royale de médecine.* Paris: J.B. Baillère.

Berrios, G.E. (1996). *The History of Mental Symptoms. Descriptive psychopathology since the nineteenth century.* Cambridge: Cambridge University Press.

Blankenburg, W. (1971). *Der Verlust der natürlichen Selbstverständlichkeit. Ein Beitrag zur Psychopathologie symptomarmer Psychosen.* Stuttgart: Enke.

Bleuler, E. (1911/1950). *Dementia Praecox or the Group of Schizophrenias*, ed. and trans. J. Zinkin. New York: International Universities Press.

Bovet, P. and **Parnas, J.** (1993). Schizophrenic delusions: a phenomenological approach. *Schizophrenia Bulletin*, **19**, 579–597.

Charbonneau, G. (2001). *Introduction à la phénoménologie des hallucinations.* Paris: Le Cercle Herméneutique.

Conrad, K. (1959). *Die Beginnende Schizophrenie.* Stuttgart: Thieme.

Damasio, A. (1999). *The feeling of What Happens.* New York: Harcourt.

De Clérambault, G.G. (1925/1992). *L'automatisme mental.* Paris: Collection les Empêcheurs de penser en rond.

Esquirol, E. (1838). *Des maladies mentales considérées sous leur rapport medical, hygiénique et medico-légal.* Paris: Librairie de l'Académie Royale de Médecine.

Ey, H. (1973). *Traité des hallucinations.* Paris: Masson.

Ford, J.M., Morris, S.E., Hoffman, R.E., et al. (2014). Studying hallucinations within the NIMH RDoC Framework. *Schizophrenia Bulletin*, **40** (suppl. 4), 295–304.

Frith, C. (1996). The role of the prefrontal cortex in self-consciousness: the case of auditory hallucinations. *Philosophical Transactions of the Royal Society of London. Series B, Biological Sciences*, **351**, 1505–1512.

Gallagher, S. and **Zahavi, D.** (2008). *The Phenomenology of the Mind.* New York: Routledge.

Gennart, M. (2011). *Corporéité et présence. Jalons pour une approche du corps dans la psychose.* Neuchâtel: Le Cercle Herméneutique.

Gross G., Huber, G., and **Klosterkötter, J.** (1992). Early diagnosis of schizophrenia. *Neurology, Psychiatry, and Brain Research*, **1**, 17–22.

Henriksen, M.G. and **Parnas, J.** (2014). Self-disorders and schizophrenia: a phenomenological reappraisal of poor insight and noncompliance. *Schizophrenia Bulletin*, **40**, 542–547.

Jaspers, K. (1963). *General Psychopathology*, 7th ed., trans. J. Hoenig and M.W. Hamilton. Chicago, IL. University of Chicago Press (originally published as *Allgemeine Psychopathologie: Ein Leitfaden für Studierende, Ärzte und Psychologen*. Berlin: Springer, 1913.

Kimura, B. (1992). *Ecrits de psychopathologie phénoménologique*. Paris: PUF.

Lanteri-Laura, G. (1991). *Les hallucinations*. Paris: Masson.

McCarthy-Jones, S (2013). *Hearing Voices: The histories, causes and meanings of auditive verbal hallucinations*. Cambridge: Cambridge University Press.

Merleau-Ponty, M. (1962). *The Phenomenology of Perception*, trans C. Smith. London: Routledge.

Minkowski, E. (1933/1995). *Le temps vécu. Etudes phénoménologiques et psychopathologiques*. Paris: Presses Universitaires de France.

Naudin, J. (1997). *Phénoménologie en psychiatrie: Les voix et la chose*. Toulouse: Presses Universitaires du Mirail.

Nordgaard, J., **Sass, L.A.**, and **Parnas, J.** (2013). The psychiatric interview: validity, structure, and subjectivity. *European Archives of Psychiatry and Clinical Neuroscience*, **263**, 353–364.

Nordgaard, J. and **Parnas, J.** (2014). Self-disorders and the schizophrenia spectrum: a study of first 100 hospitals admission. *Schizophrenia Bulletin*, **40**, 1300–1307.

Parnas, J. (2004). Belief and pathology of self-awareness: a phenomenological contribution to the classification of delusions. *Journal of Consciousness Studies*, **11**, 148–161.

Parnas, J. (2015). Delusions, epistemology and phenophobia. *World Psychiatry*, **14**, 174–175.

Parnas, J. and **Bovet, P.** (2015). Psychiatry made easy: operation(al)ism and some of its consequences. In K.S. Kendler and J. Parnas (eds.) *Philosophical Issues in Psychiatry III: The nature and sources of historical change*, pp. 190–212. Oxford, UK: Oxford University Press.

Parnas, J. and **Gallagher, S.** (2015). Phenomenology and the interpretation of psychopathologic experience. In L.J. Kirmayer, R.B. Lemelson, and C.A. Cummings (eds.). *Revisioning Psychiatry: Cultural phenomenology, critical neuroscience, and global mental health*. New York: Cambridge University Press.

Parnas, J. and **Henriksen, M.G.** (2014). Disordered self in schizophrenia spectrum: a clinical and research perspective. *Harvard Review of Psychiatry*, **22**, 251–265.

Penfield, W. and **Perot, P.** (1963). The brain record of auditory and visual experience: a final summary and discussion. *Brain*, **86**, 595–696.

Plaze, M., **Paillère-Martinot, M.L.**, **Penttilä, J.**, et al. (2011). Where do auditory hallucinations come from?—a brain morphometry study of schizophreniapatients with inner or outer space hallucinations. *Schizophrenia Bulletin*, **37**, 212–221.

Rasmussen, A.R. and **Parnas, J.** (2015). Anomalies of imagination and disordered self in schizophrenia spectrum disorders. *Psychopathology*, **48**, 317–323.

Saks, E.R. (2007). *The Center Cannot Hold: My journey through madness*. London: Virago Press.

Sass, L. (1994). *The Paradoxes of Delusion: Wittgenstein, Schreber and the schizophrenic mind*. Ithaca, NY: Cornell University Press.

Schneider, K. (1950/1959). *Klinische Psychopathologie* (3. vermehrte Auflage der Beiträge zur Psychiatrie ed.). Stuttgart: Thieme. (English version: *Clinical Psychopathology*, trans. M.W. Hamilton. New York: Grune and Stratton, 1959).

Stanghellini, G., Langer, A.I., Ambrosini, A., and **Cangas, A.J.** (2012). Quality of hallucinatory experiences: differences between a clinical and a non-clinical sample. *World Psychiatry*, **11**, 100–103.

Tatossian, A. (1997). *La phénoménologie des psychoses*. Paris: L' Art du Comprendre.

Upthegrove R., Broome M.R., Caldwell K., et al. (2016). Understanding auditory verbal hallucinations: a systematic review of current evidence. *Acta Psychiatrica Scandinavica*, **133**, 352–367.

van Tol M.J., van der Meer L., Bruggeman R., et al. (2013). Voxel-based gray and white matter morphometry correlates of hallucinations in schizophrenia: The superior temporal gyrus does not stand alone. *Neuroimage Clinical*, **4**, 249–257.

Vollmer-Larsen, A. and **Parnas, J.** (2007). Reliability of measuring of anomalous experience: the Bonn scale for the assessment of basic symptoms. *Psychopathology*, **40**, 245–248.

Chapter 27

Comment on "The ontology and epistemology of symptoms: The case of auditory verbal hallucinations in schizophrenia"

Paul Hoff

27.1 Introduction

The chapter by Parnas and Urfer-Parnas continues the longstanding debate on the definition of pivotal psychiatric terms like symptom, diagnosis, illness, disease, therapy. Ontologically confident authors, who deliberately reach beyond the scope of mere definitions, might speak of the "nature" or "essence" of psychiatric phenomena.

This debate has accompanied scientific psychiatry since its very beginnings. For example, the representatives of "romantic psychiatry," who were oriented to Friedrich Wilhelm Schelling's philosophy of nature and gained substantial influence during the first half of the nineteeth century, emphasized the subjective and biographic perspectives for understanding and treating mental illness (Marx 1990, 1991). About a century later, Karl Jaspers, in the final phase of writing his seminal *Allgemeine Psychopathologie* [General psychopathology] (1913), published a paper on "The phenomenological approach in psychiatric research" ("Die phänomenologische Forschungsrichtung in der Psychiatrie") (Jaspers 1912). Here he postulated the necessity to recognize, describe and, as far as possible, understand what the patient experiences—what it is like, how it "feels" to be paranoid or depressed or hallucinating, for example. And since all these phenomena—contrary to many clinical symptoms in somatic medicine—may neither be observed directly nor fully covered by quantitative measures, but display themselves, if at all, indirectly—e.g., by gestures, specific behavior, content of speech, or pieces of art—it became obvious for Jaspers that psychopathological and, indeed, all mental phenomena necessarily include a personal (subjective) and an interpersonal (intersubjective) dimension. He convincingly numerated the risks of unrecognized or underestimated scientific prejudices in psychiatry (Hoff 1989). That is why, for Jaspers, the phenomenological approach had to develop and maintain a critical impetus towards the unavoidable limitations of *any* scientific method.

Parnas and Urfer-Parnas basically follow these lines of thought in their chapter. Consequently, carrying forward their previous work on the relevance of phenomenology for present-day psychiatry, they now address auditory verbal hallucination (AVH) from a phenomenological perspective, contrasting it with what they call "operationalism," i.e., with the consequences of psychiatry's turn towards explicit descriptive criteria and algorithms. That process gained momentum in the 1970s, culminating in the publication of the third edition of the *Diagnostic and Statistical Manual of Mental Disorders* (DSM-III) by the American Psychiatric Association (APA) in 1980 and the tenth edition of the *International Classification of Diseases* (ICD-10) by the World Health Organization (WHO) in 1992. The authors place the recent debate on Research Domain Criteria (RDoC) (Insel et al. 2010) in exactly that tradition.

After briefly summarizing the main ideas of their chapter (from a necessarily subjective perspective, that is), I shall put forward supportive arguments along with a few questions concerning possible limitations.

27.2 **Core elements of Parnas' and Urfer-Parnas' chapter**

The authors start by challenging psychiatry to pay more attention to the conceptual basis of "signs" and "symptoms." They decribe the historical background of this debate including the peculiar "division of psychopathological labor between French and German psychiatry" in the nineteenth century, French authors focusing on hallucinations, German-speaking authors on delusion. After introducing current research strands on auditory verbal hallucinations (including RDoC, as mentioned above), Parnas and Urfer-Parnas give a detailed and informative overview of phenomenological perspectives on AVH. They criticize the DSM-5 (American Psychiatric Association 2013) and RDoC approach of defining AVH as sensory experiences with "sufficient sense of reality to resemble a veridical perception" (Ford et al. 2014).

As opposed to this, the authors delineate a number of qualitative features: The "phenomenological poverty" of AVH, their relation to the "internal space" or "interiority" of the person, even their "radical dissimilarity from normal acoustic perceptions," the person's feeling of "complete passivity and exposure" to AVH (also called their "givenness") and, finally, their foundation in the phenomenon of "alterization" which is seen as "core of the psychotic experience," as opening the door to a "privately accessible ontological dimension." In their concluding remarks they emphasize the "gestalt-prototype" of psychopathological symptoms that should be acknowledged and—in Parnas' and Urfer-Parnas' view—may well be successfully implemented into contemporary research.

27.3 **An undogmatic phenomenological perspective is a down-to-earth approach in psychiatry**

According to a regrettably widespread cliché, phenomenological psychopathology is overtly theoretical in nature, philosophy-laden, even irrelevant for clinical practice. It may therefore be surprising to call it a down-to-earth approach in psychiatry. However, that seems appropriate to me since this method strives to grasp the meanings of the patient's utterances, feelings, or behaviors in a very concret and individualized manner. As Jaspers already emphasized (at least as I read him), phenomenology is *nothing less* than a polemical rejection of strictly quantitative measures in psychiatry, e.g., in neuroscientific or epidemiological research. Quite the opposite: It fully acknowledges their relevance, as long as they refrain from claiming to be the *only*, i.e., the exhaustive, way to deal scientifically with mental issues.

In 1974, Thomas Nagel, in an epistemological context, asked the intriguing (and since then much debated) question "What is it like to be a bat?" In our present context we might reformulate it to "What is it like to be paranoid?" or, closer to Parnas' and Urfer-Parnas' topic, "What is it like to hallucinate voices?" Possible answers *cannot only* be grounded on psychopathological description or on mathematical correlations between descriptive symptoms and neurobiological measures such as blood flow changes detected by fMRI.

Therefore, in my view the most essential quality of the phenomenological attitude towards clinical psychiatry is to keep psychopathological "spaces" open, to detect problematic "tacit implications" of diagnostic procedures, and to respect the richness and complexity of subjective phenomena including their lifelong dynamic development, usually called a person's biography. Such an approach does not exclude *any* other scientific method. On the contrary, it strives to link specific, albeit heterogeneous, methods in psychiatry with the indispensable level of subjectivity.

There is one more relevant aspect, the historical one, where "historical" has a double meaning. On the one hand, phenomenological psychopathology actively includes the temporal dimension by embedding the patient's symptoms and behavior into their biography up to the present circumstances. On the other hand, to do so requires a thoroughgoing knowledge of the epistemological and historical backgrounds shaping the psychiatric concepts involved—an issue that Parnas and Urfer-Parnas rightly highlight in the last paragraph of their chapter.

27.4 **Even down-to-earth approaches in psychiatry do not come without limitations**

Phenomenology's profound relevance for psychiatry makes it advisable to avoid unnecessarily strong philosophical presuppositions. From that point of view, I suggest reflecting on two questions and one possible extension concerning Parnas' and Urfer-Parnas' approach.

27.4.1 **Ontology**

Is it essential for the phenomenological perspective to make very strong epistemological claims? This happens, for example, when the authors emphasize the "fundamental fact that the patient lives simultaneously in two different and incommensurable ontological frameworks" or when they straightforwardly identify *fundamental* differences with *ontological* ones:

> Thus many patients report feeling fundamentally (ontologically) different from other people since childhood and adolescence. This feeling of difference is difficult for the patient to specify in terms of mundane characteristics. It is a sense of difference that is prior to the awareness of "what" is different. ... The *Anderssein*-difference lies in the structure of subjectivity and the associated ontological framework.

Beyond doubt, there are clearly incommensurable subjective *perspectives* at work in the two people involved, when a severely paranoid patient tries to explain his experiences to the psychiatrist. But do these perspectives mirror fully distinct *ontological* frameworks? Might such a strong notion of difference not bear the risk of creating manifold "private ontologies" that would be even more difficult to approach scientifically?

27.4.2 Categorical specificity of schizophrenic AVH

Is there necessarily a categorical (not to say ontological) difference, a "radical dissimilarity" in Parnas' and Urfer-Parnas' wording, in the subjective quality of AVH between people suffering from schizophrenia and those with a delirious state (e.g., following abrupt alcohol withdrawal)? Furthermore, some schizophrenic patients claim that their "voices" are quite similar to those heard in an ordinary conversation. In addition, there obviously are peculiar abnormalities of perception and subjective experiences, including different types of AVH, beyond schizophrenia and even in healthy subjects.

27.4.3 The interpersonal realm

Phenomenological psychopathology strives to come as close to the patient's subjective sphere as possible, to touch it, so to speak. It does acknowledge the interpersonal realm, since clinical psychopathology, let alone therapy, is all about communication. Parnas and Urfer-Parnas make that quite clear when in the last section of their chapter they quote Karl Jaspers, who committed the psychiatrist "to know what people experience and how they experience it."

However, I suggest pushing this idea even further by regarding the concept of interpersonality not only as an additional perspective, but as one of the very principles of psychopathology or, in fact, of mental life in general. This is basically an adaptation of a Kantian and, especially, Fichtean concept: Epistemology is not only a matter of understanding how knowledge can be acquired, but emphasizes the fundamental role of interpersonality ("the other person") that is seen as prerequisite of any scientific knowledge (Hoff 1997, 2017, in press).

This may be elucidated by a close reading of the following passage of Parnas' and Urfer-Parnas' chapter:

> The phenomenon of alterization is at the core of the psychotic experience .... The psychotic experience is *primarily an intrasubjective event* having a character of revelation .... It is an emergence of *another presence, a co-presence* within the intimacy of the self. (italics by PH)

The "intrasubjective emergence of another presence, a co-presence" is a meaningful example for the hypothesis (in fact fundamental to Fichte's philosophy) that any process of generating knowledge necessarily addresses the other autonomous person in order to become effective (Williams 1984, Asmuth 2007, von Manz 2014). From this perspective, however, the epicentre of personhood is much broader than the "core self" or "minimal self" quoted by the authors (Damasio 1999, Gallagher and Zahavi 2008).

Adopting this framework of transcendental philosophy *sensu* Kant and Fichte to psychiatric issues will result in claiming a fundamental interdependence of personal and interpersonal acts—in the etiology and pathogenesis of mental illness as well as in psychiatric diagnosis, therapy, and research. Hence, Parnas' and Urfer-Parnas' statement cited above could be modified as follows: The psychotic experience is primarily an intrasubjective *and interpersonal* event. For me, this is a line of thought worth following in current psychopathology.

27.5 **Conclusion**

In my view, a substantial, i.e., non-reductive and non-eliminative, integration of the phenomenological and neuroscientific perspectives in psychopathology is not only a possible option, but also a promising one. Admittedly, the longstanding, not to say classical controversies between these two (and other) approaches may give rise to scepticism. But they should not discourage us from further developing this debate since it may well become a major issue in twenty-first-century psychiatry.

References

American Psychiatric Association (1980). *Diagnostic and Statistical Manual of Mental Disorders*, 3rd edn. Washington, DC: American Psychiatric Association.

American Psychiatric Association (2013). *Diagnostic and Statistical Manual of Mental Disorders*, 5th edn. Arlington, VA: American Psychiatric Association.

Asmuth, C. (ed.) (2007). *Transzendentalphilosophie und Person*. Bielefeld: Transcript.

Damasio, A (1999). *The Feeling of What Happens*. New York: Harcourt.

Ford, J.M., **Morris, S.E.**, **Hoffman, R.E.**, et al. (2014). Studying hallucinations within the NIMH RDoC framework. *Schizophrenia Bulletin*, **40** (suppl. 4), 295–304.

Gallagher, S. and **Zahavi, D** (2008). *The Phenomenological Mind. An introduction to philosophy of mind and cognitive science*. London: Routledge.

Hoff, P. (1989). Erkenntnistheoretische Vorurteile in der Psychiatrie—eine kritische Reflexion 75 Jahre nach Karl Jaspers' "Allgemeiner Psychopathologie." *Fundamenta Psychiatrica*, **3**, 141–150.

Hoff, P. (1997). Fichte und die psychiatrische Forschung. *Fichte-Studien*, **13**, 241–255.

Hoff, P. (2017, in press) Von Kant zu Fichte: Transzendentales Denken und die Grundlegung von Psychiatrie und Psychotherapie im 21. Jahrhundert. In M. Ivaldo, H.G. von Manz, and I. Radrizzani (eds.) *Vergegenwärtigung der Transzendentalphilosophie. Das philosophische Vermächtnis Reinhard Lauths*. Würzburg: Königshausen und Neumann.

Insel, T., Cuthbert. B., Garvey, M., et al. (2010). Research Domain Criteria (RDoC): toward a new classification framework for research on mental disorders. *American Journal of Psychiatry*, **167**, 748–751.

Jaspers, K. (1912). Die phänomenologische Forschungsrichtung in der Psychopathologie. *Zeitschrift für die gesamte Neurologie und Psychiatrie*, **9**, 391–408.

Jaspers, K. (1913). *Allgemeine Psychopathologie: ein Leitfaden für Studierende, Aerzte und Psychologen*. Berlin: Springer.

Marx, O.M. (1990). German Romantic psychiatry, Part I. *History of Psychiatry*, **1**, 351–381.

Marx, O.M. (1991). German Romantic psychiatry, Part II. *History of Psychiatry*, **2**, 1–25.

Nagel, T. (1974). What is it like to be a bat? *Philosophical Review*, **83**, 435–450.

Von Manz, H.G. (2014). *Interpersonalität und Ethik*. Würzburg: Königshausen & Neumann.

Williams, R.R. (1994) The question of the other in Fichte's thought. In D. Breazeale and T. Rockmore (eds.) *Fichte—Historical Contexts/Contemporary Controversies*, pp. 142–157. Atlantic Highlands, NJ: Humanities Press.

World Health Organization (1992). *ICD-10 Classification of Mental and Behavioural Disorders (Including Disorders of Psychological Development). Clinical Descriptions And Diagnostic Guidelines*, Chapter V (F). Geneva: World Health Organization.

Part III

Epistemic iteration

Section 10

Epistemic iteration in scientific taxonomies

Chapter 28

Introduction to "Epistemic iteration and natural kinds: Realism and pluralism in taxonomy"

Josef Parnas

This is an important chapter concerned with the mechanisms of scientific progress and written by a leading figure in the philosophy of science. The author presents his concept of epistemic iteration originally developed in the realm of the natural sciences and here applies it to the development of psychiatric classification. In his book *Inventing Temperature: Measurement and Scientific Progress* Chang describes how the concept of temperature emerged from a cumulative scientific activity which had as its starting point our phenomenological sensations of warmth and cold. Epistemic iteration is to be understood as the business of "getting on" in the absence of assured foundations. It is a process of inquiry in which "successive stages of knowledge, *each building on the preceding one*, are created in order to enhance the achievement of certain epistemic goals" (Chang 2004, p. 45).

In my understanding epistemic iteration is basically a linear cumulative improvement of our knowledge and may be contrasted with revolutionary changes of scientific paradigms such as the emergence of relativity theories and quantum mechanics (even though such changes might be a consequence of epistemic iteration). On the issue of realism–antirealism Chang declares himself a pragmatic realist:

> Traditional realism is untenable where it seeks or claims a correspondence between theory and reality, as we do not have direct access to reality. Realism needs to be refitted along pragmatist lines [. . .] Realism, as I propose to take it, is a commitment to learn the most we can about nature."

In turning his attention to psychiatry Chang bases his considerations on numerous papers by Kenneth Kendler who himself is certainly a pragmatic realist. An important aspect of the paper advocates scientific pluralism. In order to avoid a stalemate in the scientific process we need to have several systems of epistemic iteration addressing the same group of problems. This pluralism is our best line of defense against oversimplified monist assumptions which very often turn into dogma.

In psychiatric research the dogmatic execution of systems used in the third and fourth editions of the *Diagnostic and Statistical Manual of Mental Disorders* (DSM III–IV) hindered new ideas and new questions, and probably contributed to the stagnation of the science of psychiatry (Hyman 2010). One possible realization of pluralism in the domain of classification would be to have different classifications for different purposes, which would mean a more open-ended system for the use in science instead of having one monolithic system serving scientists, practitioners, politicians, and insurance companies alike.

References

Chang, H. (2004). *Inventing Temperature: Measurement and scientific progress.* New York: Oxford University Press.

Hyman, S.E. (2010). The diagnosis of mental disorders: the problem of reification. *Annual Review of Clinical Psychology,* **6**, 155–179.

Chapter 29

Epistemic iteration and natural kinds: Realism and pluralism in taxonomy

Hasok Chang

29.1 Introduction

In this paper I seek to discuss the notion of "epistemic iteration" and its implications for psychiatric nosology. In particular, I want to ask what we will have learned if we do achieve stability and convergence through an iterative process, especially in the face of the "local minimum" problem. The iterative framework is more realistic than the standard "realist" one, as it does not presume or require the availability of the one "right" classification. Epistemic iteration points to a pluralist realism. For readers who are unfamiliar with the notion of epistemic iteration, I provide an introduction in section 29.3. It is interesting to note that the original context in which I developed the idea of epistemic iteration was the development of thermometry, a very remote area of science from psychiatry. Yet there are some significant and useful resonances with current concerns in psychiatric nosology.

29.2 Preamble: Is psychiatric nosology unscientific?

A significant aspect of what I want to achieve in this paper is to reflect on what the natural sciences might helpfully suggest to psychiatry, through parallels and contrasts. In that regard, the first thing I want to stress is that psychiatrists need not be overawed by a false sense of how great things are in the physical sciences. For those who are worried that nosological categories in psychiatry change as time goes by, seemingly in a "random walk" with no discernible direction of progress, it will be useful to remember that chemists, physicists, geologists, and astronomers have also made drastic changes in their fundamental conceptual categories over the centuries. As Thomas Kuhn pointed out (1970, pp. 206–7), there has not been a clear direction of progress in this development as astronomers and physicists went from the spherical geocentric universe of Ptolemy, to the heliocentric system of Copernicus (still based on circles, with the Sun at the center), to Newton's vision of infinite absolute space and time in which there is no center at all, to the closed curved four-dimensional space-time of Einstein's cosmology. If cosmology seems like an entirely different sort of science from psychiatric nosology, take another example, specifically taxonomic: the basic ontology of matter went from the Aristotelian four elements, to an early modern system including various elements and "principles" like phlogiston and caloric, then to the set of indestructible atoms postulated by Dalton, and on to transmutable atoms made up of elementary particles regrouping themselves through nuclear fusion and fission.

If anyone should claim that such flip-flops are only a sign of immaturity that held sway in the long past of the physical sciences, it is sufficient to point to fundamental theoretical physics in the twentieth century, which has to be the most formidable phase of modern science. The century began with the ether as the fundamental substance of the universe, and electrons as structures in the ether. After the breakdown of that ontology there was a happy moment when everything in the entire universe was thought to be made up of electrons, protons, and neutrons. But that moment, still so persistent in popular imagination, never even really existed; by 1932, when the neutron was discovered, other particles were already being registered experimentally, and theoretical physics had concluded that all those particles were not little billiard balls, but quanta with their wave–particle duality and other metaphysical quandaries. And then the protons and neutrons were seen to be made up of quarks and gluons, a host of new particles were observed, and antimatter became accepted as real, but photons persisted as their own kind of things. The "particle zoo" was only brought to order into the Standard Model of elementary particle physics in the 1970s (roughly at the same time as the publication of DSM-III in 1980). And was the taxonomy of fundamental physics stable after that? No, now we have superstrings and dark matter and dark energy, the latter two allegedly making up a clear majority of "stuff" (matter–energy) in the universe. According to current wisdom the vacuum is not just emptiness but swarms with virtual particles, and there is a lively debate on whether space-time itself is a kind of substance. And what will greet us next in the wonderful world of physics? Nobody knows (cf. the "mess" discussed by Miriam Solomon in Chapter 9 of this volume).

I bring up these cases not in order to denigrate physics, but in order to dispel a false ideal of science which hampers productive thinking. Physics has surely achieved a great deal of stable and cumulative progress, but not without great turmoil and sharp disagreements. There is no obvious reason why psychiatry should not be able to do the same. But how? This is where epistemic iteration becomes relevant, as we try to find a way to render changes in psychiatric nosology cumulatively progressive. One helpful recognition is that within the physical sciences there are much more stable parts than the above examples would suggest. For example, some phenomenological laws (e.g., Snell's law of refraction, or Archimedes's law of the lever) have remained for many centuries, and found their uses in numerous situations with various refinements to suit each specific situation.[1] Mendeleev's periodic system of chemical elements has flourished for 150 years now, gaining in its order and precision while undergoing significant changes in its detailed principles

[1] See Chang (2004), p. 52, and references therein, for a discussion of this point, especially by Herbert Feigl.

of organization, and accommodating numerous newly discovered elements (see Scerri 2007). The international network of metrologists have systematically maintained the units of basic physical quantities for more than a century now, increasing the precision and reliability of measurements without creating disruptions from previous standards at each step, while updating the fundamental definitions of the quantities in question (Quinn 2012, ch. 15, 17). These, rather than the metaphysical roller-coaster of fundamental theoretical physics, are more plausible and productive models on which enterprises like psychiatric nosology can model themselves (cf. warnings by Dan Stein against premature reductionism and Paul Hoff against reification, in Chapters 8 and 14 of this volume respectively).

Healthy "physics-envy" requires a careful decision on which aspects of physics to emulate. And when we look at those aspects of the physical sciences that have developed in a truly cumulative fashion, we very often find epistemic iteration in action. In considering whether and how epistemic iteration is applicable to psychiatric nosology, there is no better place to start than one of Kenneth Kendler's papers (2009, p. 1939):

> A defining feature of the mature sciences is their cumulative nature. Knowledge progresses with research programs building on what has gone before. Should psychiatric nosology strive toward such a goal? For critics of psychiatric diagnoses who view them as social constructions, this is an incoherent project. If there is no truth out there, we cannot expect to get close to it. For those who adopt either realist or pragmatist perspectives on psychiatric nosology—that there are things or inter-related sets of things out there in the real world that correspond to individual psychiatric illnesses—it is a more rational and, I would argue, vital task. I here explicate this approach through the concept of iteration.

(Note Kendler's unusual pairing of realism and pragmatism as allied perspectives, to which I will return.)

29.3 What is epistemic iteration?

So, what is epistemic iteration? Colloquially speaking, it is the business of "getting on" in the absence of assured foundations. It is a process of inquiry in which "successive stages of knowledge, *each building on the preceding one*, are created in order to enhance the achievement of certain epistemic goals." (Chang 2004, p. 45) Epistemic iteration allows two modes of progress: "enrichment, in which the initially affirmed system is not negated but refined . . .; and self-correction, in which [it] is actually altered in its content as a result of inquiry based on itself." (Chang 2004, p. 228) Refinement is a straightforwardly cumulative pattern of progress, and self-correction can be regarded as cumulative in a weaker sense, if there is convergence in the sequence of results reached by successive iterations.

A good illustrative example of epistemic iteration is the one that led me to the general idea in the first place: how can measurement standards be established and improved, in the absence of pre-established standards by reference to which the proposed standards may be justified (Chang 2004, ch. 1, 2). Temperature measurement, for example, began by trusting bodily sensations of hot and cold to indicate something real; the rough correlation between such sensations and the expansion and contraction of various substances gave rise to crude early thermometers (or rather "thermoscopes," giving no meaningful numbers); trusting those instruments allowed the establishment of "fixed points," namely, phenomena that seemed to take place always at the same temperature; trusting the fixed points to be fixed allowed the construction of numerical scales of temperature; and so on. Having the later, more refined standards allowed the "correction" of earlier standards: even the crude thermoscopes could show that our sensations do not always reflect changes of external temperature reliably; readings of numerical thermometers containing various fluids did not agree exactly with each other, and the discrepancy led to more refined investigations, which led to modifications in the initial assumption that each of the thermometric fluids expanded linearly with real temperature. Generally, any process of building knowledge in the absence of pre-approved foundations (God-given or self-evident) would have to proceed in such an iterative manner.

It is useful to compare and contrast epistemic iteration with mathematical iteration (which is the origin of the general idea of "iteration"), defined as follows in the *Oxford English Dictionary*:

> The repetition of an operation upon its product . . . esp. the repeated application of a formula devised to provide a closer approximation to the solution of a given equation when an approximate solution is substituted in the formula, so that a series of successively closer approximations may be obtained.

For example, with "Newton's method" for finding the roots (or zeroes) of a real-valued function $f(x)$, one can start with a guess x_0 at the solution and then refine it toward the correct answer by following an algorithm that draws the tangent to the curve at $f(x_0)$, and doing the same again from x_1, where the tangent hits the x-axis, and so on (see Figure 29.1). If the initial guess is close enough, the successive approximations will converge on the correct answer.

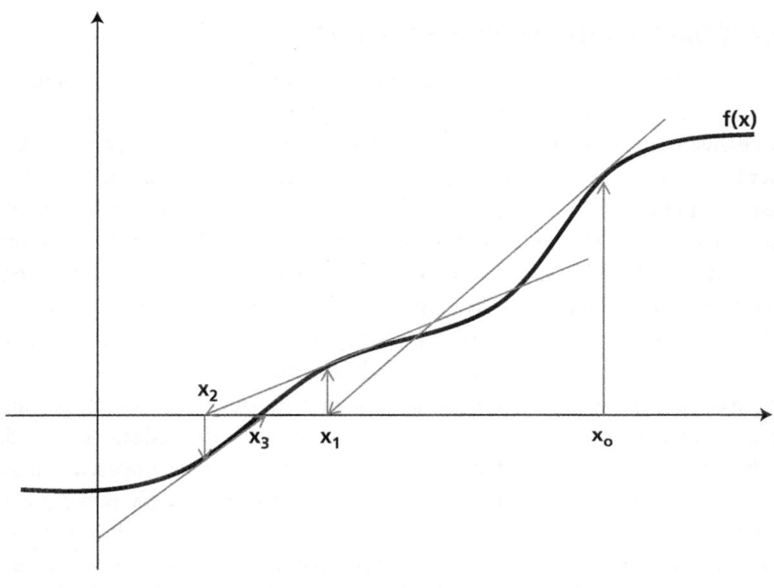

Figure 29.1 Newton's method as an example of mathematical iteration.

There are important differences between the two kinds of iteration. While mathematical iteration relies on a well-defined algorithm to produce the successive approximations, in epistemic iteration each stage is based on the previous stage but cannot be deduced from it in any straightforward sense. And while mathematical iteration approaches the correct answer that is knowable by other means, in epistemic iteration there is no guarantee that a correct answer even exists. Yet, if epistemic iteration works out, we may hope to reach a practical convergence, in which the changes get smaller and subtler as we go on and the system becomes quite stable after a while. But what exactly does such a convergence show?

29.4 **From the "local minimum" problem to pluralist realism**

For realists, the kind of stability afforded by an iterative process may not be considered good enough, as stability does not mean truth. This is a very serious problem that needs to be overcome, if we are to regard epistemic iteration as the model of cumulative progress in science. Even if we have convergence, it may merely be convergence to a "local minimum," while the real answer lies elsewhere entirely. Thinking back to mathematical iteration, one can easily imagine a situation (see Figure 29.2) in which an iterative algorithm is very effective in finding a local minimum of a curve but entirely unable to detect the global minimum which lies far away from the initial guess. It is also easy to imagine an analogue of this problem in epistemic iteration.

In another metaphor: what if the stability we reach is only a symptom of being stuck in a "box canyon?" (See Zachar, Chapter 35 of this volume, section 35.5.) If

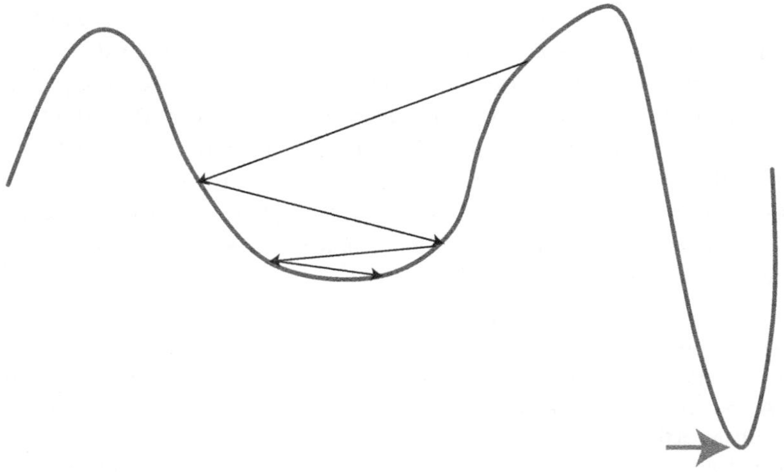

Figure 29.2 Illustration of the local minimum problem.

what we are after is the truth, what good is convergence? Kendler expresses this worry forcefully in the context of psychiatric nosology (2012, p. 317):

> Why might our disorders get stuck in a local minimum? . . . the most interesting (and worrying) possibility is that the clinical-historical syndromes that we have started this process with are not close enough to the truth about psychiatric illness for us to get there from here. This is the 'not even in the ball-park' metaphor I used previously.

So what do we do about this? Kendler again (2012, p. 318):

> The problem of local minima is a deep one. In particular, how will you know when you are in one? When do you decide that a diagnostic category is so broken that small fixes are not going to work? I cannot now provide any satisfactory answers for these questions.

To know whether we are stuck in a local minimum, we would need to have some non-iterative criteria to tell us when convergence is to a false answer. But what, other than the true answer itself, would work as such a criterion? Some theoretical word-of-God, or some set of super-validators? Neither seems plausible.

Worse yet, successful iteration may generate a false sense of security. In trusting epistemic iteration, we may be condemned to celebrate false answers that have only trapped us by deceptive convergence, like a mouse who has found the little bit of food in the mousetrap while the whole hunk of cheese is in the cupboard, now completely out of reach. Iterative convergence might build up and entrench our tentative initial guess into a dogma, and give it a force of hard-earned apparent empirical vindication. If so, convergence could easily be a curse in disguise. This seems to be a worry expressed by Jeffrey Poland (2014, p. 57) about efforts to reform the *Diagnostic and Statistical Manual of Mental Disorders* (DSM) framework.

The local minimum problem may seem like an unsolvable difficulty that will destroy any benefits of epistemic iteration. But I want to argue that addressing this problem actually gives us a great opportunity for improving the concept of epistemic iteration and getting beyond an unrealistic kind of realism. In brief, this is my main contention: all instances of successful epistemic iteration constitute cumulative progress; if there are multiple systems of practice[2] in the same domain, each of which is progressing iteratively, then all of them should be kept alive, ideally in productive interaction with each other. In other words, the key to transcending the local minimum problem is pluralism (as opposed to monism), by which I mean an ideology of science that holds that it is beneficial to create and maintain multiple systems of practice even in one field of science.

---

[2] A "system of practice" is a term I introduced in Chang (2012, pp. 15–16), to refer to "a coherent set of epistemic activities performed with a view to achieve certain aims." An "epistemic activity" is defined as "a more-or-less coherent set of mental or physical operations that are intended to contribute to the production or improvement of knowledge in a particular way, in accordance with some discernible rules."

We need to question the monist assumption that there is one right answer to a question. Even in mathematics, there may be multiple correct answers to a problem (the simplest example: $x^2 = 1$). In empirical science there are additional reasons why there may be no such thing as "the" right answer. Of clear relevance here is what Kendler calls "wobbly iteration" (2009, p. 1940). Not only do agreed validators change over time, but at any given moment people may have irreconcilable sets of weights attached to them (Kuhn 1977). And different investigators may not actually be asking exactly the same question, even if they seem to be on the surface. Science cannot count on being able to force people to ask the same questions and evaluate the answers in the same way; rather, it needs to make progress in a situation where it makes no sense demand the one right answer. How is that possible?

Here I return to Kendler's implied alliance of realism and pragmatism. Traditional realism is untenable where it seeks or claims a correspondence between theory and reality, as we do not have direct access to reality. Realism needs to be refitted along pragmatist lines. We should reclaim realism for realistic people, away from the so-called realists whose main mode of operation is speculative wishful thinking about ultimate truth. Realism, as I propose to take it, is a commitment to learn the most we can about nature. This involves creating and developing as many successful scientific systems of practice as possible. Pragmatist realism is inherently pluralist.[3]

I think much of the worry about "local minima" can be dissolved by a judicious application of pluralism: abandoning monism removes much of the angst about whether we have found the right answer. Away from that inoperable question, we can get on with the task of assessing the merits of the answers that we do have in our hands, by reference to criteria of evaluation that we do have and can use. If we re-approach scientific practice with this orientation, then we begin to see that there will be many "local minima" in a typical real problem-situation, and that there is benefit in reaching a local minimum. Don't ask how we can get out of a local minimum: why should you want to? All minima look, locally, like local minima. That is as good as it gets. The key is not to stop when we find one local minimum. If there is no one right answer, we should try to find as many good answers as possible, and develop each of them as much as we can. There is no compelling reason for scientific researchers to keep only one system, if there are multiple ones that are each progressing iteratively. Wouldn't it be more productive to let many systems spring up, keep the ones with initial plausibility, and see how far each one may develop, also looking out for the benefits that can come from the interaction between the competing systems? (In certain practical realms, such as medical diagnosis, there may be a need for one official system; that is the subject of the next section.)

What are often presented as realist worries about such thoughts as above are actually *monist* worries. It is a misconception to think that only one among

---

[3] See Chang (2012), ch. 4, 5, for a more extended account of realism and pluralism along these lines.

competing systems can be given realist credence. Significant iterative progress can be achieved only when nature does not get in the way of it. Only a small number of schemes we try out, only some starting points of attempted iteration, will be successful, yet there is no reason to assume that only one system can be successful in a given domain of study. It is important to recognize that a sense of scientific realism does not require monism. It makes perfect sense to say, for example, that both phlogiston (as conceived by Priestley and Cavendish) and oxygen (as conceived by Lavoisier) are real.[4] What do I mean by "real" there? It is a term that applies to a concept, to indicate that it is a significant part of an empirically successful system of practice. Being "successful" means achieving certain agreed aims; being a "significant" part of a successful system means playing an actual role in the success, rather than just being tacked on to other elements responsible for the success.[5] (Cf. Erik Turkheimer on "meaningful but arbitrary," in Chapter 5 of this volume.) Success comes in degrees, which means reality does, too. Repeated success is better than one-off success, and iterative success is more reassuring than success at any one stage.

But won't pluralist realism force us to accept the truth of mutually inconsistent statements? If one system says that schizophrenia is real and another system says that it is not, surely they cannot both be right? We must be more careful here. The question of truth comes up properly only if we have defined our terms so that we can make precise statements. Once the terms are defined, there will be facts of the matter about whether certain well-specified statements are true or not. "There is no such thing as schizophrenia" is not such a well-specified statement, until we are all agreed on what "schizophrenia" means (and also what the phrase "there is no such thing" should mean in practice). And if we have two systems that employ different terms, then there is always the possibility of semantic incommensurability; statements made in the different systems cannot be compared directly with each other in their contents, unless there is an unambiguous translation between the terms of the two systems. Given semantic incommensurability, the worry about contradiction evaporates.

The fear of plurality can be worse in the abstract than when we examine some real concrete cases. In order to illustrate this, I briefly recall one case of healthy plurality in science, from my earlier work on the history of thermal physics that initially gave rise to the notion of epistemic iteration (Chang 2004, ch. 4). It is well-known that Lord Kelvin (William Thomson) created the concept of absolute temperature. What is not widely known is that in fact he made *two* concepts of absolute temperature:

- Absolute temperature in 1848: In an ideal Carnot engine, a unit of heat descending from a body *A* at the temperature $T°$ of this scale, to a body *B* at the temperature $(T-1)°$, would give out the same mechanical effect, whatever the number *T*.

---

[4] For further discussion of this point, see Chang (2017).

[5] So, any concept that is genuinely part of a successful system is real, but reality is not an *explanation* of success; rather, success is the license for regarding something as real.

- Absolute temperature in 1854: $T_a/T_b = Q_a/Q_b$, where Q_a and Q_b are the amounts of heat absorbed and emitted in the two isothermal strokes of the Carnot cycle, and T_a and T_b are the temperatures at which those strokes happen.

The two concepts were very different, especially since the first concept was defined in a theoretical framework in which heat was a conserved quantity, and the second one was based on energy conservation and the interconvertibility of heat and mechanical work. The second concept became the basis of our modern temperature concept, with absolute zero determined as −273.15 °C. The operational meaning of this concept was consolidated by a very explicit process of iteration.[6] The iterative process began by assuming that gas thermometers measured absolute temperature, and continued with empirical investigations, using gas thermometers themselves and heavily aided by theory, that gave indications of how much gas-thermometer readings deviated from absolute temperature.

Kelvin's first absolute temperature concept was discarded, though it was perfectly coherent within itself in terms of Carnot's old pre-energy thermodynamic theory. It could have been preserved and developed, and it would have pointed to something real. In retrospect we say, quantitatively, that $T = \log T'$ (writing T and T' for the first and second concept), which implies that if one is a well-formed quantity then so is the other. So we can speculate with reasonable safety that an iterative development of T would also have led to convergence. Kelvin could have gone either way (or both ways!) between his two temperature concepts, without harming future generations. One of his reasons for choosing T' was the fact that it seemed to agree better than T with the readings of the gas thermometers in practical use, but that is not an absolute kind of reason. What might have happened if Kelvin's first absolute temperature concept had been kept and developed iteratively? Can we tell what might have developed? Have we lost something valuable here?[7]

29.5 **Pluralism and iteration in taxonomy**

The pluralist realism stemming from epistemic iteration is particularly germane in the realm of taxonomy, including psychiatric nosology. Taxonomy is a key part of the business of building a conceptual (or linguistic) framework. Epistemic

---

[6] This was necessarily an iterative process, because the definition of the concept was in terms of the Carnot cycle, the idealized heat engine that no one even attempted to make in reality.

[7] Another notable case of healthy plurality in science is that of the Wedgwood pyrometer (thermometer for measuring high temperatures). Josiah Wedgwood's clay pyrometer was rejected not for any absolute reason, but because it disagreed with various other standards, which agreed well enough among themselves (Chang 2004, pp. 128–141). It is difficult to say what benefits Wedgwood pyrometry might have brought, if it had been preserved and developed. In another case, that of phlogiston chemistry, the lost potential of the discarded system can be clearly recognized, because later science actually went on to recover the potential, albeit under a different name (Chang 2012, ch. 1).

iteration is a method perfectly suited for the task of creating and refining the very framework of thought and expression that we need in order to make any statements. (The situation is very different in mathematical iteration, which occurs within an already well-defined framework.) We must recognize that to ask whether a conceptual framework is "true" or "false" amounts to a category mistake. The goodness of a framework can only be judged by its fruits, by what it enables us to achieve.[8] Therefore the starting point of taxonomical work is pluralistic in a logical sense, even if it is in fact monistic due to our lack of imagination. And then, when we have multiple taxonomic systems, we can and should ask if each of those systems is a good one. For example, in nosology we may ask about the relative merits of symptom-based classifications and etiology-based classifications. (cf. Kenneth Schaffner and Kathryn Tabb, this volume, Chapter 41).

Here the notion of "natural kinds" becomes relevant, if we can divest it of traditional essentialist connotations as advocated by Harold Kincaid (2014), Peter Zachar (2014), and Rachel Cooper (2013) among others. I suggest, following these authors, that we regard a classificatory concept as a natural kind if it is sufficiently effective in aiding practices in the natural sciences (cf. Michael First on "practical kinds," Chapter 17 of this volume). Stéphanie Ruphy (2010, p. 1110) reminds us of the whole purpose of having classificatory terms in scientific practice: "coming up with kind-membership conditions that define epistemically fruitful groupings of entities . . ., rather than trying to discover the hidden essence of antecedently recognized kinds." A classificatory concept that keeps playing an obviously non-idle role in various successful systems of practice will gain increasing credence. We may express this credence in the form of a declaration that such a concept is a natural kind, as John Dupré allows (1993, p. 83):

> There is certainly no harm in calling a set of objects that are found to have a substantial number of shared properties a natural kind. The discovery of such a kind, however, provides no basis for the supposition that some particular properties can nonarbitrarily be singled out as essential.

This stance also dovetails nicely with Richard Boyd's (1991) conception of natural kinds as "homeostatic property clusters."

This view of natural kinds, combined with my notion of realism explained above, implies that concepts that are "natural" are also "real," and vice versa. Concepts prove their naturalness/reality by their ability to support successful epistemic activities. If we hit upon some stable and effective classificatory concepts in our inquiry, we should cherish them (calling them "natural kinds" would be one clear way of doing so), but without presuming that we have thereby found some eternal essences. The old familiar metaphor of "carving nature at its joints" should be replaced by a humbler motto: "suck it and see." Here the notion of epistemic iteration becomes important again. It is logically possible that there might be a static

[8] This was a clear insight from the great pragmatist philosopher C. I. Lewis (1929), now mostly forgotten.

system that serves all our purposes. More likely, however, what we need, and what we have in most successful sciences, is a steadily evolving system.

Kendler (2009, pp. 1935–7) draws an instructive parallel between psychiatric nosology and biological taxonomy. But I want to question the endpoint of his narrative, where he seems to assume that the long-standing system of classification by characteristics was iteratively improved, yet was replaced altogether in the end by the post-Darwinian system of classification by descent. I think John Dupré (1993, ch. 2, 3) has made a compelling case that it would be a mistake if biologists discarded classification by characteristics entirely, even though classification by descent is clearly superior in some respects. And the old system has in fact not been discarded completely. We should not be afraid to admit that we do in fact have two parallel systems, and we should try to form a clearer idea about how that is beneficial. Each system has its uses; we do not know how far each one will develop; and there are situations in which it is useful to be able to draw from both systems.

29.6 Developmental patterns in taxonomy

If we let our classificatory concepts develop in an iterative way, what are the positive developmental patterns we can hopefully look out for, and actively try to achieve? Here it is important that we keep our perspective broad, in two senses: we should take inspiration from positive developments found in various areas of science, and we should not restrict ourselves to the kinds of developments that monists would approve of.

29.6.1 Increase of precision

If iteration works out straightforwardly, we may be able to retain and refine our concepts. For example, having defined chemical elements by reference to atomic weight, chemists later learned to differentiate different isotopes with slightly different atomic weights, which were all classified as variants of the same element as they shared all chemical properties. Through this development, the periodic table of elements was not only retained but refined further, as chemists updated the principle of ordering from atomic weight to atomic number. Another example is the International (Practical) Temperature Scale first agreed in 1927, refined by further revisions in 1948, 1968, and 1990, in a manner somewhat reminiscent of the successive versions of the DSM. Hopefully, the development of nosology can also show an increase of precision, measured in terms of increased reliability of diagnosis.

29.6.2 Additional layers of meaning

Epistemic iteration can also lead to the enrichment of meaning by a coherent addition of layers of interpretative connections. For example, "contagion" in epidemiology was mostly a phenomenological category, until the discovery of bacteria and other disease-causing microorganisms added a micro-causal layer to its understanding. Metrologists are currently in the process of redefining the kilogram in terms of

Planck's constant, via the Josephson effect and the quantum Hall effect; this will add a new layer of meaning to the concept of mass without destroying its old meaning (Quinn 2012). This pattern is not strictly reductionist, as significant changes may be made to the original concept. For example, "oxidation" became a misnomer when it became understood as the loss of an electron by an atom (or a group of atoms), not necessarily involving oxygen as the receiver of that electron; "oxygen" (acid-maker) itself became a misnomer when Lavoisier's theory of acidity was discarded.

29.6.3 Differentiation

In the course of scientific research, what we start out considering as a unified category may turn out to be a heterogeneous one. An excellent example is diabetes, which is nowadays seen to comprise two very different conditions ("type 1" and "type 2") which have little to do with each other (Kendler, this volume, Chapter 38). Such bifurcation (or differentiation into many categories, or even a continuous "spectrum") need not get in the way of successful iteration; each branch of the concept can continue to develop iteratively. Kelvin's two concepts of absolute temperature, discussed above, could have constituted such differentiation. This may be a very important developmental pattern for psychiatry: concepts such as autism, depression, and panic disorders may all be rightly going through this process. Whether such a differentiated concept still constitutes a single concept in any meaningful sense is an interesting question.

29.6.4 Implosion

A valid outcome of an iterative process is not always convergent or constructive. Iteration may lead to a result that contradicts our starting point so fundamentally that it is judged to be untenable. In that case we need to abandon the starting point and begin somewhere else. It could be said that this was the fate that rightly greeted the Galenic four-humor theory of medicine, after many centuries of earnest development. On a smaller scale, something similar might be said about, say, the Freudian concept of the Oedipus complex. I will not enter into the debate here on whether the whole DSM-based system has reached this state, as Jeffrey Poland and Barbara von Eckardt (2013) seem to suggest.

29.6.5 Convergence and closure

A system of practice may become very stable, so that further rounds of iteration produce only small changes. In rare cases there may be a point of complete convergence, where no change seems possible. Kuhn (1970, p. 79) referred to geometric optics as such a completed paradigm, and spectroscopy in its various branches may have also reached such a stage of development. On the theoretical side, Werner Heisenberg's notion of "closed theories" may point to a similar phenomenon (see Bokulich 2008, ch. 2). When a sufficient degree of convergence has been achieved, research becomes a game of diminishing returns. At some point scientists may decide that the system is now closed, dead as a research subject but lasting as a reliable basis for applications.

26.6.6 Parallel iterations

When a system reaches convergence, some may be happy with that state of affairs. Others may think that it is not good enough, because there are some important problems that it cannot solve, or some important concerns that it does not address. Monists will see this as the "local minimum" problem, but we should try to get beyond that perspective. Without assuming that there will be some system that does everything well, we can grant that it would be worthwhile to open up another line of iterative development from a different starting point.[9] In this way, multiple systems can coexist, and productive interactions may occur. We may have such a situation in the parallel development of latent-variable analysis and network models, and of the DSM and the Research Domain Criteria (RDoC).

29.7 Pluralism under an official system

The prospect of parallel iterations might seem worrisome to practical people, such as those who have to think about the actual organization of medical care and social welfare. Don't we need one consistent and unified system in order to prevent inefficiency, confusion and chaos? Without a single *official* system of diagnostic categories, how would we be able to maintain a healthy sense of medical authority, and handle practical business such as insurance-billing (see Solomon 2015)? Don't the necessities of action demand monism, at least concerning the basic categories of discourse? This is reminiscent of the argument for unification by Otto Neurath, a leader of the Vienna Circle of logical positivism and the spearhead of the Unity of Science movement, which was based on a demand for "unity at the point of action" (see Cat et al. 1996)

While acknowledging that action ultimately needs to go in one direction rather than many in each case, I want to caution against translating that necessity into an argument for monism in scientific research. Even Neurath acknowledged that different scientific disciplines needed to flourish separately, although they needed to be brought together at the point of action. Effective monist action requires a pluralist research base. Science needs pluralism in research, in order to reap the practical benefits that will flow from successful research.

Let me make that point more concrete, in the context of taxonomic concepts. As a framework for coordinated practice, we do need an official system, such as the DSM. But that does not mean that all research should take place within that system, or that other systems cannot be tested on a trial basis in limited areas of practice, or that some people should not be allowed to opt out of the system altogether. A scientific–practical community should invest some of its resources in the development of some well-chosen parallel systems that will constitute a fertile soil for further growth of even the official system itself.

[9] This is different from differentiation, which is the result of a more refined understanding of a concept within a given system.

Even though science may be able to progress fairly well by the iterative development of one official system, there are three broader issues that we must not lose sight of.

- Potential for other or better developments may lie elsewhere, along lines of iterative development with entirely different starting points; here we return to the worry about the local minimum problem, and the role of pluralism in countering that problem.
- The iterative development of the official system may lead to the differentiation of a concept; further developing the differentiated branches of the concept may result in the creation of parallel systems.
- Epistemic iteration is a creative process, and often requires new ideas that may not easily arise from within the system; sources of new ideas may dry up if no other systems are maintained.

All three considerations point to the need to entertain and develop multiple systems at once, even while maintaining one of them as the official system. Metrologists have done this very effectively for about a century now, having learned to go beyond the once-and-for-all reforming zeal of the French Revolution (see Quinn 2012). Doubts about the official standards, whether they be the meter stick or the standard kilogram, have been dealt with by vigorous fundamental and practical research into alternatives, while maintaining the doubted official standards, until the international community could agree that new superior standards could be made. In my humble opinion, the development of the DSM is also approaching this mature model, and could go further in that direction with benefit.

So, how should the iterative development of taxonomic systems in a scientific–practical field proceed? The answer I offer, I think, is actually not so different from the account by Peter Zachar et al. (Chapters 34–36 of this volume) of how personality disorders have been dealt with in the transition from DSM-IV to DSM-5. Even though there may have been frustrations with various aspects of this episode, I think the outcome was a productive one in terms of how dissatisfaction with the official system was dealt with.

1 The essential first step, emphasized by Kendler (2009, p. 1937) is to accept the historicity of knowledge, and acknowledge the contingency of the starting point of an iterative process.

2 We also need to clarify and articulate our aims and values (which produce the relevant standards of judgment), noting any significant disagreements within our own community and across different communities. This is a key step prior to any iteration being attempted, but it also needs to be an ongoing process, partly because our aims and values may change as time goes on.

3 After the first two steps are taken we can properly attempt an iterative development, noting successes and failures as we go on. The dominant system should not be discarded unless it is judged to be a clear failure (showing the pattern of "implosion" discussed above). Flip-flopping on the choice of the official system on the basis of insufficient evidence should be strenuously avoided.

4 After some efforts, we should identify any aims that are not being met in the dominant system despite its iterative development, and identify or develop alternative systems that might do better in meeting those aims. Once alternative systems are identified, it is up to various practitioners to attempt an iterative development of each system that passes the test of initial plausibility, noting its successes and failures. We can also reap the benefits of interaction between different systems.

5 We then assess the relative overall merits of the competing systems, and assess the designation of the official system. There are several possible outcomes here:

5a Retention of the official system. This seems to be just what happened, for example, with the proposed new nosological system for personality disorders. The new system was seriously considered; it was in the end not accepted as the new official system, but recognized as a viable alternative and included in DSM-V "in a section at the back of the book" (Zachar, section 35.1).

5b Revolutionary change. One of the alternative systems may be judged to be superior to the dominant system, and chosen as the new official system. The old system is discarded, like the ancient four-elements system or the associated four-humors system of medicine. Will the same happen to currently dominant designations like schizophrenia? It has already happened to Freud's oral–anal–genital stages of development and the id–ego–superego structure of the mind, though these ideas live on unofficially.

5c Division of domain. The old official system may be maintained as superior in certain situations, but another system may be recognized as superior in another domain and become the official system there. In such a situation, areas of overlap between the two domains would need to be handled very carefully. Something similar to this can be seen in the International (Practical) Temperature Scale, which is actually a patchwork of different official standards in different segments of the whole temperature range. Various fundamental theories of physics have also been accommodated by a division of domain, though without the kind of explicit legislation that metrologists make: classical mechanics remains *de facto* the official theory of physics in the domain of everyday-size objects and much of celestial mechanics (and "rocket science" as the combination of the two); quantum mechanics handles most microlevel situations; in the borderland of "mesoscopic" phenomena, we have some very interesting and intricate mixed classical–quantum reasoning. Could something like this work in psychiatric nosology? I believe there is good sense in what I have called "conservationist pluralism": don't kill the "good-old" systems, as they are likely to continue to work in their original domains (Chang 2012, p. 218).

The outcome of step 5 should then trigger a new rendition of step 3, and thereafter a truly mature iterative phase of development can begin.

29.8 **Summary**

I have presented my view on how the method of epistemic iteration might be best applied to the development of taxonomic systems. The adoption of pluralism allows us to actualize the full potential of epistemic iteration by dissolving worries about whether we are approaching the one true system. A pluralist and pragmatist realism underlies a mature scientific attitude that allows us to recognize and promote progress in a variety of iterative developmental patterns.

References

Bokulich, A. (2008). *Reexamining the Quantum–Classical relation: Beyond reductionism and pluralism.* Cambridge: Cambridge University Press.

Boyd, R. (1991). Realism, anti-foundationalism and the enthusiasm for natural kinds. *Philosophical Studies*, **61**, 127–148.

Cat, J., **Cartwright, N.**, and **Chang, H.** (1996). Otto Neurath: Politics and the unity of science. In P. Galison and D. Stump (eds.) *The Disunity of Science*, pp. 347–369. Stanford, CA: Stanford University Press.

Chang, H. (2004). *Inventing Temperature: Measurement and scientific progress.* New York: Oxford University Press.

Chang, H. (2012). *Is Water H_2O? Evidence, realism and pluralism.* Dordrecht: Springer.

Chang, H. (2017). Is pluralism compatible with scientific realism? In J. Saatsi (ed.) *Routledge Handbook of Scientific Realism* London: Routledge (forthcoming).

Cooper, R. (2013). Natural kinds. In K.W.M. Fulford, M. Davies, R.G.T. Gipps, *et al.* (eds.) *The Oxford Handbook of Philosophy and Psychiatry*, pp. 950–965. New York: Oxford University Press.

Dupré, J. (1993). *The Disorder of Things: Metaphysical foundations for the disunity of science.* Cambridge, MA: Harvard University Press.

Kendler, K.S. (2009). An historical framework for psychiatric nosology. *Psychological Medicine*, **39**, 1935–1941.

Kendler, K.S. (2012). Epistemic iteration as a historical model for psychiatric nosology: promises and limitations. In K.S. Kendler and J. Parnas (eds.) *Philosophical Issues in Psychiatry II: Nosology*, pp. 305–322. Oxford: Oxford University Press.

Kendler, K.S. and **Parnas, J.** (eds.) (2012). *Philosophical Issues in Psychiatry II: Nosology.* Oxford: Oxford University Press.

Kincaid, H. (2014). Defensible natural kinds in the study of psychopathology. In H. Kincaid and J. Sullivan (eds.) *Classifying Psychopathology: Mental kinds and natural kinds*, pp. 145–173. Cambridge, MA: MIT Press.

Kincaid, H. and **Sullivan, J.** (ed.) (2014). *Classifying Psychopathology: Mental kinds and natural kinds.* Cambridge, MA: MIT Press.

Kuhn, T.S. (1970). *The Structure of Scientific Revolutions*, 2nd edn. Chicago: University of Chicago Press.

Kuhn, T.S. (1977). Objectivity, value judgment, and theory choice. In *The Essential Tension*, pp. 320–339. Chicago: University of Chicago Press.

Lewis, C.I. (1929). *Mind and the World-Order: Outline of a theory of knowledge.* New York: Charles Scribner's Sons.

Poland, J. (2014). Deeply rooted sources of error and bias in psychiatric classification. In H. Kincaid and J. Sullivan (eds.) *Classifying Psychopathology: Mental kinds and natural kinds*, pp. 29–63. Cambridge, MA: MIT Press.

Poland, J. and **von Eckardt, B.** (2013). Mapping the domain of mental illness. In K.W.M. Fulford, M. Davies, R.G.T. Gipps, et al. (eds.) *The Oxford Handbook of Philosophy and Psychiatry*, pp. 733–752. New York: Oxford University Press.

Quinn, T. (2012). *From Artefacts to Atoms: The BIPM and the search for ultimate measurement standards.* Oxford, UK: Oxford University Press.

Ruphy, S. (2010). Are stellar kinds natural kinds? A challenging newcomer in the monism/pluralism and realism/antirealism debate. *Philosophy of Science*, 77, 1109–1120.

Scerri, E. (2007). *The Periodic Table: Its story and its significance.* New York: Oxford University Press.

Solomon, M. (2015). *Making Medical Knowledge.* Oxford: Oxford University Press.

Zachar, P. (2014). Beyond natural kinds: Toward a "relevant" "scientific" taxonomy in psychiatry. In H. Kincaid and J. Sullivan (eds.) *Classifying Psychopathology: Mental kinds and natural kinds*, pp. 75–104. Cambridge, MA: MIT Press.

Chapter 30

Psychiatric nosology, epistemic iteration, and pluralism

Kenneth S. Kendler

This is a rich, variegated, and in many ways charming paper. It is hard not to be touched by Dr. Chang's preamble—essentially a pep talk for psychiatric nosologists and philosophers. He tells us not to lose heart and be too self-derogatory about our problems. He is correct that many of us—who know little of the history and philosophy of the hard sciences of physics and chemistry—have an idealized view of those fields. My vague view of them (e.g., the grass is greener . . .) would have been something like this, "They have solved all their basic problems and we, in psychiatry, are bumbling our way along from one confused crises to the next." For me, the pep talk worked. It was reassuring to see how many times fundamental conceptual issues have shifted in these fields and how much uncertainty there is about basic theoretical and practical questions. I especially like learning about the major shifts of our approach to defining foundational constructs like the meter. It was also a pleasure to read his clear description of the concept of epistemic iteration, which he first articulated in Chang (2004). Chang's enthusiasm for the scientific enterprise suffuses his essay as well captured by this quote:

> If we hit upon some stable and effective classificatory concepts in our inquiry, we should cherish them . . . but without presuming that we have thereby found some eternal essences. The old familiar metaphor of "carving nature at its joints" should be replaced by a humbler motto: "suck it and see."

Turning to more substantive comments, I here want to make four broad points. First, Chang proposes, in an application to psychiatric nosology, a marriage of epistemic iteration and scientific pluralism. We should not be preoccupied with having only one "target" for our epistemic iteration, he argues. Being "stuck" in a local minimum is not such a problem, as having a few potential diagnostic systems under consideration is likely to be beneficial.

Indeed, pluralism has many positive features for basic sciences. Often truth is distributed. He gives us physical examples such as the two ways to conceive of absolute temperature and the many different possible approaches to measuring temperature. It is quite convincing that having multiple perspectives compete over time is a sensible strategy. Indeed, it is rather basic to the success of the scientific method. The history of science shows that we are bad at predicting winners. Sometimes the correct view emerges from "way out in left field"—think of continental drift or prions. Who would have thought that two unknowns, Watson and Crick, would beat the great Linus Pauling in finding the correct structure of DNA? Furthermore, in psychiatry, I have been strongly committed to "empirically based pluralism" as a guiding light for psychiatric science (Kendler 2012, 2014). Why should I be concerned about applying a similar approach to diagnosis?

The answer is found in the history of psychiatry. The original cacophony of different diagnostic systems in pre-DSM times might not be well known to some readers of this volume. Studies were not comparable. The diagnosis of schizophrenia varied widely in different centers even in the same country. As the first major "somatic" therapies developed (e.g., insulin coma therapy and electroconvulsive therapy) it was nearly impossible to compare treatment results across centers because of large differences in diagnostic practice (Langfeldt 1960). It was a real mess.

Then there were the problems of forensic psychiatry. In high-profile legal cases, "experts" would disagree wildly about the diagnosis using quite different diagnostic formulations. This was permissible because there were no rules, no agreed-upon systems. (This is not the strongest of arguments because, even in the era of operationalized criteria, psychiatry has still had trouble agreeing on diagnoses in high-profile forensic cases, for example, that of Breivik in Norway; see Melle 2013.)

Then what about the hurly-burly world of clinical practice and research where psychiatry is already chronically underfunded compared to other biomedical fields? Think about a fight that a chair of psychiatry might have with a chair of surgery over resources in a hospital or medical school. The chair of surgery would never consider the question of pluralism in his or her diagnostic practice—bowel cancer, gallbladder disease, etc. Pluralism will not be part of their vocabulary. I can hear the argument now, "You want to take money from my surgeons and give it to those damn psychiatrists who can't even make up their minds about the disorders they treat?"

So, is there a space between the rigid monopoly of a single diagnostic system and the chaos of every great professor having their own diagnostic scheme? How do we find a "controlled pluralism" that can have important benefits for psychiatric nosology? Chang's examples—the two competing personality disorder systems in the fifth edition of the *Diagnostic and Statistical Manual of Mental Disorders* (DSM-5) and Research Domain Criteria (RDoC) versus DSM-5 —are good ones. Another example can be added for a positive role "nosologic pluralism." Binge eating disorder was placed in the appendix in DSM-IV to encourage further study. By the time DSM-5 came around, enough empirical data had been collected for it to "graduate" to the main volume. Our goal is to encourage robust scientific competition that prevents the premature shut-down of promising categories or diagnostic approaches but does not produce diagnostic chaos with all its negative effects. Philosophers can live in the world of thought experiments. The real world of psychiatry might impose some constraints on our ideal set of practices.

Second, Chang proposes what I might call a "blending" of scientific realism and pragmatism (with a strong dose of pluralism, as noted earlier). He writes, "Epistemic iteration points to a pluralist realism." Later he notes, "In empirical science there are additional reasons why there may be no such thing as 'the' right answer." And "This involves creating and developing as many successful scientific systems of practice as possible. Pragmatist realism is inherently pluralist." I can imagine trying to explain this perspective to a room full of hard-nosed biological psychiatrists. They are likely to be "naive realists" who would accept the commonsense correspondence theory of truth that either there is something "out there" that corresponds to schizophrenia (in some form or another) or there is not. Personally, I am quite sympathetic to this proposed blending. Coming from a very different perspective, I have elsewhere advocated a view of the nature of psychiatric disorders that might be called a pragmatically informed weak realism (Kendler 2016). Chang's key takeaway point here is that science does not give absolute and permanent answers to the questions we pose. Everything is a sketch and over time it will change and hopefully advance. Looking for a single hard, perpetual truth is unlikely to be a profitable enterprise. I think this is basically sound but this brings us to my third point about one other feature of realism which cannot I think be ignored when considering psychiatry.

That is, we need to consider this rather non-philosophical argument: In a world where the legitimacy of psychiatric illness is questioned, is there a moral obligation to advocate for the reality of psychiatric illness? The suffering is real. There remains major stigma. Care for psychiatric problems, at least in the United States, is more poorly funded than for non-mental medical disorders. Compared to the impact of these disorders on disability, research for psychiatric disorders is markedly underfunded. Do we want to contribute to this confusion by arguing that our psychiatric categories are just practical constructs for which we wish to make no claim regarding their reality? I do not have a definitive answer to this question but believe it needs to be part of this discussion.

I would be less celebratory about local minima/box canyons than Chang is. Some might turn out to be quite productive. But some really turn out to be mistakes (think humoral theory of medicine or subtypes of schizophrenia). At least for an official nosology, there can be reasons for deleting categories that perform poorly. Trimming off the dysfunctional categories can keep the system better functioning and prevent a proliferation of categories. Furthermore, Chang writes "Don't ask how we can get out of a local minimum: why should you want to?" You might want to because reformulating the category you are working on might get you "over the hump" and to a place of greater validity that would be possible with the current formulation.

Finally, Chang concludes his essay explicitly calling for "Pluralism under an official system." He offers an explicit recipe with five steps to develop such a system. As noted above, there is some pluralism in the current system (in particular, the criteria in section III of DSM-5). But he is proposing more than that. He suggests that in a mature system, like DSM:

> After some efforts, we should identify any aims that are not being met in the dominant system despite its iterative development, and identify or develop alternative systems that might do better in meeting those aims.

This is a challenging suggestion. I find it hard to imagine that the American Psychiatric Association would itself launch an "alternative DSM." Official nosologies are, after all rather "official." Such pluralism in psychiatry is more likely to emerge from research settings. For example, the last 10 years have seen a robust series of reports developing a meta-structure of psychiatric disorders based on broad psychopathological constructs—especially "internalizing" and "externalizing" disorders (Krueger et al. 2001, Kendler et al. 2011). Plans were proposed to shape the organization of disorders in DSM-5 using this approach, although this was not ultimately adopted. Competing paradigms can be stimulating for the nosologic enterprise, although as noted above, unchecked this could lead to chaos. I see it as a considerable challenge to find an optimal balance between the institutional and professional needs for an official nosology and the desire for the dynamic interactions generated by multiple possible nosologic perspectives.

In sum, I hope this interchange illustrates the positive synergism we were hoping from this meeting. You, as readers, have heard a conversation here between a deeply versed philosopher-historian of science and an active psychiatric nosologist. My hope is that we have learned enough of each other's language and concepts to have a productive interchange on what is a very interesting and important set of issues.

References

Chang, H. (2004). *Inventing Temperature: Measurement and scientific progress.* New York: Oxford University Press.

Kendler, K.S. (2012). The dappled nature of causes of psychiatric illness: replacing the organic-functional/hardware-software dichotomy with empirically based pluralism. *Molecular Psychiatry*, **17**, 377–388.

Kendler, K.S. (2014). The structure of psychiatric science. *American Journal of Psychiatry*, **171**, 931–938.

Kendler, K.S. (2016). The nature of psychiatric disorders. *World Psychiatry*, **15**, 5–12.

Kendler, K.S., Aggen, S.H., Knudsen, G.P., et al. (2011). The structure of genetic and environmental risk factors for syndromal and subsyndromal common DSM-IV Axis I and all Axis II disorders. *American Journal of Psychiatry*, **168**, 29–39.

Krueger, R.F., McGue, M., and **Iacono, W.G.** (2001). The higher-order structure of common DSM mental disorders: internalization, externalization, and their connections to personality. *Personality and Individual Differences*, **30**, 1245–1259.

Langfeldt, G. (1960). Diagnosis and prognosis of schizophrenia. *Proceedings of the Royal Society of Medicine*, **53**, 1047–1052.

Melle, I. (2013). The Breivik case and what psychiatrists can learn from it. *World Psychiatry*, **12**, 16–21.

Section 11

Problems in the validation of psychiatric diagnoses

Chapter 31

Introduction to "Validity and the causal structure of a disorder"

Kenneth S. Kendler

In this challenging and stimulating essay, John Campbell, a distinguished analytic philosopher with a long interest in psychology and psychiatry, provides a critique of the current approach to the validation of psychiatric disorders as operationalized in the *Diagnostic and Statistical Manual of Mental Disorders* (DSM) enterprise from DSM-III onward. He argues this approach, which in turn derives historically from the framework proposed by Robins and Guze (1970), is an amputated and deficient version of a full validation model. This amputation is problematic because it cuts the validation exercise free from a grounding in the "world out there." He poses the question of whether, for our psychiatric disorders, "there is anything there at all to detect or measure?" Or, to put it another way, "does the concept refer at all?" In his key figure, multiple versions of which he presents in his essay, he terms this an "external phenomenon."

In this critique, Campbell raises a number of intriguing issues only some of which I can touch on in this introductory essay. First, Campbell argues that, for all intents and purposes, the current DSM diagnostic criteria constitute the disorders they seek to define. Having a major depression is, he suggests, nothing more than meeting the relevant DSM-5 criteria. He writes, "it's assumed that our concepts of each of the disorders are exhausted by the diagnostic criteria." And, a bit later, he notes, "Are the criteria for the disorder actually constitutive of possession of the disorder?" While I agree this is an attitude often adopted by the users of DSM, it is a mistaken one based on a confusion about the nature of diagnostic criteria. Throughout medicine, diagnostic criteria have been created as practical tools to identify affected individuals with good sensitivity, specificity, and utility. That is, they have an indexical function. For example, early World Health Organization criteria for myocardial infarction (aka "heart attack" or MI) defined a definite MI as meeting these three criteria (JISFC/WHO 1979):

1 Clinical history of ischemic-type chest pain lasting for more than 20 minutes
2 Changes in serial EKG tracings
3 Rise and fall of serum cardiac biomarkers such as creatine kinase-MB fraction and troponin.

These criteria are well validated. They are good at predicting relatively definitive diagnostic tests for MI—such as a coronary angiography that directly identifies blockage in the arteries feeding the heart. They are practical. We use them because they are good at indexing who, among those with chest pain, are likely rather than unlikely to be having an MI. Diagnostic criteria should not try to list every possible important sign and symptom of a disorder. That is not their purpose. They emphasize those signs and symptoms that can be easily and reliably assessed, and that have the highest differential diagnostic value (i.e., can tell an MI from other causes of chest pain, like a muscle strain or gastric reflux). But it is a category mistake to argue that meeting these criteria constitutes "having an MI."

As I have outlined in more detail elsewhere (Kendler 2016), the problem in psychiatry is that we lack definitive tests like coronary angiography. This makes it easier for us to slide into thinking major depression is "just" the DSM criteria. But it is not. There is still a syndrome out there that clinicians diagnose and treat. It can have quite subtle symptoms (like depressive derealization) that might be important clinically but don't make sense to put into diagnostic criteria because they are hard and time-consuming to assess. Campbell is, in my view, correct in interpreting how DSM has often been seen by working psychiatrists but not how it should be used and understood.

Campbell's incisive conceptual approach to the problem of the validation of psychiatric illness could be complemented by a more overtly historical perspective. In the history of medicine, syndromes often begin as collections of signs and symptoms that are noted to frequently co-occur and often predict a certain course of illness (like recovery or rapid death). Most commonly, there is, at this stage, nothing but the vaguest ideas about etiology. Over time, with the accumulation of greater clinical expertise and more advanced scientific methods (such as the develop of specific diagnosis tools and laboratory tests), these syndromes have often been subdivided into more homogenous categories from which pathophysiology can be more clearly delineated. I have, in Chapter 38 of this volume, given a good example of this. From the syndrome of diabetes mellitus (excess sweet urine) came two quite distinct diseases (type I and type II diabetes) that we now understand to have entirely different causes, courses, and optimal treatments. But this process does not always work. Sometimes, we are left with broad multifactorial syndromes like essential hypertension or osteoporosis which resist further clean subdivisions. It is these broad syndromes our current psychiatric disorders most closely resemble.

As is often said, psychiatry lags behind much of medicine in this historical progression. Perhaps defensively, we argue, this is because our organ of focus—the brain—is a whole lot harder to understand than the heart, bone, or kidney. But, compared to many of these historical disorders of centuries past, we actually now know quite a bit about causal factors for psychiatric disorders. That is, we have rather substantial lists of risk factors that have, with varying degrees of confidence, been shown to be causally linked to the disorder in question. But Campbell is correct that we have the "Princess Elisabeth" problem in psychiatry. (She was the seventeenth-century Bohemian princess who asked Descartes to explain how causal interactions could occur between mind and body.) We lack any convincing and biologically coherent idea how psychological or social risk factors for psychiatric illness interact with biological vulnerabilities to produce disorders. But we do have many examples of "environmental" risk factors that have been shown to produce biological changes—such as childhood sexual abuse predicting reduction in the size of the hippocampus (Stein et al. 1997) and trauma producing changes in DNA methylation (Vinkers et al. 2015).

There is one more way we could argue that there is an "outside" in the psychiatric validating process. Campbell writes

> . . . and the very idea of an external phenomenon out there, to which we are causally responding and to which we are referring, is doing no work in the picture.

It is the validators rather than the ideal construct of the disorder which are doing the work. If you begin with a clinical set of diagnostic criteria, how can you ground those—learn if they are at all informative about the patients they describe? Campbell argues that validations for psychiatric disorders are "entirely in terms of correlations." If by this he means we have not well worked out complete causal pathways from putative validators to the disorders, he is on firm ground. But that is a quite demanding standard. For genetic risk factors, the molecular basis of which is starting to be identified for some disorders, we know biological pathways must exist from these variants to the disorders. But they are far outside of our ability to now articulate in anything beyond the sketchiest forms. For a lot of what we do in medicine, correlations work just fine. Indeed, double-blind studies that have so influenced modern treatment are based on correlations. We know they are likely causal because of the randomization process, but these studies typically provide no insight into the intervening mechanisms.

In this essay, Campbell provides a challenging critique for key issue in modern psychiatric nosology of validation. He is surely correct that our process is imperfect. In my view, these imperfections are an inevitable consequence of the nature of our disorders. When viewed historically, I do not think the picture is as grim as Campbell paints it. If we were making thermometers for the mass market, we could validate our product against a high-quality research instrument. That is a grounded validation process far beyond what we can now conceive in psychiatry. Instead, we need to settle for a gradual historical process of iteration, of pulling ourselves slowly up by our bootstraps in successive approximations. I don't claim this is an ideal situation. It is rather messy and vague around the borders. But it is one that other aspects of medicine have passed through. Only our task is that much more complex because of the very complex nature of our phenotypes as well as the mind–body problem which forces us to consider etiological models crossing ontological categories. I do not see how this process could be done any other way. So my view is that there is an "outside" there in Campbell's framework. It is not as robust an entity as one would wish or find in some other areas of medicine. But the difference is a quantitative and not a qualitative one.

References

JISFC/WHO. (1979). Nomenclature and criteria for diagnosis of ischemic heart disease. Report of the Joint International Society and Federation of Cardiology/World Health Organization task force on standardization of clinical nomenclature. *Circulation*, **59**, (3) 607–609.

Kendler, K.S. (2016). The phenomenology of major depression and the representativeness and nature of DSM criteria. *American Journal of Psychiatry*, **173**, 771–780.

Robins, E. and **Guze, S.B.** (1970). Establishment of diagnostic validity in psychiatric illness: its application to schizophrenia. *American Journal of Psychiatry*, **126**, 983–987.

Stein, M.B., Koverola, C., Hanna, C., et al. (1997). Hippocampal volume in women victimized by childhood sexual abuse. *Psychological Medicine*, **27**, 951–959.

Vinkers, C.H., Kalafateli, A.L., Rutten, B.P., et al. (2015). Traumatic stress and human DNA methylation: a critical review. *Epigenomics*, 7, 593–608.

Chapter 32

Validity and the causal structure of a disorder

John Campbell

32.1 Causal Counterfactuals and Processes

This paper looks at the problem raised by there being both psychological and biological causes for disorders. I argue that the position is methodologically relatively straightforward so long as we think of causation merely in terms of intervention counterfactuals or probabilistic relations. Once we think in terms of causal processes, however, it becomes much more difficult to interpret the causal structures here. There are mental processes and there are physical processes, but there does not seem to be any way of connecting the two.

I think that this puzzle forms the background to some of the uncertainty we naturally feel about the validity of psychiatric classifications. The problem is that to have the question of the validity of a classification properly posed, we have to have at least a hypothesis about the causal structure of the disorder. Our uncertainty as to causal structures here means that it is difficult to know how to pose the problem of validity in any particular case.

32.2 The "Princess Elisabeth" problem in psychiatry

There appear to be both environmental and genetic risk factors for many disorders. There has to be an understanding of how those risk factors are transduced into proximal aspects of the individual that generate those disorders. And at the moment, for many of the environmental risk factors, there is only a psychological understanding to be had of their implications for the individual. Consider, for example, divorce or bereavement, which are risk factors for major depression. There is no neurobiology of divorce or bereavement. On the other hand, consider the transduction of genetic risk factors for a disorder. These typically have only a biological transduction into proximal causal factors for a disorder. So the general situation is as diagrammed in Figure 32.1 for the case of major depression.

At the moment, there is no particular evidence to support the idea that the psychological factors will of themselves coalesce into a progression, comprehensible in purely psychological terms, leading to major depression and its symptoms. The purely biological risk factors may be ineliminable. But nor is there any evidence to

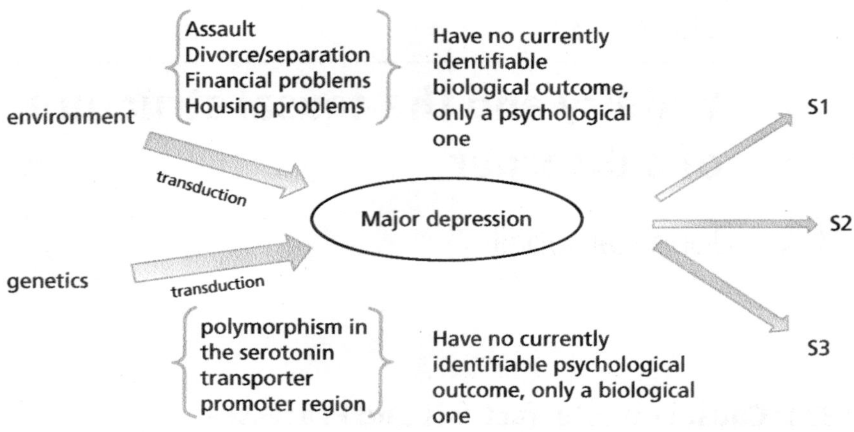

Figure 32.1. Schematic diagram of one possible causal structure for major depression. Environmental risk factors characteristically have a psychological transduction. Genetic risk factors characteristically have a biological transduction.

support the idea that the psychological interpretations of the environmental risk factors will ultimately be eliminable in favor of purely biological causal factors.

You might argue that the psychological and the purely biological causal structures here are relatively insulated from one another: the psychological factors generate psychological upshots and psychological symptoms, the purely biological factors generate purely biological upshots and purely biological symptoms. But that hardly seems credible as an interpretation. In general, biological factors are relevant to the psychological symptoms of a disorder.

It thus appears that at the moment, understanding the causal structure of a disorder will, in general, require understanding the causal relations between psychological and biological factors. Now there are another two ways in which you might try to get round the need to do this.

- You might argue that ultimately, there are only biological causal factors here. All the causation is to be understood at the biological level. At the moment, admittedly, we have to work with psychological factors. But that is only a reflection of our currently limited knowledge of brain biology. In the future, our understanding of the causal structures of disorders will be entirely at the biological level; talk of psychological risk factors is something we have to do only because of the current limitations on our knowledge.
- You might argue that all the biological risk factors for disorders can ultimately be interpreted in psychological terms. Perhaps serotonin imbalances can be interpreted in terms of some psychological construct like psychological resilience, for example, and ultimately the causal structures of disorders can be interpreted entirely in psychological terms.

At the moment, both of these pictures are science fiction. Of course our knowledge of brain biology seems bound to improve. But it is merely speculation to suppose that this will enable us to eliminate talk of psychological risk factors for disorders. It therefore seems worth looking at the difficulties we face if we have to regard psychiatric disorders as having both psychological and biological factors implicated in their etiology.

To focus directly on the theoretical question here, let's simplify the empirical picture. Suppose we look directly at just two risk factors for major depression. Suppose we consider social humiliation as our example of a psychological factor that we take to be not reducible to biology. And suppose we consider genetically based irregularities in serotonin transport as our example of a biological factor that may have no psychological interpretation. Perhaps the example will turn out to be badly chosen, perhaps there will turn out to be a biological reduction of humiliation, and perhaps there will turn out to be a psychological interpretation of serotonin irregularities. As I said, my point is only to investigate the implications of there not being a wholesale biological reduction of the psychological risk factors for disorders, or it not generally being possible to give a psychological interpretation of the biological risk factors for a disorder; so let's take it for the moment that there is no biological reduction of humiliation and no psychological interpretation of serotonin imbalance. So the situation, for this simple example, is as shown in Figure 32.2.

Now so long as we think only in terms of correlations, the situation here is relatively unproblematic. Certainly there could, in principle, be correlations between humiliation and depression, and between serotonin imbalance and depression. Indeed the correlations might be such that it is only when we have both humiliation and serotonin imbalance that we have an increased risk for depression. We have, though, to consider the case in which humiliation and serotonin imbalance are joint causes of depression. The problem comes when we try to think through the mechanisms or processes that might be involved in their joint production of the outcome. On the one hand we might suppose that we have a biological reduction of humiliation, so that we can explain the mechanism by which they jointly produce their outcome in entirely biological terms. But we are trying to explore the consequences of supposing that biological reductions are not always available.

To try to make vivid the theoretical perspective I am suggesting here, consider the position of a social psychologist investigating the consequences of a "don't ask, don't tell" policy in the military, or the causes of voting behavior—why do people vote for a particular candidate? The beliefs and preferences of the population are

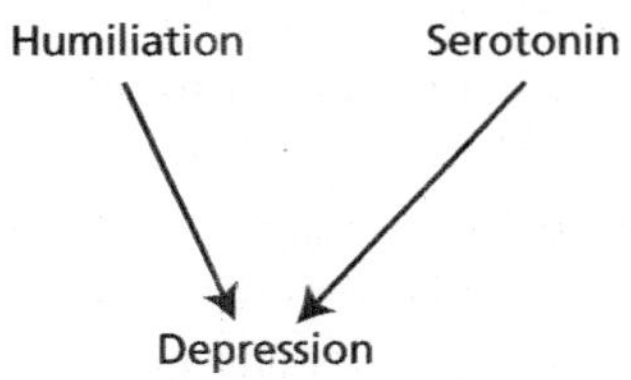

Figure 32.2. A "mixed" pair of causal factors for major depression.

likely to figure among the causes of behaviors. But the demand for a biological reduction of those beliefs and preferences is likely to strike our social psychologist as idle. Similarly, you might take the view that psychological factors such as social humiliation figure among the causes of disorders. But you might equally feel that the demand for a biological reduction of those factors is, for the moment at any rate, idle.

On the other hand we might suppose that there is a purely psychological mechanism available here, that there is some psychological interpretation of serotonin imbalance that will allow us to understand, in psychological terms, how depression is generated. But we are exploring the consequences of supposing that psychological interpretations of the biological are not always available. This leaves us, I think, without any understanding at all of how there could be a mechanism by which humiliation and serotonin jointly produce depression.

To explain our ordinary notions of mechanism and process, we first need the distinction between general and singular causation. General causation is exemplified by claims such as "smoking causes cancer," or "humiliation causes depression." It relates variables, such a "level of smoking" and "risk of cancer," which may take different values. Singular causation, on the other hand, is exemplified by claims such as "Sally's smoking caused her cancer," or "Bill's humiliation caused his depression." These claims relate particular things—Sally's smoking, Bill's depression—rather than variables.

Let's start by focusing on singular causation. In many cases, singular causation is a matter of there being a *process* connecting cause and effect. In the physical case, we have a reasonably firm grasp of what constitutes a causal process: at bottom, it's something like what Locke (1690/1975) called "the transmission of motion by impulse," what Fair (1979) called the "transfer of energy," or that Dowe (2000) talks of in terms of "exchange of conserved quantities." Something like that is the basic idea of a physical process. Biological processes can generally be seen as particularly complex versions of underlying physical processes, conceived in this way. In the psychological case, on the other hand, we think of mental processes as normatively guided sequences of psychological states. So for example, if you are trying to decide whether to apply for a particular job, your "mental processes" will involve the recruitment of your current knowledge and beliefs, and your objectives, with the goal of trying to make the right decision. Jaspers (1923/1963, p. 301) famously drew a distinction between (1) "subjective" and (2) "objective" psychopathology as follows:

1 We sink ourselves into the psychic situation and *understand genetically by empathy* how one psychic event emerges from another.

2 We find by repeated experience that a number of phenomena are regularly linked together, and on this basis we *explain causally.*

Now understanding "genetically by empathy" is what provides us with our grasp of a mental process—a psychological causal process. It's the basis of our understanding of singular causation in the psychological case. This is how we achieve our knowledge of how "one psychic event emerges from another," of how Bill's being attacked gives rise to his defensiveness, for example. As Hoerl (2013) argues, the distinction Jaspers is really after here seems to be a distinction between singular causation in the psychological case, which is known about by empathy, and general causation, which can be studied by looking at correlations and experiments across a population.

Now the trouble with thinking of both humiliation and serotonin imbalance as being, in a particular case, the interactive causes of someone's depression, is that we have no idea what a process might be in which these two factors are combined to generate the depression. If we try to think in terms of a purely biological process that generates the outcome, we run into the problem that this leaves out the humiliation. On the other hand if we try to understand the causation in this particular case purely in terms of empathetic understanding, we leave out the serotonin imbalance.

The notion of "mechanism" stands to general causation somewhat as the notion of "process" stands to singular causation. If you are told that Sally's smoking caused her cancer, you can ask what the process was by which it did so. If you are told that in general, "smoking causes cancer," you can ask, "What's the mechanism?," where what you are looking for is something like: the structure that sustains a particular type of process. So if we are told that humiliation and serotonin combine to generate depression, we can ask, "What's the mechanism?" And then we find that we have no idea at all how we might think of those two factors combining to generate the outcome.

It is very often the case that we can establish general causation without knowing anything about the mechanism by which it works. John Snow (1965) famously demonstrated that the water supply could be a cause of cholera while having only the haziest idea of the mechanism by which contaminated water produces cholera. In a randomized controlled trial of a drug, to find for example whether it prevents breast cancer, if the trial is well executed then it can provide knowledge of the causal connection even if the experimenters' conjecture as to the mechanism by which the drug is working turns out to be wrong.

Similarly, a randomized controlled trial can demonstrate definitively that the drug is, for example, preventing breast cancer, even though it does not allow one to say, of any one participant in the study, "The drug was responsible for this person's not getting breast cancer." The trial works across the population, it does not allow you to identify any one case as one in which it was the action of the drug that had this outcome.

This opens the possibility that, looking at trials across a population, we could find that both humiliation and serotonin imbalances were correlated with the outcome of depression. In fact, by exploiting the possibility of "natural experiments," we could demonstrate a causal connection between these two factors and depression as outcome. We could do this without having the slightest idea how to go about thinking of a "mechanism" by which these two factors might combine to generate the outcome. And we could do this without having demonstrated, for any particular case, that humiliation and serotonin imbalance caused *this* individual's depression.

Elisabeth, Princess of Bohemia, famously challenged Descartes as to there could be causal interactions between mind and body, given his dualist conception of mind and body as different substances (see Mattern (1978) for references and overview). As an undergraduate, this problem always struck me as fake; hadn't Hume (1740/1975) shown that causation was constant conjunction? And of course there can be correlations between mental and bodily states. The problem arises, however, when we think of causation in terms of mechanism and process. We know about mental mechanisms and processes, and we know about physical mechanisms and processes. But we have absolutely no understanding of how there could be mechanisms and processes linking mental and physical. My point in this introductory section has been that the "Princess Elisabeth" problem is written large in psychiatry. It means that we do not have a clear conception of the causal structures our diagnostic procedures are trying to identify. If we think of causality in terms of mechanism and process, then we cannot work with a mixed set of psychological and physical variables in specifying the causal structures we are trying to identify. But we have only optimism supporting the idea that we will be able to give a purely psychological account of the relevant causal structures; and similarly it is only optimism that supports the idea that we will be able to eliminate the mental and give a purely physical account of the relevant causal structures.

32.3 **Validity as reference versus assessment of ways of finding out**

The idea of validity, as it is usually used in connection with scientific constructs, has two dimensions. One kind of case is when we have a phenomenon, some characteristic of objects such as mass or temperature, and we want to know if a particular way of identifying its presence or measuring it is any good. So, for example, we might all agree that there is such a thing as "general intelligence" in humans, and we have some idea of how it is caused and what differences it makes, but we argue about whether particular types of IQ test provide good ways of quantifying it. Perhaps, for example, these tests might be challenged as subject to some cultural bias, so that results are affected by the specifics of one's general knowledge in a way that IQ itself is thought to be indifferent to. Here, let's suppose, the existence of the thing, intelligence, may not be in question, but particular ways of detecting or measuring it are up for assessment as more or less valid ways of measuring that thing.

The other, more radical dimension of the idea of the validity of a construct has to do with whether there is anything there at all to detect or measure. So, for example, the category "neurasthenia" might be declared to be "invalid" not because any one measure of it is somehow incorrect, but because there is no such thing at all. Similarly, in physical chemistry the category "phlogiston" could be declared to be invalid, not because any measure of it is incorrect, but because it does not exist. This can happen even when we are not working with a fully explicit characterization of the variables in the relevant causal structure, but are, for example, thinking of "phlogiston" as merely a latent variable playing a specified causal role. There may be no latent variable with that causal role.

These two ways of thinking about validity are in practice often twined together, because if you consider the categories used in the *Diagnostic and Statistical Manual of Mental Disorders* (DSM), often in practice no distinction is made between the concept and the ways we use to detect and measure the characteristic. If you ask for the meaning of "schizophrenia," you will be sent to the diagnostic criteria. That can make it seem puzzling how there could be a distinction between the question whether the concept is "valid" in the sense that those criteria correctly measure the thing, and whether the concept is "valid" in the sense that it stands for something.

Nonetheless, I think it is important to try to hold on to this distinction, because it gives us a fixed structure we need in addressing the deeply puzzling question of the validity of our diagnostic categories in psychiatry. Let's begin with the question: what more is there to the validity of a concept, in the sense of it standing for something, rather than merely the value of the diagnostic criteria associated with it? Now straight off I think that there are two things we can specify here:

1 In order for there to be such a thing as schizophrenia, for example, there must be the external phenomenon to which we are causally responding in using the term. There must be something "out there" we are responding to. That is the condition we're talking about. This is where it seems relevant to talk about a particular type of causal structure, such as, for example, an essentialist structure with a hidden essence causally generating various symptoms.

This condition states a kind of minimal realism that seems to me implicit in talking about the validity of categories in the first place. It's a substantive condition, often denied by people who say that they take a "pragmatic" or "instrumentalist" approach to psychiatry. I'll amplify on this in a moment, but for now I want only to remark that the metaphysical slant these authors put on their discussion usually seems better recast as an epistemic one. These writers are generally moved by a kind of epistemic modesty, a concern that we should not be claiming to know more than we do about the phenomena of mental illness out there. This kind of modesty is better served by realism about disorders coupled with an appreciation of how slender our knowledge of these categories is, rather than by attempting to cut down the reality of mental disorders to fit our current epistemic capacities.

The second thing about concepts standing for something is this:

2 We have to have some conception of what structure it is out there that we're causally responding to. This "governing conception" that we associate with a term is a picture or model of the kind of phenomenon that we are causally responding to when we use the term.

Richard Boyd explained this idea in a now-famous paper, "Metaphor and theory change" (1979), in which he gave some examples of "theory-constitutive" metaphors, which cannot be eliminated from the practice of science, and which can "accomplish non-definitional reference-fixing." Examples he gave from psychology included:

> the suggestion that certain information is "encoded" or "indexed" in "memory store" by "labeling," whereas other information is "stored" in "images";

disputes about the extent to which developmental "stages" are produced by the maturation of new "programmed" "subroutines," as opposed to the acquisition of learned "heuristic routines," or the development of greater "memory storage capacities" or better "information retrieval procedures";

the view that learning is an adaptive response of a "self-organizing machine" (Boyd 1979, p. 360)

Boyd's point was that these kinds of ideas play a role in determining what's being referred to when a scientist talks about "iconic memory," for example. The conception being used to fix reference here need not be detailed, and insofar as it is detailed it need not be more than roughly accurate. It's a matter of having a working model, a picture, a metaphor that can be developed in many different ways. Particularly, it will offer some insight into the causal structure of the phenomenon, by suggesting that the causal structure of one domain can be modeled on the causal structure of another.

Now Boyd confined his remarks to "relatively mature sciences" (Boyd 1979, p. 482). You might say that psychiatry does not fall under this head. But it seems to me that in practice psychiatrists are typically working with quite rich "governing conceptions" of the disorders they name, even if those metaphors do not explicitly make it into the DSM. The governing conception associated with "hysteria," for example, can shift over time. And if it finally emerged that clinicians in classifying people as falling or not falling under this category had been responding to the presence or absence of some specific form of post-traumatic stress disorder (PTSD), then we might say: "Yes, there is such a thing as hysteria, it turned to be. . . ." On the other hand, if it emerged that what clinicians had been responding to was a purely neurological condition, with no significant psychological etiology, we might be more inclined to say: "People who formerly were classified as 'hysterical' are now thought to have neurological condition X; properly speaking there is no such thing as hysteria." (See Ahn and Kim (2008) for a review of ways in which clinicians conceptualize the causal structures of disorders.)

These two aspects of a diagnostic concept, the existence of an external phenomenon to which it is a response, and that thing fitting, more or less, our "governing conception" of what kind of phenomenon that is, seem required if we are to have a diagnostic concept that refers to anything at all. And it is only once our diagnostic concept can be said to be referring to something that it even makes sense to inquire into the validity of our ways of determining whether the characteristic is present in any given case, or of measuring different features of the condition. We might diagram the situation as in Figure 32.3.

Within philosophy this kind of picture is not unremarkable; many authors would endorse something like this structure (see e.g., Evans 1982, Fodor 1987, Peacocke 1992, though not all put it in just this way, e.g. Fodor does not explicitly accept a role for anything like "governing conception"). For our purposes the key point is that a discussion of the validity of a category should be set up in two stages: there is first the question of reference, "Is there any such thing as X?," does the concept refer at all? If the concept is valid in the sense that there is something it refers to, then we can move to the second stage. Here we can look at particular

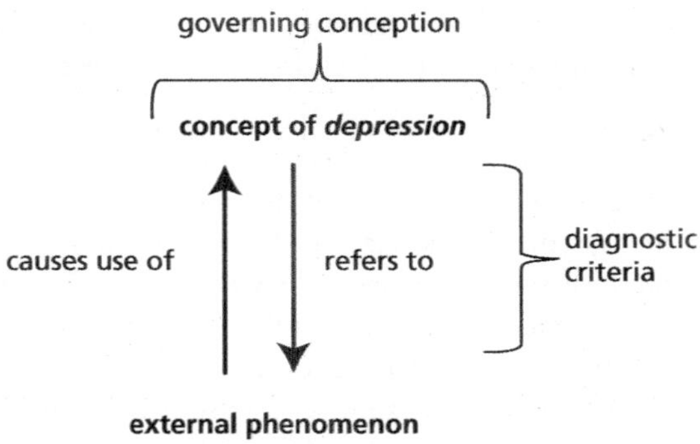

Figure 32.3. A realist picture of the relation between the concept for a disorder, the external phenomenon it names, and the diagnostic criteria for that disorder.

ways of finding whether something has the characteristic in question, and ask whether they are good ways of doing that.

One thing that is mildly confusing about using this picture in practice is that talk about the "diagnostic criteria" comes in not only at the second stage, when we are asking whether the criteria are any good. Diagnostic criteria will also matter at the first stage, when we are asking whether there is an external phenomenon out there causing our use of the concept, and to which the concept therefore refers. For the "causation" of our use of the concept by the external phenomenon will typically be a matter of it triggering our use of the concept by our applying the diagnostic criteria. That does not eliminate the distinction between the two levels. After all, a condition might trigger our use of the concept of "neurasthenia" when we apply standard diagnostic criteria for neurasthenia; we could therefore say, "this is the condition we were talking about when we used that category." It is still open that we might give favorable or unfavorable assessments of how good or bad those criteria are as ways of finding out about that condition. The role of diagnostic criteria in fixing the reference of a concept does not mean that those criteria must automatically be assessed as good ways of finding whether the concept applies.

Let me relate this way of thinking about validity to the way the idea is usually explained to students in science. The concept of validity is often informally explained in terms of the functioning of a gunsight. A well-functioning gunsight allows you to identify the target you want to hit, and you can use it to get a bullet to the target. Analogously, an ordinary concept has associated some idea of what it is you are referring to when you use it, and ways of determining when the concept applies.

In the case of a gunsight, there are different ways in which the thing might go wrong. Suppose there are a number of possible targets in front of you, and after firing, you can verify how well you have done. Suppose you select a single target using the gunsight, and take several shots at that thing. There are two questions you can raise:

1 Do all your bullets land in the same place as one another (whether or not that's the spot occupied by the target)?

2 On the whole, do your bullets tend to cluster round the intended target, or is the average landing spot for them biased in some direction away from the target?

The first question has to do with whether there is any statistical uncertainty in where use of the gunsight will get bullets to land; the second has to do with whether there is any systematic uncertainty in where the bullets will land. Or as it is sometimes put, the first question has to do with the precision of the gunsight, the second has to do with its accuracy. Or, finally, the first is a question about the reliability of the gunsight, the second is a question about its validity.

How does this picture apply to, for example, our use of a concept like depression? Well, there is the characteristic out there—the target—that we are responding to, and there are the different ways we have of determining whether the phenomenon is present in a particular case. The whole approach depends on supposing that there is some target that is the thing we are aiming at. Once that is in place, we can ask whether the criteria we are using are good ways of getting onto it, or if one set of criteria is better than another. In the case of a concept like depression, I have in effect been saying that what determines the target is this: which real-world property is it that usually triggers our applying the concept, when we use our current diagnostic criteria? But it is not that we have only the blank fact of our causally responding to that phenomenon: we also have the "governing conception" that informs our understanding of what we are talking about, and constrains what the concept can be said to be referring to. Getting the right external property in place is the analog of fixing a target; once that is done, we can assess ways of getting onto it as more or less valid. So we can add to our previous picture a step of validating the criteria we use, as ways of getting onto the intended external phenomenon. This is shown in Figure 32.4.

So far, this is just like the gunsight example. The great difference is that in the most basic cases in science, it sometimes seems that we do not have any analog

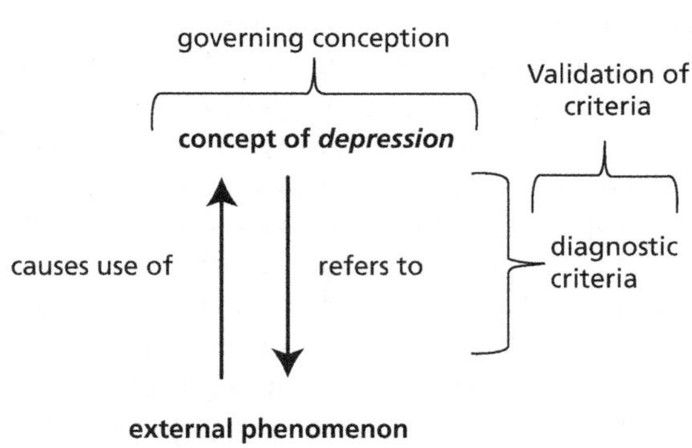

Figure 32.4. The place of validation of criteria, on a realist picture. The aim of validation is to determine (a) whether the concept identifies any external phenomenon at all, and (b) if so, whether the diagnostic criteria provide a good way of detecting that thing.

of looking at the scene directly, without the benefit of the gunsight. We typically do not have any way, external to the use of the gunsight itself, of identifying the target or determining how closely our shots have landed. If you think about what the implications of this would be for the assessment of an ordinary gunsight, they seem radical indeed. On the face of it, we would have no way of assessing reliability or validity. This is the situation quite dramatically in psychiatry, where there is no way, independent of the DSM criteria themselves (or rival criteria that are not, currently, in any significantly better an epistemic position) of assessing when we really have found someone with, say, schizophrenia. So let's look at how validation of a DSM category goes in practice.

32.4 **Validation in DSM**

From the perspective of those remarks, the central problem with the approach to validation used in DSM is that for the purposes of the exercise of validation, it is assumed that our concepts of each disorder are exhausted by the diagnostic criteria. DSM does not appeal to the idea of the phenomenon to which we are causally responding, or to our "governing conception" of the disorder. This is problematic, because it is not enough to fix the references of the names of the disorders. And if we have not even attempted to fix the references of the terms, we cannot make sense of validity as a distinction between terms that refer and terms that do not, or good ways and not so good ways of spotting the presence or absence of the referent of the term.

To anyone familiar with the way of thinking of validators used in DSM, at least since Robins and Guze (1970), my remarks so far may seem alien to the point of unintelligibility. The guidelines for changes to DSM proposed for the fifth edition (DSM-5) included a list of types of validators, with the most important asterisked (Table 32.1).

Now one thing that is striking about the list in Table 32.1 is that, on the surface at any rate, it proceeds entirely in terms of correlations. We are looking what correlates we can find with someone's having been established to have a disorder, by means of a particular set of diagnostic criteria. The validity of the disorder has to do with the number and strength of those correlations. And as remarked, different weights may be given to different types of validator in this process.

This is an intuitive approach: it would hardly have been so widely accepted if it were not. And I am not going to suggest that there is anything fundamentally wrong-headed about it. But my first point is that it masks the distinction I made above, between (1) establishing that there is something to which the concept refers (that there is any target there at all), and (2) determining how good or bad our ways are of detecting the presence of that thing, or measuring it.

My second point is that this approach does not explicitly give any place to an analysis of the causal structure of the disorder in determining the validity of a diagnosis. And yet, intelligent use of these criteria of validation seems to depend on some interpretation of causal structure. There are different ways in which we can think of the use of DSM criteria. One is roughly analogous to the way we think

Table 32.1 Proposed types of validators

I Antecedent Validators
A.*Familial aggregation and/or co-aggregation (i.e., family, twin or adoption studies)
B. Socio-Demographic and Cultural Factors
C. Environmental Risk Factors
D. Prior Psychiatric History
II Concurrent Validators
A. Cognitive, emotional, temperament, and personality correlates (unrelated to the diagnostic criteria)
B. Biological Markers, e.g., molecular genetics, neural substrates
C. Patterns of Comorbidity
[Note - while categories A and B would most typically be assessed after illness onset, they also could be assessed prior to illness onset as pre-morbid characteristics]
III Predictive Validators
A. *Diagnostic Stability
B. *Course of Illness
C. *Response to Treatment

Reproduced from Kendler Kenneth S., D. Kupfer, W. Narrow, K. Phillips and J. Fawcett. 2009. 'Guidelines for Making Changes to DSM-V'. Washington, DC: American Psychiatric Association. Unpublished manuscript.

of criteria for giving someone a job, such as "exam qualifications," "commitment," "relevant social skills," and so on. Here we need not be thinking that there is some one underlying condition to which all these indicators point. But it would be perfectly possible to assess the validity of a particular picture of a "strong applicant" by looking at the antecedent, concurrent, and predictive validators of the tests that are actually being applied by interviewers; indeed, something like that is how these tests actually are evaluated. On the other hand, you could be thinking of "the disorder" as something that is the causal outcome of the antecedent validators, which is expressed in the concurrent validators, and has as a causal outcome the way things go with the predictive validators. This is quite different to the case of criteria for a successful job application. On the face of it, it seems entirely possible that one conception of the causal structure here may lead to a quite different weighting of validators than does the other conception of causal structure. It is hard to see how the discussion of validation in DSM can really operate at the level of correlations, without at least implicitly bringing in some picture of the causal structure of the disorder.

So I have made two comments about the Robins and Guze-style criteria. One is about the need to separate out the "reference-fixing" dimension of validity—does the term refer to anything at all?—from the other dimension: given that the term refers to something, how could are our diagnostic criteria for detecting the presence of that thing? The other comment was about the need to operate with some picture of the causal structure of the disorder—are the criteria for the disorder actually constitutive of possession of the disorder, for example, or are they intended to point to some further inner condition? But these two comments are, I think, not independent. The "governing conception" that we have of a disorder will in the first instance be an interpretation of the causal structure of the disorder. Until we have determined what kind of causal structure we are looking for, we have not identified a condition at all. To put the point in a more confrontational way, the current combination of a DSM that merely lists diagnostic criteria, coupled with a Robins and Guze-style approach to validation, cannot actually succeed in fixing references for the names of disorders at all. If that is all we have to go on as fixing the reference of a term like "major depression," for example, then what does it take to be depressed? Is it enough if one merely meets the diagnostic criteria? Or is there some further condition that one has to have, so that one could in principle meet the diagnostic criteria and yet not in fact be depressed (just as one could have the symptoms of a viral illness yet not have the virus)? If you try to keep the chips up on that kind of question, claiming that our knowledge is as yet insufficient, then you have not fixed a reference for the term "major depression" at all. You have missed out a crucial component in the attempt to fix a reference for your term. Consequently, there is no saying whether there is or is not such a thing as "depression." And there is little point in trying to raise the question of whether your current tests are good indicators of the presence of that thing. What thing?

In fact, the evidence seems to be that clinicians do not interpret disorders in ways that stay out of the question as to their causal structures. Ahn and Kim (2008) found that clinicians generally had clear causal structures associated with the diagnostic criteria for disorders, and hypothesized that "symptoms that cause many other symptoms (i.e., causally central) would be treated as being more important than symptoms that cause few other symptoms (i.e., causally peripheral)" (2008, pp. 4–5). They remark,

> In contrast [in DSM], the system is set up, with a few explicit exceptions, so that all symptoms in a given disorder are equally weighted. For instance, the four symptoms with boldface boxes in Figure 2 [Figure 32.5] must *all* be present to warrant a diagnosis of Anorexia nervosa, making all four symptoms equally important for classification. However, according to the clinicians' data collected in our experiments, "distorted body image" was most causally central in the clinicians' theories, whereas "absence of the period (in women) for more than 3 menstrual cycles" was rated the most causally peripheral. Furthermore, "distorted body image" was considered to be the most diagnostically important of the criteria, and "absence of the period (in women) for more than 3 menstrual cycles," though also a DSM diagnostic criterion for Anorexia nervosa, was considered to be the least diagnostically important. We obtained similar patterns of results across eight other mental disorders . . ..

Ahn and Kim (2008, p. 7) suggest that

> instead of sticking with a purely descriptive approach, incorporating a causalist approach, whenever possible and wherever reasonable, may actually encourage

clinicians to rely more on the DSM. As we suggested, incorporating causal information at the symptom-to-symptom level might be a reasonable place to start. Attempting to adhere solely to a descriptive approach in the DSM may not necessarily lead to better reliability in clinicians' diagnoses.

These points, if well-taken, imply that it is not as if there is some pragmatic value in keeping causal information out of DSM. And what I have been saying previously is that unless causal information is allowed into what I have been calling our "governing conception" for a disorder, we simply cannot claim to have uniquely specified any real-world phenomenon. I think it is this failure of the DSM names, if strictly and literally interpreted merely in terms of their associated criteria, to actually identify any particular condition that makes the whole question of their validation so confusing. It is also what encourages the frequent claims by people reflecting on DSM that the diagnostic categories are merely "social constructs." If the terms do not refer to anything "out there," then perhaps they do only have to do with some projections of the theorists. But that is a mistake. The problem is that the terms are being interpreted so that they do not refer at all, rather than that they refer to "social constructs," whatever they are.

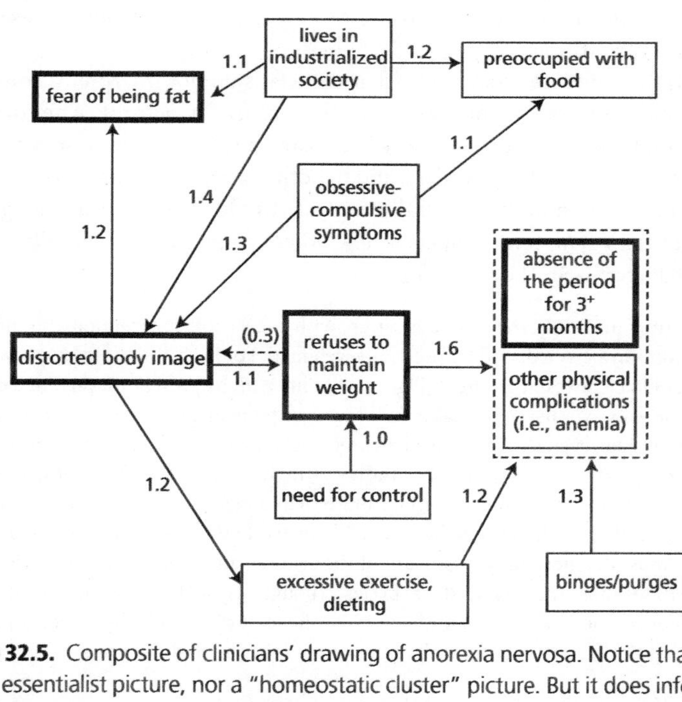

Figure 32.5. Composite of clinicians' drawing of anorexia nervosa. Notice that this is not an essentialist picture, nor a "homeostatic cluster" picture. But it does inform the understanding and use of the diagnostic criteria.

Reproduced from Woo-kyoung Ahn and Nancy S. Kim, Causal Theories of Mental Disorder Concepts, *Psychological Science Agenda*, 22, pp. 3–8, Figure 2 © 2016 American Psychological Association.

I think that the official picture of validation in DSM can be seen as a kind of amputated form of the picture of validation that I gave in section 32.2. Let me be explicit that I think the amputation was well-motivated: the motive was great, and well-grounded, epistemic caution. But I think it has now been completely forgotten that this was an amputation of the usual picture of validation. We can diagram the DSM picture of validation as in Figure 32.6.

Compare this to Figure 32.4. From this picture, anything about our "governing conception" of the causal structure of the disorder has been dropped. And the very idea of an external phenomenon out there, to which we are causally responding and to which we are referring, is doing no work in the picture. We saw that a common explanation of the usual scientific picture of validation is as a matter of determining how good the gunsight is, whether we are getting onto a target with it at all, and if so, how good the gunsight is at doing that. The official DSM picture is like that, only the very idea of the target has been dropped, and the idea of the shooter having sight of the target, so that they know which thing they are trying to hit, has been abandoned. All we have are correlations with signs that the gun is about to be used, concurrent and predictive corrrelations with the use of the sight. If these all seem to pan out, then we say that the gunsight has been validated.

Now the point about the amputated conception of validity is that it ultimately makes sense only when you realize that it is an amputation. The whole point of the validating criteria is to try to find when you are getting onto the external phenomenon. You might be cautious about what you claim to know about the validation of the gunsight, but the whole point of the exercise is in the end to find out whether you are hitting anything. If you do not keep in mind that this is ultimately what is going on, then it is likely to seem to you that the whole business of gunsight validation is nothing more than a "social construct" or something like it, because what on earth is this ritual of validation about, if it isn't about finding out whether you're hitting something?

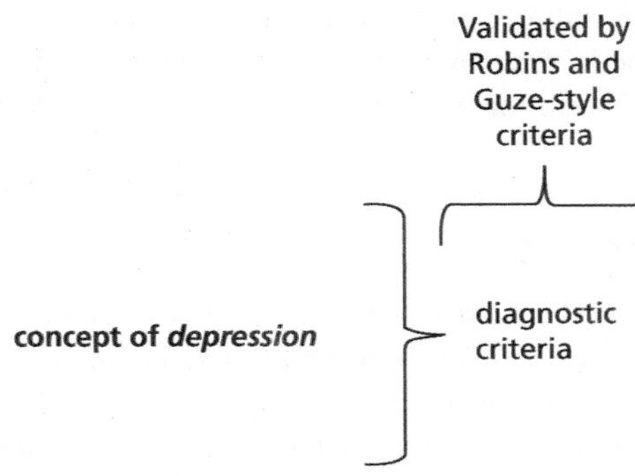

Figure 32.6. A picture of validation that tries to do without the idea of the "external phenomenon" to which the concept refers, so that we do not think of validation as involving either (a) determining that there is such a thing, or (b) whether the diagnostic criteria are good ways of detecting it.

Psychiatry has been using Robins and Guze-style validators for decades, and a vast body of important knowledge has been developed using them. You can live within this world. But that means that when you ask: do I need the notion of "the disorder itself," the external phenomenon to which we're causally responding and to which I'm referring?, well, that notion does not seem to be part of the official validation process. So at this point you might say: do I need the notion at all? Perhaps all it comes to that "there is such a thing" as schizophrenia, for example, is that the validation exercise has passed our diagnostic criteria as valid. There isn't any further question. Our concept of schizophrenia, on this way of thinking about it, is exhausted by the diagnostic checklist, and its validity is simply a matter of the Robins and Guze criteria being met. There is no more to the existence and nature of schizophrenia than that. It is only a "social construct," a product of our diagnostic and validatory practices. There is something quite paradoxical about this position. Remember that it began with great epistemic caution, a sense that we do not know much about the disorders. But now the amputation of our validatory practices leads us to a picture on which there is no more to know about schizophrenia, for example, than what we currently know. After all, if the thing is merely a social construct, a product of our diagnostic and validatory practices, how could there be any more to know about it than those practices themselves generate? We have lost the very picture of the disorder "out there," the thing about which we know little, that is what motivated the original amputation of our process of validation.

It should be evident that this is all a by-product of losing sight of the bigger picture that can alone make sense of validation. We need the idea of the thing out there to which we are referring, if we are to make sense of what we are doing in validation. That means that we have to reckon in to our concept of schizophrenia not just the diagnostic criteria, but our "governing conception" of the thing, our grasp of its causal structure, and the disorder out there to which we are causally responding in giving diagnoses. As we have seen, that would already reflect good clinical practice. The trouble is that when we try to think how we would go beyond the approach of Kim and Ahn to find true causal models of disorders, we run into the "Princess Elisabeth" problem. We do not know what kinds of mechanism and process we should be thinking in terms of when we reflect on the causal structures of disorders.

Acknowledgement

Such understanding of these issues as I have, I owe almost entirely to Ken Kendler. I was also helped by discussion of an earlier draft at the Copenhagen meeting and by Dominic Murphy's comments there. In my understanding of how reliability and validity are thought of in the physical and social sciences, I have been helped by discussions with Robert MacCoun and Saul Perlmutter.

References

Ahn, W-K. and **Kim, N.S.** (2008). Causal theories of mental disorder concepts. *Psychological Science Agenda*, **22**, 3–8.

Boyd, R. (1979). Metaphor and theory change. In A. Ortony (ed.), *Metaphor and Thought*, pp. 356–408. Cambridge, UK: Cambridge University Press.

Dowe, P. (2000). *Physical Causation*. Cambridge: Cambridge University Press.

Evans, G. (1982). *The Varieties of Reference*. Oxford: Oxford University Press.

Fair, D. (1979). Causation and the flow of energy. *Erkenntnis*, **14**, 219–250.

Fodor, J. (1987). *Psychosemantics*. Cambridge, MA: MIT Press.

Hoerl, C. (2013). Jaspers on explaining and understanding in psychiatry. In T. Fuchs and G. Stanghellini (eds.) *One Century of Karl Jaspers' General Psychopathology*, pp. 107–120. Oxford, UK: Oxford University Press.

Hume, D. (1740/1975). *A Treatise of Human Nature*, ed. L. A. Selby-Bigge, 2nd edn rev. P. H. Nidditch. Oxford: Oxford University Press.

Jaspers, K. (1923/1963). *General Psychopathology*. Chicago: University of Chicago Press.

Kendler K.S., Kupfer D., Narrow W., et al. (2009). Guidelines for making changes to DSM-V. Washington, DC: American Psychiatric Association. Unpublished manuscript.

Locke, J. (1690/1975). *An Essay Concerning Human Understanding*, ed. P.H. Nidditch. Oxford: Oxford University Press.

Mattern, R. (1978). Descartes's correspondence with Elisabeth: Concerning both the union and distinction of mind and body. In Michael Hooker (ed.) *Descartes: Critical and interpretive essays*, pp. 212–222. Baltimore, MD: Johns Hopkins University Press.

Peacocke, C. (1992). *A Study of Concepts*. Cambridge, MA: MIT Press.

Robins, E. and **Guze, S.B.** (1970). Establishment of diagnostic validity in psychiatric illness: its application to schizophrenia. *American Journal of Psychiatry*, **126**, 983–987.

Snow, J. (1965). *Snow on Cholera: Being a reprint of two papers by John Snow with a biographical memoir*. New York: Hafner.

Chapter 33

Saving the explananda

Georg Repnikov and Dominic Murphy

The law that nosology precedes etiology is not easily broken.

(Cattell 1943, p. 560)

33.1 Introduction

Do our diagnostic terms refer? If they do not, what implications does this have for our understanding of the practice of validation in psychiatry? These are the questions raised and addressed in the main part of John Campbell's contribution to this volume, and the ones we will focus on in our reply. While we are sympathetic to Campbell's contentions that the *Diagnostic and Statistical Manual of Mental Disorders* (DSM) style of validation needs reassessment, and that causality should play a more prominent role in nosological revisions, we think his picture of reference and validation is misconceived. In this short comment, we first address Campbell's question about the reference of our diagnostic terms, before briefly sketching an alternative view of validation.

33.2 Two questions about reference

Questions about reference can be read in either of two ways. On the reading that Campbell has in mind, we are asking whether there *exists* something (e.g. some entity or attribute) in the physical world that our terms refer to. This is a natural reading, but it presupposes that an affirmative answer has already been given to a logically prior question that could be phrased in exactly the same way. On this second version, we are asking whether the reference of the terms has already been "fixed," whether there is anything reasonably determinate that we are talking about. While the first reading yields an empirical question, the second reading leaves us with a semantic question. Obviously, the second question needs to have an affirmative answer before it even makes sense to ask the first question. For unless a term like "aa," say, refers to *something* (e.g., a specific kind of basaltic lava) it makes no sense to go out in the world in order to determine whether aa actually exists or not, since we would not know *what* it is we are looking *for*.

Campbell clearly recognizes the logical priority of the semantic question. He observes, for instance, that unless you have fixed the reference for the term "depression," "there is no saying whether there is or is not such a thing as 'depression'" (section 32.4). We may generalize this insight. Unless it has been specified what *counts* as a case of a given mental disorder, it makes no sense to ask whether there exist any cases of *that* mental disorder. *What* mental disorder?

Once the logical priority of the semantic question has been recognized, however, it becomes obvious that we should not *start* with the empirical question of whether our diagnostic terms refer. Rather, we should ask to *what*, if anything, our diagnostic terms refer. We should also ask how it is that the reference of our diagnostic terms comes to be "fixed," as Campbell puts it. We will take these questions in turn. It is by comparing Campbell's answers to our own that the first fundamental disagreements come into plain sight.

33.3 **Syndromes and causal structures as possible referents**

So, let us ask, to what do our diagnostic terms refer? Here are two possibilities. First, a diagnostic term could be used "descriptively" to refer to a specific *syndrome*—a characteristic pattern of co-occurring observed signs and reported symptoms affecting patients. This, we take it, is the standard use of diagnostic terms in psychiatry. It invokes no causal-explanatory notions. Now you may not be *happy* about the fact that—after more than a hundred years of intense biomedical research—we are still largely stuck with purely descriptive syndromal diagnoses in psychiatry. For the moment, however, there is no escaping the neo-Kraepelinian world we live in.

Second, diagnostic terms *may* be used "explanatorily" to refer to hypothetical *causal structures*, as Campbell would call them. Models correctly describing these causal structures could be either network models (Borsboom and Cramer 2013), "essentialist" common cause models (e.g., the dopamine hypothesis of schizophrenia; Kendler and Schaffner 2011), or something more complicated. Observed signs and reported symptoms would be incorporated into these models either as effects of a common cause or as mutually interacting and reinforcing causes. If one of these models accurately represented the relevant causal structure in any given case, it would provide us with an explanation of the genesis of its clinical presentation. The important point to note is that the reference of the diagnostic term here "goes beyond" the clinical presentation, and includes causes or causal relationships of some kind.

Now, according to Campbell we *always* use diagnostic terms to refer to causal structures if we refer to anything at all. As we read him, he seems to deny the possibility that we could use diagnostic terms to refer to syndromes. However, suppose we do take our diagnostic terms to refer to syndromes, but that supposition is actually wrong. Then what *do* our current diagnostic terms refer to? Nothing, according to Campbell:

> it is this failure of the DSM names, if strictly and literally interpreted merely in terms of their associated criteria, to actually identify any particular condition that makes the whole question of their validation so confusing (section 32.4).

We disagree. If there *is* anything wrong with current validation practices, *this* is not it. In order to make our case we need to pick apart the account of "reference-fixing" that is the backbone of his argument.

33.4 Fixing the reference

So how is the reference of our diagnostic terms "fixed?" According to Campbell, two conditions must be fulfilled for our diagnostic terms to successfully refer to *something*:

> These two aspects of a diagnostic concept, the existence of an external phenomenon to which it is a response, and that thing fitting, more or less, our "governing conception" of what kind of phenomenon that is, seem required if we are to have a diagnostic concept that refers to anything at all (section 32.3).

We will discuss these two conditions in turn. The first, "the existence of an external phenomenon to which it is a response," is obviously a sufficient condition for the *successful* reference of our terms, as Campbell construes it. For asking about the reference of our terms, in the *empirical* sense we noted above, just *is* asking about the existence of the referents of our terms. But is it a necessary condition for the "fixity of reference?"

Campbell seems to suggest it is. For he writes that "[d]iagnostic criteria will also matter at the first stage, when we are asking whether there is an external phenomenon out there *causing our use of the concept, and to which the concept therefore refers*" (section 32.3; our emphasis). Let us try to clarify this point. If we understand him correctly, Campbell here suggests that what causes our use of a concept is *therefore* the referent of the concept. But we can certainly refer to numbers and rules, fictional characters and future events, without any of these "things" *causing* our use of the corresponding concepts. Whatever physical phenomena cause our use of the words that express those concepts, these physical causes are certainly not the referents of those concepts. In that sense, the external phenomena to which our "use" of a diagnostic term is a causally triggered response may simply be *irrelevant* to the "fixity of reference" of our diagnostic terms—even if a concept is, among other things, a means of categorizing the world.

Campbell seems to think that the first condition is necessary for the "fixity of reference," but acknowledges that it is, by itself, not sufficient. There is, according to him, at least one further condition that has to be fulfilled for the reference of our diagnostic terms to be "fixed." As he puts it,

> it is not that we have only the blank fact of our causally responding to that phenomenon: we also have the 'governing conception' that informs our understanding of what we're talking about, and constrains what the concept can be said to be referring to (section 32.3).

Only if we have a "governing conception" of the phenomenon incorporated into our diagnostic concepts, and the phenomenon actually fits that "governing conception," can our diagnostic concepts be said to refer to anything.

According to Campbell, "the 'governing conception' . . . that we have of a disorder will in the first instance be an interpretation of the causal structure of the disorder". It is "a working model, a picture, a metaphor that [. . .] will offer some insight into the causal structure of the phenomenon" (section 32.3). Depression, for instance, could be pictured, or mathematically modelled, as either a network of causally interacting signs and symptoms or as an underlying biological condition which causes the overt signs and symptoms. In either case, depression is conceptualized as a particular kind of causal structure. This conceptualization is supposed to be a necessary condition for our diagnostic term "depression" to have a fixed reference, for unless "we have determined what kind of causal structure we are looking for, we have not identified a condition at all" (section 32.3).

Again, we deny that this is a necessary condition. There are perfectly legitimate uses of diagnostic terms where their reference has been "fixed" *without* the invocation of any "governing conception," as Campbell construes it.

33.5 **Reference, fixed**

What a word (e.g., a common noun like "schizophrenia") refers to or stands for—what is conventionally *meant* by a word—may be neither determined by some putative causal connection between an external phenomenon and our utterances of that word, nor "fixed" by some kind of picture we have in mind whenever we think about the word and what it might stand for. Instead, the reference of a word is determined by the *meaning* of the word.[1] What is the meaning of a word? The meaning of a word is what is given in an explanation of what the word means. What we give in an explanation of the meaning of a word are rules for the correct use of that word, rules that provide a standard of correctness for the application of the word. In explaining the meaning of a word, we do not describe the meaning of the word—as if it was an entity of some kind. Rather, we state rules that specify what the word means, that tell us how it is to be used correctly.

What are the rules that guide our applications of diagnostic terms such as "depression" and "schizophrenia?" What are the rules that provide the "criteria of identity" for these conditions, that tell us what actually *counts* as a case of schizophrenia or depression? For DSM-defined disorders, the answer is, of course, that we can find these rules in the relevant *diagnostic criteria*. As Campbell himself puts it: "If you ask for the meaning of 'schizophrenia,' you will be sent to the diagnostic criteria."

The diagnostic criteria for any given disorder tell us what currently counts as a case of that disorder. For most disorders in the DSM-5, though by no means all, this is done by specifying the sort of temporal pattern of observed signs and reported symptoms that has to be present for a correct diagnosis of the disorder to be made.[2] It should be noted that, insofar as the presence of a particular kind of cause, or combination of causal relations, is not a necessary condition for a diagnosis to be made, according to the diagnostic criteria, the reference of the relevant

---

[1] Of course, when it comes to the determination of so-called "speaker's reference" (i.e., what a particular speaker, on a given occasion, refers an audience to through the use of a word), features of the speaker and the linguistic context she finds herself in become crucially important.

[2] Caffeine-induced sleep disorder (American Psychiatric Association 2013, p. 417) is a good example of a disorder that is not merely a syndrome, but a causal structure describable in terms of a common cause model.

diagnostic term is not "fixed" to a "causal structure" of any kind. We agree with Campbell on this. This does not mean, however, that the diagnostic terms refer to nothing at all. Quite to the contrary, it will obviously refer to a specific *syndrome*—a particular kind of clinical presentation *in need of a causal explanation*. In other words, the clinical manifestations we refer to with our current diagnostic terms are the *explananda* for which the etiologies and pathophysiological mechanism we are actively trying to discover would provide the *explanantia*.

What about the "governing conception" of the disorder? Could we not at least *add* one to the current diagnostic criteria in order to turn the referent of the diagnostic term from a syndrome into a disorder with a particular causal structure? Indeed, we could. However, insofar as the causes, or causal mechanisms, are merely *hypothetical*, the diagnostic term only refers to a hypothetical causal structure. Although we do not, in principle, condemn using diagnostic terms to refer to hypothetical causal structures, using the *same* term to refer to both a syndrome and a hypothetical causal structure can, and typically will, lead to unnecessary confusion—especially as the hypothetical structure referred to changes in step with theoretical change.

33.6 **Successful reference**

Having clarified and answered the semantic question about the reference of our diagnostic terms, we can now turn our attention to the empirical question about the reference of our diagnostic terms. What is needed for our use of diagnostic terms to be "referentially successful?"

Again, a full answer will differ slightly for syndromes and causal structures. The basic answer, however, is the same for both types of medical conditions. A particular condition *exists* insofar as there are true cases of the condition. A true case of a condition is a case that meets the relevant "gold standard" for the correct application of the diagnosis. A true case of any given DSM-5 syndrome will be a patient presenting with a particular kind of clinical picture, meeting the relevant diagnostic criteria and additional constraints on the correct application of the diagnosis. For a true case of any given causal structure condition to exist, a specific type of cause, or combination of causal relationships, has to be present in a patient, in addition to—or even instead of—the associated symptomatology.

Let us briefly illustrate the points just made by looking at two examples. First, consider *paralytic poliomyelitis*, an infectious disease caused by the poliovirus. To suffer from paralytic poliomyelitis is to experience acute flaccid paralysis due to an infection with the poliovirus. If the paralysis is not due to an infection with the poliovirus, it is not paralytic poliomyelitis. If the presence of the poliovirus causes no symptoms in a patient, the patient is not suffering from paralytic poliomyelitis, but merely from an asymptomatic polio infection. Does paralytic poliomyelitis, or polio, *exist*? According to the World Health Organization:

> Polio does still exist, although polio cases have decreased by over 99% since 1988, from an estimated more than 350,000 cases to 359 reported cases in 2014. This reduction is the result of the global effort to eradicate the disease (World Health Organization 2016).

Polio is a disease that exists insofar as there are cases of the disease. It can go out of existence, or exist only in a few countries, and it can be eradicated for good if we prevent future cases.

For our second example, let us introduce a new term—"bogus syndrome," say. We can now specify the rules that guide the correct application of the term through a stipulative definition. Someone "suffers" from bogus syndrome, we might stipulate, if and only if that person is living in Australia, weighs less than 60 kg, works in a shopping mall, and loves to eat cheese. With the reference of the term "fixed" in this way, we can ask whether bogus syndrome exists. Again, the answer will be in the affirmative insofar as there is anyone living in Australia who weighs less than 60 kg, works in a shopping mall, and loves to eat cheese.

"But," someone might interject, "doesn't this commit you to being a *realist* about bogus syndrome? Surely you don't want to say that bogus syndrome is a *real* condition, *on a par* with paralytic poliomyelitis?" Our response to this is, of course, that it depends on what you mean by "real," "on a par," and "being a realist about something." If by "being a realist about something" you mean that one accepts this something as "real," *and* by "real" you simply mean "existing," then yes, bogus syndrome is real insofar as there are actually people who meet the criteria. This might not sound like a metaphysically interesting conclusion, but, viewed from the "deflationary" perspective we are advocating, there is nothing metaphysically interesting going on when we say that *polio* is real, either.

The more interesting question is whether bogus syndrome is "on a par" with paralytic poliomyelitis. Similar questions have been asked repeatedly about mental disorders and medical diseases. But what do these questions amount to? In our view, they usually raise one of two different types of concerns. First, one might be worried about the *normative status* of bogus syndrome. Is it really *pathological* in the same way that polio is? No, obviously. But this is a normative judgment, not a scientific discovery. Second, even if we deemed bogus syndrome pathological, we might still question whether it could be a proper object of biomedical investigations. Will we ever be able to find neat causal explanations of how people typically develop bogus syndrome? Is there a "cure" to be found for the syndrome? And will knowledge of the fact that someone suffers from bogus syndrome ever be useful in predicting other features of that person's biology and behaviour? We predict not, of course. But these questions are all empirical. If we really wanted to know the answer to each of these questions, we would have to go out in the world, find people with bogus syndrome, and see whether they have anything interesting in common. If we were to do that, however, we could be said to be embarking on a quest for the *validation* of bogus syndrome, a quest similar to the one first proposed by Robins and Guze (1970) in their famous paper on the establishment of diagnostic *validity* for psychiatric disorders.

We now conclude our discussion by briefly "addressing the deeply puzzling question of the validity of our diagnostic categories in psychiatry" (section 32.3).

33.7 Validity and validation

There are many points worth making about validity and validation, but we will mention just two. First, we agree with Campbell that current DSM validation practice, as described, for instance, in the *Guidelines for Making Changes to DSM-V* (Kendler et al. 2009), is still, for the most part, concerned with establishing the *external validity* of psychiatric diagnoses (Kendler 1990)—that is, with showing whether, and to what degree, they are statistically associated with specific validators (e.g., course of illness, response to treatment, and so on). What we take exception to, though, is his contention that this practice is based on an "amputated conception of validity" (section 32.4). In Campbell's view, the DSM conception of validity and validation is amputated because "the very idea of an external phenomenon out there, to which we are causally responding and to which we are referring, is doing no work in the picture." However, as we have already argued at length above, the names of DSM disorders *do* refer—namely to *syndromes.* It is these syndromes that are the objects of both study and intervention, it is these clinical manifestations that psychiatrists and others work relentlessly to understand and mitigate.

Second, we think Campbell's picture of validity and validation should be replaced. Instead of thinking about classification systems as entity-detection devices, it is better to think of them as conceptual schemes, or technical vocabularies, introduced to allow the delimitation and demarcation of various forms of psychopathology. Accordingly, instead of picturing validity as a measure of entity-detection capabilities, one should think of validation as the evaluation of the pragmatic value, or usefulness, of different ways of classifying the domain of psychopathology.

The pragmatic value of a classification is, in part, determined by its predictive utility—especially, though not exclusively, with respect to the currently accepted validators. How well a given psychiatric diagnosis performs on these validators is an empirical question. What validators we choose, or consider as more important, is *not.* The choice between two alternative classifications, based on their differential performance on various validators, is not a choice between truth and falsity, but the expression of a value judgment—a judgment about what kind of classification we want, given the goals that we have, and the situation we find ourselves in.

References

American Psychiatric Association. (2013). *Diagnostic and Statistical Manual of Mental Disorders*, 5th edn. Washington, DC: American Psychiatric Association.

Borsboom, D. and **Cramer, A.** (2013). Network analysis: an integrative approach to the structure of psychopathology. *Annual Review of Clinical Psychology*, **9**, 91–121.

Cattell, R. (1943). The description of personality. I. Foundations of trait measurement. *Psychological Review*, **50**, 559–594.

Kendler, K. (1990). Toward a scientific psychiatric nosology. *Archives of General Psychiatry*, **47**, 969.

Kendler, K., **Kupfer, D.**, **Narrow, W.**, et al. (2009). Guidelines for making changes to DSM-V. http://www.dsm5.org/ProgressReports/Documents/Guidelines-for-Making-Changes-to-DSM_1.pdf. Retrieved 23 March 2016

Kendler, K. and **Schaffner, K.** (2011). The dopamine hypothesis of schizophrenia: an historical and philosophical analysis. *Philosophy, Psychiatry, and Psychology*, **18**, 41–63.

Robins, E. and **Guze, S.** (1970). Establishment of diagnostic validity in psychiatric illness: its application to schizophrenia. *American Journal of Psychiatry*, **126**, 983–987.

World Health Organization. (2016). *Does polio still exist? Is it curable? World Health Organization*. http://www.who.int/features/qa/07/en/. Retrieved 23 March 2016

Section 12

Personality disorders in DSM-5

Chapter 34

Introduction to "Epistemic iteration or paradigm shift: The case of personality disorder"

Kenneth S. Kendler

In this thoughtful and well-informed essay, Peter Zachar—a frequent and important contributor to the psychiatry–philosophy dialog—tackles what is widely regarded as the single most controversial outcome in the fifth edition of the *Diagnostic and Statistical Manual of Mental Disorders* (DSM-5)—the rejection of the major changes proposed by the Personality and Personality Disorder Work Group (PPDWG). The DSM-IV system was basically maintained and the PPDWG proposal placed in an appendix so as to be available for future study. I cannot here claim to be a neutral historian. Indeed, as chair of the Scientific Review Committee, I was in the thick of things and Zachar clearly outlines my point of view on the process.

Rather than again going over controversial ground, I want to make three more general comments. The first is to advocate for exactly the kind of philosophically informed history of the DSM process that Zachar is practicing here. Given the importance of the DSM process, the field of scholars who have been involved directly or indirectly in the work has, in my view, an obligation to provide informed historical accounts of the process. Given the amount of work that went into the PPDWG proposal, the field needs to make a genuine effort to learn from this and so reduce the chances of a repetition in the future. If those with some sympathy and knowledge of the process do not write the histories, then the only histories we will have will be written by outsiders who are often (but not always) critics, many of whom have little interest in producing a generative account of the processes that might aid those who will lead a revision effort in the future.

Second, I believe that one of the many themes engaged in the PPDWG dispute was the deep differences in the science cultures in psychiatry versus psychology. Psychiatry is a branch of medicine and all of us in the club put on our white coats and spent years of our life in medical school and residency caring for people with a range of medical and psychiatric problems. There is a part of medical training which is immediate and practical. You have to make decisions, and you have to do things, sometimes very quickly. It is therefore no accident that the Robins and Guze culture of "validation" of diagnostic criteria fits well in a psychiatric world view. We want our diagnosis to do practical things in the world—predict outcome and treatment and be linked to palpable etiologic factors—genetic variants—or changes in an MRI scan that shows us brain tissue. The world of psychometrics and exploratory and confirmatory factor analysis that is so prominent in the psychological world of personality theory has much less appeal to the medically minded and seems rather divorced from the practical world we want to inhabit. I say this as someone who commonly uses psychometric approaches in my own research. There are also relevant differences in the clinical cultures of psychology and psychiatry. Clinical psychology has the strong tradition of psychological testing which typically generates quantitative scores. Psychiatrists, as physicians, are trained to make diagnoses—and so are more comfortable living in the world of categories.

Third, the box canyon problem goes down to bedrock. Nearly everyone working in psychiatric nosology feels that we are in some sort of "middle game." We have a broad consensus about our syndromes and a working set of criteria which, though far from perfect, do at least get the job done. But we all hope we can see, dimly, over the historical horizon something different and more definitive—a nosology based, in some way that we can barely conceive, on etiology. We know if will not be the "single cause" kind that we have for Mendelian genetic disorders or for our one true success—general paresis of the insane. So maybe it will be some common final pathway or really strong link to endophenotypes. Along that way there is likely to be a transformation of our nosologic system. Maybe we get to throw out all of our current validators and simplify the list to a few, much better measured, constructs. Maybe complex mathematical models will reveal a clarity we cannot now see. But if there is to be a change, how we will know it is time? When do we know we are really stuck and have to do a reboot? What is the evidential base we will need to make the jump? What should our level of tolerance be for multiple competing systems—the kind of "nosologic pluralism" which Hasok Chang advocates in Chapter 29 of this book?

Reboots will be painful. Diagnostic criteria will likely need to be entirely relearned from scratch—not just a change of a criteria here or there. Too much caution may cause our nosology to ossify. Too little caution could produce false solutions and "bridges to nowhere"—a reboot that really solves no problems or just exchanges one set for another equally problematic set. Having multiple competing systems will certainly be stimulating to the field, but we do not want to regress to the pre-DSM days of nosologic chaos where study results were not comparable across centers.

It is these and other important nosologic issues that are the subject of this essay. These issues are, on the one hand, eminently practical questions confronted and debated in the DSM-5 process by real people in real time and with real emotions and, on the other hand, raise challenging conceptual and philosophical issues to which clear and self-evident solutions are not always at hand.

Chapter 35

Epistemic iteration or paradigm shift: The case of personality disorder

Peter Zachar

35.1 The Alternative DSM-5 Model of Personality Disorder: a scientific controversy

In the late fall of 2012, the Board of Trustees of the American Psychiatric Association (APA) rejected a model of personality disorder that was newly proposed for the fifth edition of the *Diagnostic and Statistical Manual of Mental Disorders* (DSM-5). Instead, the previous DSM-IV model of personality disorder was reprinted in the main text of the manual. The proposed DSM-5 model was placed in a section at the back of the book and named the "Alternative DSM-5 Model of Personality Disorder."

The old DSM-IV model classified ten personality disorders types (or categories) that were identified by means of diagnostic criteria. To elucidate, for the category of narcissistic personality disorder there were nine diagnostic criteria such as "grandiose sense of self-importance." Criteria, utilized like symptoms, were rated as either present or absent. Anyone who met five of the nine criteria for this disorder could be diagnosed. In contrast, the alternative DSM-5 model includes both categories and dimensions. An example of a dimensional rating is *degree* of grandiosity—from very low to very high.

The diagnostician's job in making a personality disorder diagnosis using this new model can be divided into three tasks:

- First, *assess each patient's self and interpersonal functioning* on a four-point scale ranging from no impairment to severe impairment. Moderate or severe impairment in two or more dimensions of self and interpersonal functioning is required to make a personality disorder diagnosis. For example, a lack of identity and feelings of emptiness represent severe impairments in self-functioning.
- Second, *document the presence of one or more pathological personality traits.* There are five primary trait dimensions: negative affect, detachment, antagonism, disinhibition, and psychoticism. These five domain level traits can be further decomposed into 25 facet-level traits such as grandiosity and manipulativeness.

- Third, *assign a specific personality disorder diagnosis.* There are two options for this task. The first option is to diagnosis one of the DSM-IV personality disorder types. Only six of the diagnostic categories from DSM-IV have been retained in the alternative model: borderline, antisocial, narcissistic, avoidant, obsessive-compulsive, and schizotypal.
- The DSM-IV diagnostic criteria, however, have been replaced with (a) a specification of the self and interpersonal deficits associated with each personality disorder type and (b) the major pathological traits that constitute that type. To illustrate, for narcissistic personality disorder one of the impairments in self-functioning is exaggerated self-appraisal, either inflated or deflated. The important primary domain level trait is antagonism, which can be further subdivided into the facet-level traits of grandiosity and attention-seeking.
- For the second option, if patients match more than one type or match no type at all, they are diagnosed as "personality disorder—trait specified." In theory, each patient could then have a profile of the elevated pathological personality traits that characterize her or his personality.

As described by Zachar et al. (2016), there was a great deal of controversy about both the proposal itself and its rejection by the Board of Trustees. According to its advocates, the proposed model represented an unambiguous scientific advance and had promising clinical utility. According to its opponents, the evidence for increased validity was inadequate and there were serious concerns about its clinical utility.

As the gap in the assessment of what the research supported was quite large, I will examine this dispute by looking upon it as a scientific controversy. Intense disagreements during a period of controversy are common in the history of science (Engelhardt and Caplan 1987, Machamer et al. 2000). For example, for nearly a century there were large gaps in how the evidence in physics was interpreted by the Cartesians compared to the Newtonians. We look back from the standpoint of current knowledge and readily notice the errors made by the losing side, but in doing so often magnify the scientific credentials of the victors. We see the Cartesians as being mistaken about the impossibility of a vacuum and their vortex theory of planetary motion, but ignore that Newton believed that God had to occasionally intervene to keep the solar system running.

The question is: how should we think about progress when trying to understand ongoing controversies between legitimate experts when we do not have the advantage of historical hindsight? One way is through the lens of epistemic iteration.

35.2 **Epistemic iteration—and empiricism**

The concept of epistemic iteration was introduced by Hasok Chang (2004) in *Inventing Temperature* (and see Chapter 29 in this volume). According to Chang, measurement in science often begins with an intuitive awareness of some phenomena. This awareness can be thought of as an imperfect gauge of that phenomenon. For example, measurement of temperature began with the sensations of warm and cold. These sensations were the sole initial basis for a trajectory of gradual improvements in measurement resulting in the amazingly precise thermometers of today. Scientists can currently measure the temperature of objects that are within a billionth of a degree of absolute zero. That is a long way from sensing that ice is colder than water.

One interesting aspect of Chang's work is his approach to the operationalism of Percy Bridgman (1927). In contrast to the general disparagement of Bridgman that has become almost a truism, especially in psychology, Chang offers a positive reading. He is able to do this by being sympathetic to an important aspect of Bridgeman's empiricism, i.e., Bridgman's awareness of the fluidity of abstract concepts such as length when we generalize them to domains that lie outside everyday experience.

> It will never be possible to give a clean-cut logical analysis of the conceptual situation, for the nature of our concepts, according to our operational point of view, is the same as the nature of experimental knowledge, which is often hazy (Bridgman, 1927, p. 25).

We readily use the concept of length to measure objects of everyday experience. But what happens if we apply that concept to the measurement of something far outside and remote from our possible experience, like the quantum realm. According to Bridgman, because our experience does not extend into that realm, and how we measure length at the quantum level is so different from everyday measurement, we cannot unthinkingly assume that the concept remains the same. Chang agrees that the concept has evolved, but he charitably emphasizes continuity with past practices.

Let us dig a little deeper into this aspect of empiricism by looking back at its introduction in the work of John Locke. After doing so, with this perspective on concepts in the background, in the remainder of the chapter I offer a historically grounded examination of the debate about personality disorder, validity, and progress that occurred during the development of the DSM-5—and make some tentative suggestions about the future.

The early empiricists Locke and Hume were suspicious of metaphysical inferences about abstract concepts such as substance, essence, and self. They considered each of these concepts to be pseudo-explanations for coherent patterns in our experience of the world.

In the process of abstraction, particular features of phenomena are omitted in order to arrive at a general concept. The more abstract a concept becomes, the more remote it is from the phenomenon it represents. This view of concepts is called nominalism. The early empiricists favored nominalism. For them, nominalism was a corrective to our intellectual attraction to playing with abstract words and concepts. Platonic philosophy and scholasticism were egregious examples of word play for the empiricists. At its worst word play results in a veneer of knowledge and fruitless arguments that do not lead to progress.

> Vague and insignificant forms of speech . . . have for so long passed for mysteries of science; and hard or misapplied words, with little or no meaning, have, by prescription, such a right to be mistaken for deep learning . . . that it will not be easy to persuade, either those who speak or those who hear them, that they are but the covers of ignorance, and hindrance of true knowledge (Locke 1689/1997, p. 11).

This nominalist dimension of empiricism is often minimized or even ignored in favor of the empiricist's emphasis on knowledge as grounded in sensory experience. In a slight variation on the traditional view on empiricism, one could argue that Locke's emphasis on sensory experience in human understanding was an attempt to make progress on the problem of empty abstractions—and the problem of abstractions is what unifies Locke's *Essay*.

In agreement with some basic principles advocated for in the scientific revolution, empiricists can accept a concept of the world as existing independent of how we happen to conceptualize it or as existing whether or not it is measured. They accept this because concepts and measures are incomplete, and there are always aspects of phenomena that elude them (Zachar 2014). For empiricists the concepts and the measures can be fiddled with in many ways. They can be made broader, made more precise, and so on and thus are what Locke called the workmanship of human understanding. That is one way to take the "inventing" in inventing temperature.

Another way to see "inventing" is in reference to knowledge generation as something that we actively do. *Inventing temperature* does not mean that the phenomenon of water boiling when enough heat is present was an invention. The *concept* of a fixed boiling point, however, is a different matter. Measurement of such depended on specifying the experimental conditions to fix a boiling point, including the use of very pure water and controlled air pressure. Alter the purity of the water or the air pressure and you alter the boiling point. "Inventing" refers to all the things scientists had to do to assign numerical values to a concept they introduced to the world.[1]

35.3 **Epistemic iteration in clinical psychology and psychiatry**

35.3.1 **In psychology**

In their groundbreaking article on construct validity, Cronbach and Meehl (1955), like Chang, observed how progress was made in measuring temperature by beginning with the sensory experience of some things feeling warmer than others, but they did so to understand not thermometry, but psychological testing. Rather than epistemic iteration, they wrote about the *bootstrap effect*. According to them, a test that is validated on a criterion can in time become more valid than the original criterion itself. A cycle of gradual improvements can begin without the benefit of a better validator. All that is needed is another imperfect validator that represents different aspects of the phenomena being measured.

---

[1] Another important aspect of this alternative view on empiricism is to see it as an incipient pragmatism. Pragmatist features enter the picture whenever an empiricist goes beyond the passive reception of sensation to an application of knowledge that emphasizes problem-solving and interaction with the phenomena in question, i.e., *workmanship*. Peirce (1878/1992) and James (1909/1975) transformed this emphasis on workmanship into a larger theory about the meaning of abstract concepts such as truth.

For example, in the early 1900s intelligence tests were originally validated on schoolteacher evaluations of student abilities. Currently, if a student obtains a high score on an intelligence test and her teachers claim she lacks academic ability, we would likely try to understand what factors are incorrectly distorting the schoolteachers' evaluations of this student. The intelligence test has become more valid than its original validator, but this improvement did not depend on raising the validity of the test by means of a more accurate measure of intelligence. Instead, the intelligence test itself has become our gold standard because it has been gradually calibrated to cohere with a large number of imperfect validators—often guided by changing concepts of intelligence.

As Meehl was a clinical psychologist who contributed to the early development of the *Minnesota Multiphasic Personality Inventory*, clinical/psychiatric concepts such as psychopathic deviate were in the forefront of his thinking about construct validity. One can readily view bootstrapping/epistemic iteration as a story of how improvements in measurement techniques can lead to increasingly better approximations of clinical reality—which is arguably how Meehl and many clinical psychologists saw it.[2]

35.3.2 **In psychiatry**

In addition to psychological measurement, epistemic iteration has also been applied to psychiatric classification. To understand its potential role here requires some historical background. The committees that developed the DSM-III and the DSM-II-R were very liberal about making changes. In time, they came to believe that minor alterations to criteria could have unforeseen negative consequences. As a result, those psychiatrists who developed the DSM-IV were more conservative about making alterations—seeking incremental improvements supported by evidence (Frances 2013). Many of those involved in constructing the DSM-IV had not changed their minds about the virtues of incremental changes when it came time to produce the DSM-5.

In the years leading up to the development of the DSM-5, there was considerable worry that scientific progress in psychiatry was being hindered by the use of invalid DSM categories (Rounsaville et al. 2002, Hyman 2010). In contrast to the approach taken by the previous task force, the DSM-5 leadership did not want to make incremental improvements; rather, they were looking for some kind of paradigm shift. They rejected the DSM-IV leadership's strong commitment to gradual iteration.

The conflict between the iteration versus paradigm shift had become a major issue by the time of the second Copenhagen conference in fall 2010. This conference was attended by important members of the DSM-IV and the DSM-5 committees.

---

[2] Brian Hood (2009) emphasizes that Meehl also remained committed to an empiricist view on construct validity in which test scores were treated as tools for making inferences. Construct validation consisted in presenting the evidence that justified the inferences made from test scores.

At this conference, Kenneth Kendler (2012) asked the audience to assume that the classification task that nosologists are working on has a correct, unambiguous solution which can be more closely approximated over time, i.e., that disease syndromes are out there waiting to be correctly classified. So framed, this is closer to Meehl's view than to Chang's—although influenced by Chang's claim that iteration is a *self-correcting* process.[3]

Kendler's own position was indefinite between advocating for such a realist vision based on scientific common sense and believing that realist views oversimplify psychiatric phenomenon. From this open perspective, he explored various ways that iteration could fail in psychiatry. He identified three barriers to successful iteration which I will describe with respect to the classification of personality disorder. These are the modified random walk, the nosological box canyon, and wobbly iteration.

35.4 The modified random walk

A random walk is a sequence of discrete random movements. For epistemic iteration a random walk would correspond to a situation where there is no fixed and stable phenomenon to increasingly approximate. There can be change, but change would be non-systematic—often covering the same territory over again. Kendler's example of a modified random walk is the changing length of women's skirts from 1605 to 1936.

The notion of "modified" refers to the fact that in psychiatry the starting points for the iterative process may shift and not be fully random. With respect to personality disorder, such shifts might follow changing preferences for various authoritative systems over time. For instance, Table 35.1 compares the personality disorder classifications of Kurt Schneider (1923/1950), the *Minnesota Multiphasic Personality Inventory* from Hathaway and McKinley (1940), William Menninger's dynamic perspective (Menninger et al. 1963), and the DSM-III of 1987.

Not only can many different personality types be described, but what counts as a personality construct (paranoid) versus a syndromal entity (schizophrenia) has been fluid. Prior to the DSM-III, for many psychodynamic thinkers much of psychiatric nosology was personality-like (Rapaport et al. 1945, Horney 1964, Shapiro 1965, Arieti 1978). From the standpoint of empiricism, personality, personality disorder, and personality types are abstract concepts—so some fluidity should be expected.

The iteration perspective on progress asks us to be charitable and accept that all these constructs may be clinically informative in some way. Any one of them could be subjected to an iterative process.

A member of previous DSM committees himself, Kendler (1990, 2009) was concerned that the lack of progress was due a history of making changes without

---

[3] Part of what Chang means by self-correcting is that concepts and measures reveal their own inadequacies.

Table 35.1 Four personality disorder classifications

Schneider	MMPI	Mennigner	DSM-III
Affectionless	Depression	Aggressive	Antisocial
Asthenic	Hypochondriasis	Antisocial	Atypical
Attention-seeking	Hysteria	Cyclothymic	Avoidant
Depressive	Mania	Emotionally unstable	Borderline
Explosive	Paranoia	Immature	Compulsive
Fanatic	Psychasthenia	Inadequate	Dependent
Hyperthymic	Psychopathic deviate	Paranoid	Histrionic
Insecure	Schizophrenia	Passive-dependent	Mixed
Labile	Social introversion	Schizoid	Narcissistic
Weak-willed		Sexual deviate	Paranoid
			Passive-aggressive
			Schizoid
			Schizotypal

adequate scientific support for increased validity. In psychiatry the menu of constructs has shifted as different "great professors" such as Schneider and their way of carving up the personality disorder domain have become fashionable for a time, only to be replaced with an alternative. Arguably these shifts relied heavily on what Miriam Solomon (2001) termed non-empirical factors—including peer pressure, competitiveness, and deference to authority. If the menu of constructs that is the focus of the discipline's research efforts shifts to a different menu based on non-empirical considerations, the whole specialty area could approximate a modified random walk.

35.5 **The nosological box canyon**

A box canyon is the geographical analogue of a dead-end street. Once you enter the canyon there is no way out the other side. An analogue in the domain of personality disorder is the view that the categories/types used in the DSM-III and DSM-IV are nosological dead-end streets. According to this view the diagnostic categories of the old DSM approach are so flawed that they are beyond improvement by gradual iteration. Instead, what is needed is a paradigm shift (Kupfer et al. 2002, Helzer et al. 2008).

When philosophers or historians of science hear about a paradigm shift, they are likely to think in Kuhnian terms of a revolution in which a ruling paradigm is abandoned in favor of a new paradigm. However, rather than revolution, the DSM-5 leadership's notion of a paradigm shift was better described as a paradigm transition in which dimensional models would be added to the DSM alongside the categories (Regier et al. 2009). They were not interested in making incremental changes to the categories, but neither were they seeking to replace them all at once. This is reflected in the term *hybrid model*. It referred to a hybrid of categories and dimensions and was the working name for the alternative DSM-5 model during its development.

In contrast to the DSM-5 leadership, some advocates for the dimensional model approach were open to a full-blown revolution in which all the personality disorder categories would be fully replaced with empirically derived dimensions (Costa 2006, Widiger et al. 2009). One of the members of the DSM-5 Personality and Personality Disorder Work Group (PPDWG), John Livesley, resigned from the group because he could not abide a system that maintained links back to what the he considered the invalid categories of the DSM-IV (Livesley 2010, 2012).

Concern in the APA leadership (above the level of the DSM-5 Task Force) about how to systematically evaluate newly proposed changes led to the establishment of the Scientific Review Committee (SRC; Kendler, 2013). The SRC was one of several DSM-5 oversight committees. Its task was to evaluate proposed changes to the manual and, ideally, to limit changes to only those that were scientifically justified.

Kenneth Kendler was the chair of this committee and his perspective was related to his work on epistemic iteration (Kendler 2009, 2012). If changes to the manual were made based upon a consensus opinion in committees of experts, psychiatric nosology might be vulnerable to becoming a modified random walk as described above—with the consensus changing as committee membership changed.

The SRC tried to alter the culture of the DSM development to one that was based upon high-quality research and substantial evidential support rather than a cycling through of diagnostic fashions. They also utilized a shared set of standards that would be applied equally to all proposals (Kendler et al. 2009). However, much to the eventual chagrin of the PPDWG, these standards were an expansion of the famous Robins and Guze (1970) program for validating *diagnostic categories* which, in combination with the introduction of diagnostic criteria, was the inspiration for the DSM-III revolution (Feighner et al. 1972, Decker 2013). After being supplemented by the additional goal of enhancing clinical utility, this model became the paradigm for producing the DSM-III-R in 1987 and the DSM-IV in 2000.

The irony is that this attempt to alter the culture to establish a more dominant role for scientific considerations ended up clashing with the scientifically minded proponents of dimensional models in the domain of personality disorder. The proponents of dimensional models readily agreed with the SRC that allowing changes to be made based on expert clinical opinion should cease, but according to them expert clinical opinion is what produced diagnostic categories rather than dimensions.

With respect to the box canyon notion, Kendler and First (2010) acknowledged that if the categorical approach is not correct, iterating the categories is a poor strategy for seeking improvement. However, they also claimed that it would be better if the competitive advantages of a new paradigm became more evident before being implemented in an official nosology such as the DSM. They were especially concerned about implementing a major change on the artificial timeline adopted for a DSM revision as opposed to allowing it to happen more organically and of its own accord.

In contrast, the advocates for the alternative model believed that the SRC criteria for making changes reified the DSM-IV personality disorder types and made them the exclusive target of iterative improvement. In their view, change was needed to assertively pave the way for future developments. In some of the interviews conducted for Zachar et al. (2016), advocates for the alternative model expressed strong disagreement about what they saw as a conservative, even reactionary opposition to change. In their view the consequence of conservatism was to maintain a taxonomic system that has been shown not to work. To not write change into the DSM, they believed, would be to actively preserve the status quo.

35.6 **Wobbly iteration**

Earlier I noted that Kendler's own view was indefinite with respect to scientific realism. After sitting through many hours of discussions on DSM committees, Kendler (1990) had an insight about the potential fluidity of concepts for disorders. Take schizophrenia for instance. Assume that our background theory for schizophrenia is that "genuine" schizophrenic illness has a deteriorating course. If that feature is used to validate the diagnostic construct, then what we demarcate as schizophrenia would be a narrow category characterized by early onset, chronicity, and prominent psychotic and negative symptoms. What if our background theory says schizophrenia is genetically based and runs in families? If that feature is used to validate the diagnostic construct then what we demarcate as schizophrenia would be a broader category that includes odd and eccentric personality types and briefer psychotic syndromes with better prognosis.

Both of these demarcations empirically fit the family of phenomenon that have historically been classified under the name schizophrenia.[4] Therefore, according to Kendler, whether what we name "schizophrenia" is a narrow deteriorating condition or a broad genetic condition involves non-empirical considerations regarding *selection of validators*. In those cases where justifying the selection of validators relies upon auxiliary assumptions, there will be a potential for fluidity in validated constructs over time. Among these non-empirical auxiliaries are metaphysical assumptions such as "real disorders are diseases" and "same disorder means same etiology and pathogenesis."

In Chang's formulation of epistemic iteration, scientists propose some standard of evaluation or a criterion for improvement—such as more precise

[4] Currently deteriorating course would not be considered a viable validator because even for cases with early onset and prominent psychotic symptoms outcome can be variable (Jablensky 2010).

measurement—and iterate toward that goal. Wobbly iteration is what would occur when the criteria/validators shift moderately over time (in contrast, radical changes in validators would produce something like a random walk).

Lack of a shared vision on the choice of standards for validating disorder concepts was one of the most important reasons that the alternative model was rejected at the level of the Board of Trustees. For instance, among the goals employed by the PPDWG are the following:

- Eliminate the non-informative diagnosis of "personality disorder not otherwise specified."
- Increase the within-category homogeneity of personality disorder constructs (i.e., increase factorial validity).
- Eliminate the perception that there is a discrete threshold between disorder and non-disordered personality.
- Comprehensively model the domain of personality pathology in an empirically based way (i.e., increase structural validity).

From the standpoint of the work group members, their proposal was calibrated to achieve all of these goals. Indeed, if one examines the alternative model and the DSM-IV model with respect to these goals, the alternative model is superior on every criterion.

However, the SRC and the PPDWG had different standards for assessing validity. As noted, the SRC was seeking incremental improvements of diagnostic categories. For large changes they required especially strong and unambiguous evidence. In contrast, the work group had no intention of iterating categories. Their charge from the DSM-5 leadership was to implement the dimensional approach that had become paradigmatic among clinical psychologists specializing in the scientific study of psychopathology. The SRC and the work group were not on the same page.

There was little dispute that the problems targeted by the work group were genuine problems, but not everyone involved agreed that they were overriding problems. For instance, there was grave concern among prominent clinicians outside of the DSM-5 process that knowledge about specific personality disorders built up over the years would be lost with the new set of dimensional concepts (Shedler et al. 2010, Gunderson 2013). Retaining what they considered hard-won knowledge became an overriding concern for them.

Two groups internal to the DSM-5 process, the Clinical and Public Health Committee and the APA Assembly (Zachar et al. 2016), believed that clinician acceptability should play a predominant role in the revision process. The new components of the alternative model such as replacing the uninformative diagnosis of "personality disorder not otherwise specified" with a listing of each patient's pathological personality traits can readily been seen as an improvement. The same can be said for assessing self and interpersonal dysfunction. Yet, making sense of trait profiles would require new skills for those without training in psychological assessment (Zachar and First 2015). Assessing self and interpersonal dysfunction is highly inferential (Gunderson 2013). In the view of these committees, the alternative model introduced too many new components and was too complicated and time-consuming for routine clinical use.

It is probably not possible for a single model to address the plurality of scientific and clinical goals that have been articulated in recent years. It seems unavoidable that if agreement on a small set of goals cannot be reached and maintained for more than one generation, the classification of personality disorder will wobble.

35.7 The conceptual space of personality disorder

Elsewhere I have described how the domain of psychiatry was unified when the problems encountered in inpatient and outpatient settings were linked together by a collection of premorbid and residual symptoms that lie on the edge of psychosis (Zachar 2014). In keeping with this theme, the domain of personality disorder began life as a set of personality features that tended to occur in cases with multiple psychiatric complaints that were resistant to treatment. Over time, cases that were not as complex were included in this slowly evolving domain if similar personality features were present. Indeed, adding these cases—drawn from the population of outpatient psychotherapy clients—solidified the personality disorder domain as it has been understood since the publication of the DSM-III.

Personality disorders are certainly unique animals within the psychiatric zoo. They are different from the psychoses, mood disorders, and anxiety disorders because as lifelong patterns they do not typically involve a decline in functioning. Nor are they gross violations of expected developmental trajectories such as autism spectrum disorder. As Schneider (1923/1950) noted, personality disorders are not morbid illnesses. Instead, he proposed that people with personality disorders have character traits that deviate from the group average, and because of this deviation they either suffer personally or make others suffer.

Karl Jaspers (1923/1963) conceived of personality disorders as ideal types. Ideal types are concepts under which collections of particular phenomena are *seen as* being the same kind of thing (Schwartz et al. 1995). Ideal types are inherently conceptual and do not represent things in the world literally. Every particular referent of an ideal type varies in numerous ways from the abstract concept.

There is a clear similarity between the Germanic notion of ideal types and the nominalism of the British empiricists. Indeed, Locke also contended that the notion of the same *kind* (which he called a species) is an invention and creature of human understanding. As Locke's view applies to concepts for both types and dimensions, let me expand upon it here.

Two diverse kinds of species were important for Locke's thinking. An example of the first is water. Water is a self-subsisting entity in the world. It is held together by shared causal processes. Humans and cats and dogs all know about water. An example of the second kind of species is murder. According to Locke, had murder never been committed, humans could still entertain the idea of murder. It does not need to exist to be thought about. Also, our decisions play some role in what features to include in the kind, for example, we say killing another human is murder but squishing an ant is not. We also add and subtract features creating distinctions such as homicide, patricide, killing during warfare, and manslaughter. Cats and dogs do not know about different kinds of murder.

What about personality disorders? They are in-between kinds of things. Personality disorders are considered to be the products of causal processes. They are not quite self-subsisting entities, but still coherent and regular phenomena in the world. They are also, potentially, fluid concepts. For example, the DSM-IV narrowed the concept of narcissistic personality disorder by making it more extroverted and attention-seeking, de-emphasizing features such as narcissistic vulnerability and shame.

The fluidity in how we demarcate concepts may influence what we take to be the important causal processes. For instance, highlighting the trait of attention-seeking in pathological narcissism influences what would count as an empirically adequate causal model of narcissism. Adding back in narcissistic features such as shame, vulnerability, and withdrawal into fantasy would broaden the concept (Pincus et al. 2009, Pincus and Roche 2011). It would also alter what would count as an empirically adequate causal model.

35.8 **Progress in the domain of personality disorder as an epistemic iterationist might view it**

With recent history in mind, and having elaborated upon an empiricist's view of epistemic iteration and the fluidity of concepts, how should we think about progress—or future prospects for progress—in personality disorder research? Is progress even possible if personality disorder concepts are fluid? I would say yes—and yes because of the fluidity not in spite of it.

The future will be determined by many unanticipated events and none of us have a crystal ball to see what those will be. Still, four features of Chang's (2004, 2012) epistemic iteration model are helpful to keep in mind with respect to working toward progress in the domain of personality disorder.

The first feature is to *be charitable about the past* and see the continuity that exists. In some sense, whether we see iteration or paradigm shift turns on a choice to emphasize what is the same or emphasize what is different during a transition (Zachar 2012). This charitable view conflicts with a historically popular strategy in psychiatry of denigrating the past and proclaiming that a revolutionary change is needed.

By charitable I mean more than seeing the continuity contained in a categorical-dimensional hybrid. Instead, we can see the continuity between a dimensional model and what preceded it. For example, Schneider's system was an attempt to subsume the theories of earlier thinkers such as Koch, Kretschmer, and Kraepelin. He influenced the developers of DSM-I and the MMPI who tried to improve on some of his concepts. The DSM-III model of personality disorder benefited greatly from an integration around the early 1970s of 50 years of largely disparate work on character disorder in the psychodynamic tradition (Kernberg 1969, 1975, Kohut, 1971).

From this charitable perspective, the alternative model is an attempt to implement in the DSM-5 an empirically based structure for the symptom space as that space is demarcated in the DSM-IV approach to personality disorder. The developers of the dimensional system implemented in the alternative model were actively seeking to recapture the symptom space defined by the DSM-IV personality disorder types, as were the two earlier models of Livesley and Clark (Clark and Livesley 1994).

In this one respect, the revolutionary nature of a dimensional model rests on seeing the endpoint of a longer process and ignoring many intervening steps. Rather than construing the categories as complete dead ends, it might be better to just say that it is not possible to iterate from categories to dimensions in one step.

Second, one iterates toward goals. The fluidity of personality disorder constructs means that wobbling is an ongoing possibility. It is fruitless to seek a privileged, single correct concept for something abstract like pathological narcissism. Such concepts do not work that way. That does not mean, however, that we cannot commit to criteria for improvement and work toward them.

The problem in the DSM-5 was that there were recognized experts both within and outside the process who did not agree on the goals. The various goals articulated, in turn, rested on many auxiliary assumptions. These include assumptions about what is meant by "validator," the nature of expertise, and what counts as clinical utility. There needs to be some conceptual work in getting auxiliary assumptions more aligned if there is going to be agreement on goals.

Third, progress is about improving on the past. Ideally progress allows us to do or know about something that was unimaginable to previous generations. In psychiatry progress in the clinical sense would include treatment goals.

In this respect, placing a traditional categorical model, a hierarchical dimensional model like the DSM-5 alternative model, and what looks to be a very minimalist dimensional model for the ICD-11 in competition with each other could be fruitful. Having three "official" options would focus the psychiatric community's attention better than would a libertine plurality of models. I might be inclined to wait a decade or more to see what this competition produces clinically rather than making changes in the next few years.

Fourth, the higher standard for iteration involves seeking coherence—which is about bringing different sectors of our knowledge into alignment. Let me suggest that seeking coherence is a goal for which scientific psychology might be helpful. Criteria such as reducing comorbidity and increasing unidimensionality were highly marketed goals for dimensional models, but not the long-term goal. What dimensional models are supposed to offer psychiatry ultimately is an anchoring of personality disorder concepts in scientific theories about both normal personality and normal development as the background for understanding the abnormal. This is a goal that Freud would have heartily endorsed, despite having very different ideas about what qualifies as a scientific theory.

References

Arieti, S. (1978). *On Schizophrenia, Phobias, Depression, Psychotherapy and the Farther Shores of Psychiatry.* New York: Brunner/Mazel.

Bridgman, P.W. (1927). *The Logic of Modern Physics*. New York: Macmillan.

Chang, H. (2004). *Inventing Temperature: Measurement and scientific progress.* New York: Oxford University Press.

Chang, H. (2012). *Is Water H_2O?: Evidence, realism, and pluralism.* Dordrecht: Springer.

Clark, L.A. and **Livesley, W.J.** (1994). Two approaches to identifying the dimensions of personality disorder: Convergence on the five-factor model. In P.T. Costa, Jr. and T.A. Widiger (eds.) *Personality Disorders and the Five-Factor Model of Personality*, pp. 261–277. Washington, DC: American Psychological Association.

Costa, P., Jr. (2006). Commentary on Trull: Just do it: Replace axis II with a diagnostic system based on the five-factor model of personality. In T.A. Widiger, E. Simonsen, P.J. Sirovatka, et al. (eds.) *Dimensional Models of Personality Disorders: Refining the research agenda for DSM-V*, pp. 195–198. Arlington, VA: American Psychiatric Association.

Cronbach, L.J. and **Meehl, P.E.** (1955). Construct validity in psychological tests. *Psychological Bulletin*, 52, 281–302.

Decker, H.S. (2013). *The Making of DSM-III®: A diagnostic manual's conquest of American psychiatry.* New York: Oxford University Press.

Engelhardt, H.T. and **Caplan, A.L.** (1987). *Scientific Controversies: Case studies in the resolution and closure of disputes in science and technology.* New York: Cambridge University Press.

Feighner, J.P., **Robins, E.**, **Guze, S.B.**, et al. (1972). Diagnostic criteria for use in psychiatric research. *Archives of General Psychiatry*, **26**(57–63).

Frances, A. (2013). *Saving Normal.* New York: William Morrow.

Gunderson, J.G. (2013). Seeking clarity for future revisions of the personality disorders in DSM-5. *Personality Disorders: Theory, Research, and Treatment*, **4**, 368–376.

Hathaway, S.R. and **McKinley, J.C.** (1940). A multiphasic personality schedule (Minnesota): I. Construction of the schedule. *Journal of Psychology*, **10**, 249–254.

Helzer, J.E., **Kraemer, H.C.**, **Krueger, R.F.**, et al. (2008). *Dimensional Approaches In Diagnostic Classification: Refining the research agenda for DSM-V.* Arlington, VA: American Psychiatric Association.

Hood, S.B. (2009). Validity in psychological testing and scientific realism. *Theory and Psychology*, **19**, 451–473.

Horney, K. (1964). *The Neurotic Personality of Our Time.* New York: W.W. Norton.

Hyman, S.E. (2010). The diagnosis of mental disorders: The problem of reification. *Annual Review of Clinical Psychology*, **6**, 155–179.

Jablensky, A. (2010). The diagnostic concept of schizophrenia: its history, evolution, and future prospects. *Dialogues in Clinical Neuroscience*, **12**, 271–287.

James, W. (1909/1975). *The Meaning of Truth: A sequel to pragmatism.* Cambridge, MA: Harvard University Press.

Jaspers, K. (1923/1963). *General Psychopathology*, trans. J. Hoenig and M. W. Hamilton. Chicago: University of Chicago Press.

Kendler, K.S. (1990). Toward a scientific psychiatric nosology. *Archives of General Psychiatry*, **47**, 969–973.

Kendler, K.S. (2009). An historical framework for psychiatric nosology. *Psychological Medicine*, **39**, 1935–1941.

Kendler, K.S. (2012). Epistemic iteration as a historical model for psychiatric nosology: promises and limitations. In K.S. Kendler and J. Parnas (eds.) *Philosophical Issues in Psychiatry II: Nosology—definition of illness, history, validity, and prospects*, pp. 305–322. Oxford, UK: Oxford University Press.

Kendler, K.S. (2013). A history of the DSM-5 scientific review committee. *Psychological Medicine*, **43**, 1793–1800.

Kendler, K.S. and **First, M.B.** (2010). Alternative futures for the DSM revision process: iteration v. paradigm shift. *British Journal of Psychiatry*, **197**, 263–265.

Kendler, K.S., Kupfer, D.J., Narrow, W., et al. (2009). Guidlines for making changes to DSM-5, revised 10/21/09. http://www.dsm5.org/ProgressReports/Documents/Guidelines-for-Making-Changes-to-DSM_1.pdf.

Kernberg, O.F. (1969). Factors in the psychoanalytic treatment of narcissistic personalities. *Bulletin of the Menninger Clinic*, **33**, 191–196.

Kernberg, O.F. (1975). *Borderline Conditions and Pathological Narcissism*. New York: Jason Aronson.

Kohut, H. (1971). *The Analysis of the Self: A systematic psychoanalytic approach to the treatment of narcissistic personality disorders*. New York: International Universities Press.

Kupfer, D.J., First, M.B., and **Regier, D.A.** (2002). *A Research Agenda for DSM-V*. Washington, DC: American Psychiatric Association.

Livesley, J. (2010). Confusion and incoherence in the classification of personality disorder. *Psychological Injury and Law*, **3**, 304–313.

Livesley, W.J. (2012). Tradition versus empiricism in the current DSM-5 proposal for revising the classification of personality disorders. *Criminal Behavior and Mental Health*, **22**, 81–91.

Locke, J. (1689/1997). *An Essay Concerning Human Understanding*. London: Penguin Books.

Machamer, P., Pera, M., and **Baltas, A.** (2000). *Scientific Controversies*. New York: Oxford University Press.

Menninger, K., Mayman, M., and **Pruyser, P.** (1963). *The Vital Balance*. New York: Viking Press.

Peirce, C. S. (1878/1992). How to make our ideas clear. In N. Houser and C. Kloesel (eds.) *The Essential Peirce: Selected philosophical writings: Volume 1 (1867–1893)*, pp. 124–141. Bloomington, IN: Indiana University Press.

Pincus, A.L., Ansell, E.B., Pimentel, C.A., et al. (2009). Initial construction and validation of the pathological narcissism inventory. *Psychological Assessment*, **21**, 365–379.

Pincus, A.L., and **Roche, M.J.** (2011). Narcissistic grandiosity and narcissistic vulnerability. In W.K. Campbell and J.D. Miller (eds.) *The Handbook of Narcissism and Narcissistic Personality Disorder*, pp. 31–40. Hoboken, NJ: John Wiley & Sons.

Rapaport, D., Gill, M.M., and **Schafer, R.** (1945). *Diagnostic Psychological Testing*, Vol. **1**. Chicago: Yearbook Publishers.

Regier, D.A., Narrow, W.E., Kuhl, E.A., and **Kupfer, D.J.** (2009). The conceptual development of DSM-V. *American Journal of Psychiatry*, **166**, 645–650.

Robins, E., and **Guze, S.B.** (1970). Establishment of diagnostic validity in psychiatric illness: Its application to schizophrenia. *American Journal of Psychiatry*, **126**, 983–986.

Rounsaville, B.J., Alarcon, R.D., Andrews, G., et al. (2002). Basic nomenclature issues for DSM-V. In *A Research Agenda for DSM-V*, pp. 1–29. Washington, DC: American Psychiatric Association.

Schneider, K. (1923/1950). *Psychopathic Personalities*, trans M.W. Hamilton. London: Cassell.

Schwartz, M.A., **Wiggins, O.P.**, and **Norko, M.A.** (1995). Prototypes, ideal types, and personality disorders: The return to classical phenomenology. In W.J. Livesley (ed.) *The DSM-IV Personality Disorders*, pp. 417–432. New York: Guilford Press.

Shapiro, D. (1965). *Neurotic Styles*. New York: Basic Books.

Shedler, J., **Beck, A.**, **Fonagy, P.**, et al. (2010). Personality disorders in DSM-5. *American Journal of Psychiatry*, **167**, 1026–1028.

Solomon, M. (2001). *Social Empiricism*. Cambridge, MA: MIT Press.

Widiger, T.A., **Livesley, W.J.**, and **Clark, L.A.** (2009). An integrative dimensional classification of personality disorder. *Psychological Assessment*, **21**, 243–255.

Zachar, P. (2012). Progress and the calibration of scientific constructs: The role of comparative validity. In K.S. Kendler and J. Parnas (eds.) *Philosophical Issues in Psychiatry II: Nosology—definition of illness, history, validity, and prospects*, pp. 21–34. Oxford, UK: Oxford University Press.

Zachar, P. (2014). *A Metaphysics of Psychopathology*. Cambridge, MA: MIT Press.

Zachar, P. and **First, M.B.** (2015). Transitioning to a dimensional model of personality disorder in DSM 5.1 and beyond. *Current Opinion in Psychiatry*, **28**, 66–72.

Zachar, P., **Krueger, R.F.**, and **Kendler, K.S.** (2016). Personality disorder in the DSM-5: An oral history. *Psychological Medicine*, **46**, 1–10.

Chapter 36

Why we should be realists about psychiatric disorders—reply to Peter Zachar

John Campbell

36.1 Epistemic modesty is not a reason to reject realism

Resistance to realism about psychiatric disorders is, I think, generated mainly by a reasonable epistemic modesty about how far we can claim to have reached definitive conclusions about the right ways to carve up the disorders. But the resistance is, I argue, a mistake. We ought to keep the epistemic modesty while insisting that a principal aim of psychiatry is to find the correct ways to carve up disorders, realistically understood.

The mistake I will try to identify is moving from the epistemic claim—we do not know much for sure about how to classify the disorders—to a metaphysical one: there really is no more to the disorders than is revealed by our current diagnostic categories. In physics, a parallel mistake would have been to say, in 1800 or so, "Well, we don't know much about the ways in which atoms are structured, and perhaps we never will," and concluding, "there's no more to the reality about atoms than is revealed by our current tests."

What is really untenable is to try to hold on to the idea of "epistemic iteration" of our diagnostic classifications—broadly, the idea that the development of diagnostic classification should be cumulative—while abandoning a realist picture of what we are aiming to get at with those classifications. Epistemic iteration makes perfect sense if you think of it as a matter of improving our ways of getting onto a structure of disorders "out there." If you have made the mistake of abandoning realism because of modesty about our current level of knowledge, then you have no way of explaining the sense in which one set of diagnostic procedures might be "better" than another. I think that the significance of the mistake is well brought out by Peter Zachar's insightful discussion.

Incidentally, you might be concerned that I am putting questions in terms of "realism" without saying much about what that is. As we will see, the big issues here, as I understand them at any rate, do not actually require any elaborate stage-setting. For present purposes, the central question is whether psychiatric diagnosis should be thought of as aiming to identify a causal structure that implicates the symptoms of a disorder, or if diagnostic procedures have no such interest in identifying particular causal structures.

36.2 Framework assumptions in validation

In his illuminating paper, Zachar is concerned with the assessment of diagnostic classifications, how we determine whether a proposed change to a category in the *Diagnostic and Statistical Manual of Mental Disorders* (DSM) is an improvement. His key point is that any procedure for validating categories must itself depend on "non-empirical" assumptions. The problem is to know what to make of disputes over which non-empirical assumptions to employ.

His example is the argument over the entry on personality disorders in DSM-5. Proponents of the "alternative model" of personality disorders had wanted to transition from thinking in terms of categories and criteria (such as "grandiose sense of self-importance"), which are binary—either one falls into the category or one does not, either one meets the criterion or one does not—to thinking also in terms of dimensions, such as "degree of grandiosity," measures that can be used to place the patient on a scale with many possible values.

The Scientific Review Committee (SRC) wanted to provide a framework for the validation of psychiatric classifications. Rather than a reliance on "expert clinical opinion" there was to be an explicit methodology for determining validity. However, Zachar remarks, much to the "eventual chagrin" of the proponents of the dimensional approach, the SRC framework was "an expansion of the famous Robins and Guze (1970) program for validating *diagnostic categories* [categories being two-valued]. . . ." (section 35.5). Zachar's key point is:

> The irony is that this attempt to alter the culture to establish a more dominant role for scientific considerations ended up clashing with the scientifically minded proponents of dimensional models in the domain of personality disorder. The proponents of dimensional models readily agreed with the SRC that allowing changes to be made based on expert clinical opinion should cease, but according to them expert clinical opinion is what led to diagnostic categories rather than dimensions.

The trouble is that the framework for validation used by the SRC already presupposes that validation must proceed in terms of categories and criteria rather than dimensions. It would, of course, be possible to shift to a framework that proceeds in terms of dimensions. But that shift would not itself be scientifically grounded in terms of either framework.

Zachar makes a similar point about the "Lack of a shared vision on the choice of standards for validating disorder concepts" between proponents of the alternative model and the SRC. The alternative model was intended to satisfy a number of methodological goals, none of which were prioritized by the SRC. (For example, "Eliminate the non-informative diagnosis of 'personality disorder not otherwise specified,'" "Increase the within-category homogeneity of personality disorder constructs. . . .," "Eliminate the perception that there is a discrete threshold between disordered and non-disordered personality," and "Comprehensively model the domain of personality pathology in an empirically based way. . . ."(section 35.6)

Zachar, as I understand him, does not think of this difference as being open to empirical resolution, merely recording "the plurality of scientific and clinical goals that have been articulated in recent years" (p. 12).

Zachar connects his point to a well-known passage from Kendler (1990):

> Validation of a psychiatric disorder cannot, therefore, occur in a vacuum. While empirical data can provide answers, the most important questions to be asked derive from the construct of the psychiatric disorder under consideration. Therefore, one important limitation of a scientific nosology is that it cannot address the validity of a psychiatric disorder where there is disagreement about its proper construct. That is, data can only provide an answer if there is an agreement about what the question is.
>
> This problem may be clarified by an example. Since the publication of DSM-III, there has been an ongoing debate about the proper construct for schizotypal personality disorder. Two positions have been articulated, which may be termed "familial" and "clinical." The familial position defines schizotypal personality disorder as a nonpsychotic schizophrenialike syndrome that occurs commonly in relatives of schizophrenics and uncommonly in other individuals. The most valid criteria for this construct, then, would be those that best discriminate relatives of schizophrenics from relatives of controls.
>
> The clinical construct for schizotypal personality disorder assumes that this syndrome should describe patients seen in the clinic who, despite the absence of classic symptoms of psychosis, nonetheless have substantial schizophrenialike symptoms. While this construct for schizotypal personality disorder less clearly dictates a single key validator, it suggests that one important test for proposed criteria would be their reliability vis-à-vis a "gold standard" clinician with extensive clinical experience in the assessment and treatment of such cases.
>
> Thus, these two constructs for schizotypal personality disorder require two different hierarchies of validators. In fact, the clinical and research literature suggests that the familial and clinical constructs of schizotypal personality disorder do not define the same syndrome. Moreover, empirical data cannot determine which of the two is better, for this decision is essentially a value judgment as to which construct of the disorder is more conceptually appealing (Kendler 1990, p. 970).

The bombshell in this passage is in the last sentence. Zachar (section 35.6) describes the framework assumptions required in determining validation as "non-empirical," while Kendler here describes them as "essentially a value judgment" relating to what is most "conceptually appealing." But if this picture is correct, on which psychiatry requires framework assumptions that cannot themselves be empirically grounded, then the prospects for a scientific psychiatry seem bleak. The use of data and experiment, statistical analysis, and clinical testing seem like distractions from the main point, that the procedures depend on assumptions that are themselves incapable of being established scientifically.

36.3 **Doing without non-empirical framework assumptions**

The idea of a science as depending on framework assumptions that are not themselves empirically testable will be familiar to most philosophers, whether or not they know anything about psychiatry (Carnap 1950). But it is not the only way to analyze the situation, whether in other sciences or in psychiatry (Quine 1953). It is true that in any context of scientific testing, we can make a distinction between the propositions that are being taken for granted in this context and those that are currently up for assessment. But that does not mean that there are any propositions that cannot be established or refuted by empirical methods. There may not be any non-empirical propositions, certainly none with the substance of "personality disorders are best assessed using dimensional terms in diagnosis," or "schizophrenia is fundamentally a genetic disorder" (cf. Zachar and Kendler 2007 for sympathy with this point).

I will look a little further at how you might elaborate the picture of the "non-empirical framework" in the next section. Right now, I want to briefly sketch a well-known alternative picture and how it might apply in psychiatry. Consider the development of models of the electron. In his famous exposition, Hilary Putnam suggested that what is going on as successive models of the electron are developed is this. Out there is a phenomenon, the electron and its various behaviors, that is causally affecting us. That's what Bohr was talking about when he said "electron." Successive models of the electron are attempting to provide ever better descriptions of "that thing," the thing to which we are causally responding in framing those models. Now why should we not have this picture of what is going on in psychiatry, with successive diagnostic procedures for a particular disorder simply being intended to be better and better ways of getting on to "that thing?"

On this view, we should have no need for "non-empirical" framework assumptions in establishing the validity of a diagnostic procedure for a disorder. We may have to make conjectural assumptions that we do not yet know how to test, just as physicists often do, but that is a long way from supposing that those assumptions are inherently "non-empirical" or "subjective." For example, current work on the rate of expansion of the universe depends on the assumptions that the rate of change of distance between the galaxies we can observe is a fair sample of the rate of change of distance between galaxies generally; I do not know how we might establish that, but that is not to say that the assumption is "non-empirical" or "subjective." The correct way to think of it is rather to say that with continued ingenuity we continue to find new ways of determining factual questions that we could not settle before. (For example, further findings about the Big Bang might affect our view as to whether we have a uniform rate of expansion throughout the universe.) Whether personality disorders are best assessed by a dimensional approach, or whether schizophrenia is fundamentally a genetic disorder, seem to be empirical questions, whether or not they can be readily settled by our present techniques.

Realism about psychiatric disorders seems sometimes to be identified with the idea that there is a single latent variable, "depression," or "schizophrenia," that is causally presumed to be causing the principal symptoms. But of course realism as such has no commitment to that kind of essentialist structure. The idea of a disorder as a "homeostatic cluster" of symptoms causally holding one another in place is just as much a realist picture of the disorder as is an essentialist analysis (cf. Kendler et al. 2011, Borsboom and Cramer 2013). And of course, these are only the simplest possible models of the causal structure of a disorder. Variously different causal models of disorders, with latent variables postulated at different locations, are possible (cf. Ahn and Kim 2008). And of course, a hypothesis about the causal structure of a disorder is not non-empirical. Such hypotheses are always in principle testable, and can be expected to have an impact on what method we use to validate a diagnostic procedure for the disorder in question.

36.4 **Operationalism in psychiatry**

Let's look at operationalism, the relevant alternative to realism here. As Bridgman put it, operationalism is the view that "we mean by any concept nothing more than a set of operations; the concept is synonymous with the corresponding set of operations" (Bridgman 1927, p. 5). Applied to intelligence testing, for example, operationalism is the view that all that we mean by "intelligence" is the ability to achieve a particular score on intelligence tests. On this view, it is quite difficult to see what could be meant by saying that one type of intelligence test is "better than," or an improvement upon, another. Each type of test measures what it does perfectly well (namely, the ability to do well on that test). Operationalism is not a particularly convincing account of the aims of intelligence testing. People engaged in intelligence testing have generally taken themselves to be trying to measure some underlying magnitude that also plays a role in many important aspects of people's lives. So it has usually been thought to be possible to make progress in intelligence testing, by filtering out the impact on test scores of, for example, such irrelevant factors as local cultural knowledge, which are thought to be extraneous to the presumed underlying magnitude. Or again, improvement in intelligence testing can be established by showing better correlation between success on the tests and other outcomes, such as professional or educational achievement, that cannot be simply accounted for by factors such as socioeconomic status that are, again, thought to be extraneous to the presumed underlying magnitude.

Of course, you might question whether there is any such underlying magnitude, "g," to be measured. But that is not as yet an endorsement of operationalism. It is, rather, a challenge to the usual concept of intelligence: it accepts that the concept is intended to identify something that is causally responsible for the ability to do well on intelligence tests, but denies that there is any such thing. So the right thing to do would be to throw out the concept, rather than keeping it and giving an operationalist interpretation of it.

Operationalism may seem more attractive for psychiatric disorders than for intelligence testing. No one cares about the ability to do well on intelligence tests for its own sake, so the idea that this is all that the tests are intended to detect has little appeal. But in the case of disorders, the symptoms that are being used in diagnosis are characteristically of great significance in their own right. Given simply that someone has a particular collection of those diagnostic symptoms, before we make any attempt at diagnosis, you might say: "Well, I'm not sure what, specifically, is wrong with this person, but it's quite evident that they need medical help." So there is some kind of initial plausibility here that is entirely lacking in the case of intelligence testing, to the idea that the whole point of the diagnosis is simply to report what symptoms the patient has. And you might push the point by saying, well all we really care about here is making people better. The realist says:

> What matters in diagnosis is identifying the causal structure, implicating the symptoms, that a patient has.

The operationalist sets aside any such concern with causal structures, and may say that all that matters is sorting patients into groups for which this or that treatment will work. Of course, on this approach, the diagnosis of patients may be expected to vary unpredictably over time. Patients which had traditionally been sorted into two separate groups, given two quite different types of treatment, may suddenly find themselves being sorted into the same group as new broad-spectrum drug treatments become available.

On this operationalist approach, you might still try to motivate something that looks like the epistemic iteration found in sciences that do concern themselves with causes and effects. You might argue for an incrementalist approach to change in diagnostic procedures, because of the enormous costs of retraining clinicians. Somewhat similarly, to adapt Kendler's (2012) example, a cartel of fashion houses might decide to go for only incremental changes in fashions, year on year, because of the costs associated with radical changes in fashion. So you could motivate something like incrementalism, without appealing to the idea of some causal structure "out there" that you are trying to get onto.

I cannot help thinking, however, that to go down this line would be to abandon all that we hope for from a scientific psychiatry. A scientific psychiatry ought to be interested in causes and effects. In diagnosing disorders, a scientific psychiatry ought to be trying to identify the causal structures that generate and sustain disorders. To say that "we know so little that we ought to confine ourselves to interpreting talk of disorders operationally" is to abandon this enterprise. It would mean accepting the status of treatments for disorders as potions or spells, that we have found to work by trial and error, but into whose action we expect no insight. That is what it means to resist realism about psychiatric disorders, but I think that once it is made explicit there would be relatively few who would really endorse this.

An operationalist account of disorders would make sense of the idea that there are "non-empirical" assumptions driving the use of one diagnostic procedure rather than another. If the diagnostic procedure is something carried out for its own sake, rather than to establish the presence of a causal structure out there, then differences between those who prefer different diagnostic procedures can only be "subjective," rather than empirically grounded. What I am suggesting is that we ought to throw out this operationalism, and we should accept that methods of validation should themselves be empirically grounded.

36.5 Epistemic iteration or paradigm shift?

Peter Zachar expounds a line of thought in Kenneth Kendler's (2012) work that lists three "barriers to successful [epistemic] iteration" (section 35.3). According to Zachar, this line of thought is consistent with resistance to realism: "Kendler's own position was indefinite between advocating for such a realist vision based on scientific common sense and believing that realist views oversimplify psychiatric phenomena." But I think it is very hard to know what is going on here unless "successful [epistemic] iteration" is explained in terms of convergence on accurate identification of a particular disorder by different diagnostic procedures. To see this, let's look at the three in turn:

1 The modified random walk (section 35.4). "For epistemic iteration a random walk would correspond to a situation where there is no fixed and stable phenomenon to increasingly approximate. There can be change, but change would be non-systematic—often covering the same territory over again." Put like this, the point seems to be that if there is a "fixed and stable" phenomenon out there that our diagnostic criteria are trying to lock on to, then we ought to have incrementalism. If our diagnostic procedures are causally sensitive to the disorder itself then we will find ourselves converging on a way of identifying it.

2 The nosological box canyon (section 35.5). "The diagnostic categories of the old DSM approach are so flawed that they are beyond improvement by gradual iteration. Instead what is needed is a paradigm shift." Notice, though, that the correlative notions of "flawed" and "improvement" here seem simply to presuppose a realist picture of disorders. If we do not have some conception of a disorder as "the causal structure out there that we are trying to detect," then in what sense might our procedures be said to be "flawed," or "beyond improvement?" The very analogy of the "box canyon" suggests there is some destination we would like to get to, from which we are barred by having wound up in this dead end.

3 Wobbly iteration. (section 35.6). "In Chang's formulation of epistemic iteration, scientists propose some standard of evaluation or a criterion for improvement—such as more precise measurement—and iterate toward that goal. Wobbly iteration is what would occur when the criteria/validators shift." Here Zachar seems to be appealing to his picture of shift of validators as a fundamentally non-empirical matter. So "wobbly iteration" is when there are these empirically ungrounded shifts in criteria/validators. Why should this kind of thing be a barrier to successful [epistemic] iteration? Well, so far as I can see, only because the empirically ungrounded nature of the shifts themselves means that they cannot be represented as a matter of us managing to home in, better than we have previously, on the causal structure we are trying to identify.

None of this addresses the details of the dispute over personality disorders that Zachar describes. I have focused instead on two ideas in his discussion: the idea that the difference over validators is non-empirical, and correlatively, the idea that we should hold off from endorsing realism about psychiatric disorders. I think these ideas can seem tempting, but as I have said, the price of embracing them is the abandonment of a scientific psychiatry.

References

Ahn, W-K. and **Kim, N.S.** (2008). Causal theories of mental disorder concepts. *Psychological Science Agenda*, **22**, 3–8.

Borsboom, D. and **Cramer, A.O.J.** (2013). Network analysis: an integrative approach to the structure of psychopathology. *Annual Review of Clinical Psychology*, **9**, 91–121.

Bridgman, P.W. (1927). *The Logic of Modern Physics*. New York: Macmillan.

Carnap, R. (1950). Empiricism, semantics, and ontology. *Revue Internationale de Philosophie*, **4**, 40–50.

Chang, H. (2004). *Inventing Temperature: Measurement and scientific progress*. New York: Oxford University Press.

Kendler, K.S. (1990). Toward a scientific psychiatric nosology. *Archives of General Psychiatry*, **47**, 969–973.

Kendler, K.S. (2012). Epistemic iteration as a historical model for psychiatric nosology: promises and limitations. In K.S. Kendler and J. Parnas (eds.) *Philosophical Issues in Psychiatry II: Nosology*, pp. 305–322. Oxford, UK: Oxford University Press.

Kendler, K.S., **Zachar, P.** and **Craver, C.** (2011). What kinds of things are psychiatric disorders? *Psychological Medicine*, **41**, 1143–1150.

Putnam, H. (1975). Explanation and reference. Chapter 11 in *Mind, Language and Reality*, pp. 196–214. Cambridge, UK: Cambridge University Press.

Quine, W.V.O. (1953). Two dogmas of empiricism. Chapter II in *From a Logical Point of View*, pp. 20–46. Cambridge, MA: Harvard University Press.

Robins, E. and **Guze, S.B.** (1970). Establishment of diagnostic validity in psychiatric illness: its application to schizophrenia. *American Journal of Psychiatry*, **126**, 983–986.

Zachar, P. and **Kendler K S.** (2007). Psychiatric disorders: a conceptual taxonomy. *American Journal of Psychiatry*, **164**, 557–565.

Section 13

The progressive validation of medical and psychiatric disorders

Chapter 37

Introduction to "Progressive validation of psychiatric syndromes: The example of panic disorder"

Josef Parnas

In this chapter Kenneth Kendler continues to articulate his interest in the mechanisms of the progress of science. He examines two phenomena: the concept of the so-called epistemic iteration (see Chapter 29 by Hasok Chang) and Lakatos's classification of research programmes. Epistemic iteration, put in layman's terms, amounts to an ongoing and rigorous improving of (for example) diagnostic criteria by continuous and repetitive empirical studies of such criteria. Kendler's approach in this chapter is historical and he examines diabetes, anxiety disorders, and subtypes of schizophrenia. He tries to determine whether the research programmes in these domains were, in Lakatos's terms, progressive (i.e., yielding increasing useful results) or degenerative (i.e., leading nowhere). Thus the division of diabetes into insulin-sensitive and non-sensitive subtypes was extremely fruitful. The separation of panic disorder from generalized anxiety disorder happened largely on the basis of an initial study by Klein of imipramine response in a sample of different patients. Kendler examines the validity of this separation and finds its validity modest but nonetheless considers this research programme a progressive one. On the contrary multiple validators (e.g., a lack of temporal stability) have not lent support to the subtyping of schizophrenia initially used by Kraepelin and these categories have largely ceased to be used in clinical work. Kendler emphasizes that studying validity must importantly involve a temporal diachronic dimension and not only consist of cross-sectional snapshots.

This introduction is not the place for a discussion of alternative views of scientific progress. However, Kendler's idea of incremental progress based on continuous empirical research is perhaps problematized by the fact that all major psychiatric treatments (convulsive therapy, antipsychotics, antidepressants) were discovered by chance and not as part of a research programme.

Chapter 38

Progressive validation of psychiatric syndromes: The example of panic disorder

Kenneth S. Kendler

38.1 Validation in psychiatric nosology

Validity has been an important concept in the evaluation of psychiatric disorders since the seminal contribution of Robins and Guze (1970). In more recent editions of the *Diagnostic and Statistical Manual of Mental Disorders* (DSM), especially in DSM-5 (American Psychiatric Association 2013), validity has played an increasingly central role in deciding whether to accept or reject proposed changes (Kendler 2013). As implemented by the Scientific Review Committee of DSM-5 and in earlier iterations of DSM, the assessment of validation was essentially synchronic. The relevant data were typically summarized in tables that might list the year of publication, but its historical unfolding was ignored (Kendler 2013).

In this essay, I explore the implications of adding a temporal dimension to the concept of diagnostic validation in psychiatry—that is, considering it in a diachronic fashion. I was prompted to consider this approach by an essay by Hasok Chang in which he recounts the historical developments of key chemical concepts (such as "element" and "acid"), proposing that they improve over time through a process of iteration (Chang 2015). From this I was stimulated to consider the concept of a research programme developed by Imre Lakatos[1] (Lakatos 1970). Lakatos suggested that research programmes can be progressive or degenerative. I suggest that Lakatos's concept be applied to diagnostic concepts in medicine. That is, they also can be progressive or degenerative. "Progressive," for our purposes, can be roughly defined as "continuing to yield new insights into etiology, course

[1] There are many features of Lakatos's theory that I do not consider in this essay. For example, he distinguished between a "hard core" of a research programme and its "protective belt" as well as "positive" and "negative" heuristics. As pointed out by Schaffner and Tabb in the accompanying comment, it is fair to say that I am here taking a rather superficial version of Lakatos's subtle theory—my main focus being only on its diachronic approach to evaluation of success and, in particular, the proposed division between progressive and degenerative programs.

and treatment." I will take up the concept of "degenerative" diagnostic concepts later and more superficially. At the end of the essay, I will comment on the degree to which these historical changes might reflect the iterative process articulated by Chang.

38.2 Type 1 and type 2 diabetes mellitus

I start with a paradigmatic example from general medicine of a progressive diagnostic concept: the division of diabetes mellitus (DM) into two main subtypes of type 1 (juvenile onset or insulin dependent) and type 2 (adult-onset or insulin resistant). As a syndrome characterized by excess urination and loss of weight, what we now call DM is described in ancient Egyptian texts from around 1500 BCE. The term "mellitus," reflecting the fact that the urine of those affected had a sweet taste, was first used by the Greek physician Aretaeus (*c.*80 to 138 CE). Flies were attracted to this urine and physicians used to make the diagnosis by tasting the urine (hence early physicians were sometimes called "piss-prophets").

Early historical descriptions of DM were nearly all of what we would now call type 1. No effective treatment was known and its presentation was dramatic. DM was uniformly fatal within weeks to months after its diagnosis. Patients would literally melt away and die in ketoacidosis. The seminal event in the history of DM was the isolation and purification of insulin, and its first administration as a life-saving treatment for DM by the Canadians Frederick Banting and Charles Herbert Best in 1921–1922.

For our story, however, the breakthrough came in a 1936 article published in the *Lancet* by Himsworth, entitled "Diabetes mellitus: Its differentiation into insulin-sensitive and insulin-insensitive types"(Himsworth 1936/2013). Himsworth used a simple procedure on patients with DM. After an overnight fast, the patients received a standardized dose of intravenous insulin and then were given orally a glucose containing drink. Himsworth begins his results section as follows:

> The work had not proceeded far before it became clear that by means of this test, diabetics can be differentiated into two types: those in whom the injected insulin produces an immediate suppression of the hyperglycæmia [elevated blood sugar] which normally follows ingestion of glucose alone; and those in whom the insulin has little or no effect in suppressing this hyperglycæmia (Himsworth 2013, pp. 1594–1595).

No p values or standard errors were presented—just the results of four patients in two figures. The first is seen in Figure 38.1. Patient I—a 60-year-old woman on low-dose insulin—showed substantial insulin resistance. One of insulin's main jobs is to help transport glucose into cells from the blood. In this patient, however, the blood sugar rises markedly despite the pretreatment with insulin that should have allowed the cells to take up the glucose. Patient II—a 21-year-old woman on a much higher dose of insulin—shows the more normal curve in which insulin prevents the rise of blood glucose by increasing the uptake of glucose into cells.

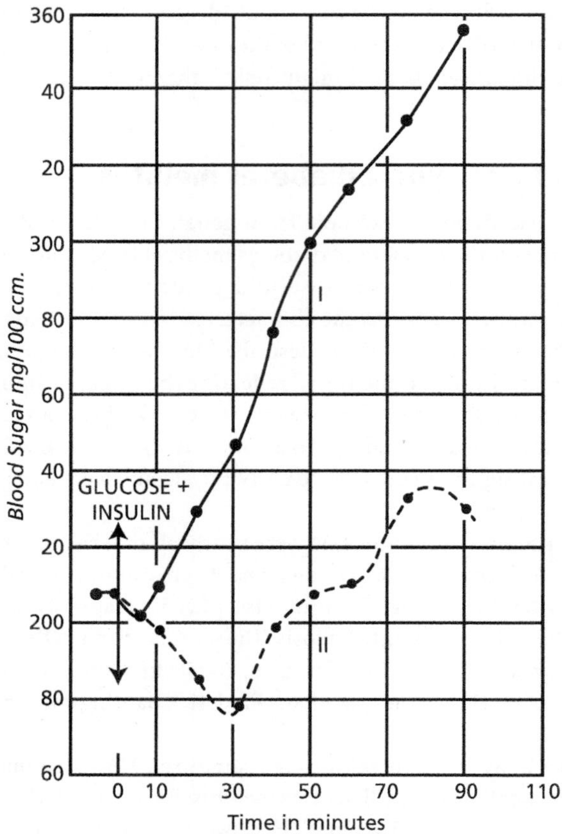

Figure 38.1 *Simultaneous glucose and insulin test.* Capillary blood-sugar curves. *Patient 1*—Insulin-insensitive. Women, aged 60, on a diet of 1500 calories containing carbohydrate 150 g, protein 80 g, fat 66 g, and 35 units of insulin daily. Passing small amounts of sugar. Received 7.3 units of insulin intravenously aged 43.8 g of glucose orally. Fasting blood-sugar 208 mg/100 ccm. *Patient 2—Insulin-sensitive.* Woman, aged 21, on a diet of 2000 calories containing carbohydrate 208 g, protein 80 g, fat 94 g, and 95 units of insulin daily. Sugar-free. No hypoglycæmic attacks. Received 7 units of insulin intravenously and 41 g of glucose orally. Fasting blood-sugar 244 mg/100 ccm. The curves have been charted so as to start at the same resting blood-sugar level.

Reprinted from *The Lancet*, 227 (5864), H.P. Himsworth, Diabetes Mellitus: Its differentiation into insulin-sensitive and insulin-insensitive types, pp. 127–30, Copyright(1936), with permission from Elsevier.

In a lovely section on "clinical observations," Himsworth makes cogent connections, subsequently confirmed, between the clinical features of diabetic patients and the two types he has observed in his small study. He writes:

> A general relationship appears to exist between the type of onset of the disease and the type of diabetes. The onset of insulin-sensitive patients is as a rule acute; the onset in

> insulin-insensitive patients is insidious . . . The insulin-insensitive type is more common in but not confined to the elderly, whilst the insulin-sensitive type is commoner in the young (Himsworth 1936/2013, pp. 1596–1597).

He then makes the prescient prediction:

> As diabetes mellitus becomes more frequent with increasing age it would appear probable—and my experience so far supports this deduction—that the commonest type of diabetes mellitus will eventually prove to be that which is not essentially due to insulin deficiency (Himsworth 2013, p. 1597).

In the United States and Europe, around 90% of the cases of DM are now type 2.

Himsworth's division has proven over time to be scientifically and clinically quite fertile. I review here only a tiny fraction of the relevant literature. For a recent summary of the now established differences between these two subtypes of diabetes see Table 38.1. Family studies have shown that these two forms of DM largely assort independently in families (Cheta et al. 1990). Treatment of the two forms of DM are now entirely different. Insulin is almost always needed for type 1 DM. By contrast, first line treatment for type 2 DM is weight loss (which is entirely ineffective for type 1 DM), followed by a range of oral hypoglycemic agents and then insulin as a last resort.

Understanding of etiology has shown that these disorders are fundamentally distinct. Autoimmune processes are critical in the large majority of cases of type 1 diabetes where antibodies destroy the beta cells of the islets of Langerhans—the insulin-producing cells of the pancreas. This usually occurs in childhood or adolescence. Sensitivity and responsiveness to insulin are usually normal in these cases. By contrast, type 2 diabetes is associated with resistance in key cells to the effects of insulin—that is, to increase uptake of glucose. Type 2 diabetes is now understood to be closely related to obesity and to the so-called metabolic syndrome.

Table 38.1 Recognized key features of type 1 and type 2 diabetes circa 2015

	Type 1 diabetes	**Type 2 diabetes**
Etiology	Autoimmune	Peripheral insulin resistance
Age of onset	Younger	Older
Obesity	Rare	Common
Family history	Rare	Common
HLA association / genetic association	Yes	No
Ketosis	Yes	No
Insulin resistance	No	Yes
Adequate levels of the body's own insulin	No	Yes
Responds to oral agents	No	Yes

Adapted from Ananya Mandal, Diabetes Pathophysiology, *News Medical: Life Sciences and Medicine*, December 2015, Copyright 2000–2016, AZoM.com Limited.

Other subtypes of DM are now known, albeit relatively rare. For example, latent autoimmune diabetes of adults is a condition in which type 1 DM develops in adults. DM can arise in alcoholics who destroy their insulin-producing cells through repeated bouts of inflammation of the pancreas due to the direct effects of alcohol.

As an example of a "difference that keeps on giving," we can look at a key 2007 paper demonstrating definitively the viability of the method of genome-wide association studies applied to common complex biomedical disorders (Wellcome Trust Case Control Consortium 2009). Types 1 and 2 DM were among the seven disorders studied. Five significant findings were observed for type 1 DM and three for type 2 DM. None were overlapping. Consistent with prior studies, a very strong signal was found in the HLA region for type 1 DM (suggested by the known role of autoimmunity in the etiology of type 1 DM). No signal in that region emerged from type 2 DM. In molecular genetic studies of type 2 DM, genes that impact on obesity emerge as risk factors. These are not seen for type 1 DM.

38.3 **Panic disorder**

> The current (fashionable) view that "crises of anxiety" ("panic disorder") constitute a separate disease is very new. Since the 1900s, such attacks have been considered as part of the anxiety neurosis; before then they were associated with conditions such as neurasthenia and psychasthenia, and even before considered to be cardiovascular or inner ear disorders (Berrios 1996, p. 264).

German Berrios, in this quote, succinctly summarizes the early history of what we now call panic disorder (PD). We focus here on its modern history which begins in 1962 with a seminal paper by Donald Klein entitled, "Psychiatric reaction patterns to imipramine" (Klein and Fink 1962). The introduction includes the following:

> In this report various patterns of behavioral response to imipramine are described; and the relationship to such factors as age, sex, pretreatment behavioral pattern, hospital diagnosis, and hospital discharge evaluation are assessed (Klein and Fink 1962, p. 432).

Working at Hillside Hospital on Long Island, New York, Klein was able to administer recently developed medications—in this case the classic tricyclic antidepressant imipramine—to a wide variety of patients. In this paper, he describes the responses of 180 patients treated between October 1958 and July 1961. They had a range of diagnoses, with 67 having some form of a mood disorder and 102 schizophrenia.

Klein observed six behavioral responses to imipramine among these patients (and a category of "non-response"). We are interested in his fourth category, "Reduction episodic anxiety" which was met by 14 patients. He describes the "before treatment" features of these patients as follows:

> Typically, subjects noted the sudden onset of inexplicable "panic" attacks, accompanied by rapid breathing, palpitations, weakness, and a feeling of impending death. Their activities became progressively constricted, until they were no longer able to travel alone for fear of being suddenly rendered helpless while isolated from help. . . .

They engaged in prolonged outpatient psychotherapy, usually devoted to the exploration of unconscious sexual and aggressive impulses, with the interpretation of the phobically barred areas as situations of forbidden symbolic temptation (Klein and Fink 1962, pp. 435–436).

He then describes the development "with treatment":

Under imipramine treatment the "panic" attacks ceased, although both phenothiazines [first-generation antipsychotic drugs including chlorpromazine or thorazine] and sedatives had been previously ineffective. However, the patients were reluctant to change their phobic behavior pattern and required much persuasion, direction and support. Their social interaction increased markedly . . . (Klein and Fink 1962, p. 436).

He then makes the following comments which presage his later claim for "pharmacologic dissection":

The reaction to imipramine is of considerable interest since the "anxiety" of the panic attack is sharply diminished while expectant "anxiety" related to the "phobic" patterns remains. The use of the common term "anxiety" may thus obscure an underlying difference in these processes. (Klein and Fink 1962, p. 436).

In a follow-up paper, Klein (1964) described a small double-blind controlled study showing that imipramine produced significantly greater symptom improvement in this group of "phobic-anxious" patients than placebo. Klein concludes that article as follows:

The use of patterns of drug response as dissecting tools . . . within psychiatric subpopulations is emphasized.

At the time Klein was doing this work, the official psychiatric nosologic system in the United States was DSM-I which defined "anxiety reaction" as follows (American Psychiatric Association 1952):

In this kind of reaction the anxiety is diffuse and not restricted to definite situations or objects, as in the case of phobic reactions. It is not controlled by any specific psychological defense mechanism as in other psychoneurotic reactions. This reaction is characterized by anxious expectation and frequently associated with somatic symptomatology.

This provides little symptomatic detail although the use of the word "diffuse" does not well describe the panic-like syndromes that Klein had been studying. In 1968, DSM-II was published with the following definition of anxiety neurosis (300.0) (American Psychiatric Association 1968):

This neurosis is characterized by anxious over-concern extending to panic and frequently associated with somatic symptoms. Unlike Phobic neurosis (q.v.), anxiety may occur under any circumstances and is not restricted to specific situations or objects. This disorder must be distinguished from normal apprehension or fear, which occurs in realistically dangerous situations.

Again, details are scant but the broad diagnosis seems to cover syndromes characterized by "anxious over-concern" as well as "panic."

38.4 Brief nosologic history of panic disorder after DSM-II

In the 1970s, Klein emerged as a prominent first-generation psychopharmacologist in the United States. He was the co-author of an influential early textbook (*Diagnosis and Drug Treatment in Psychiatric Disorders*), published in 1969, that became something of a bible for the early neo-Kraepelinians in the United States (Klein 1969). He was on the faculty of Columbia University, then as now one of the leading departments of psychiatry. Bob Spitzer—who led the development of DSM-III (Decker 2013)—was also at Columbia. Don Klein was one of the 14 members of the Task Force led by Bob Spitzer that produced DSM-III (American Psychiatric Association 1980).

Klein told me (interview 7/23/15) that when he proposed the addition of PD to the DSM-III Task Force, Bob Spitzer was strongly in favor of the proposal. The supporting literature—much of it produced by Klein and his colleagues—was well known to the members of the committee, he said. No reports or summaries were required as there was a general consensus that this was a valid disorder.

But there was a problem. What should be done with the anxiety neurosis patients from DSM-II who did not meet criteria for PD? It was from this discussion again by consensus that the concept of "generalized anxiety disorder" (GAD) emerged as a new DSM category. Klein recalls that the term "generalized" referred mainly to its temporal dimension. While PD was characterized by brief episodes of severe anxiety or terror (i.e., panic), anxiety in GAD was chronic and present most of the time—hence "generalized." Having PD accepted in DSM-III substantially influenced its credibility in the field and further helped propel research. This also permitted pharmaceutical companies to develop medications specifically for PD. For example, there are now two benzodiazepines (alprazolam and clonazepam) and four serotonin-specific reuptake inhibitors (SSRIs) (fluoxetine, paroxetine, sertraline, and venlafaxine) that have won Food and Drug Authority (FDA) approval as treatments for PD in the United States.

Detailed operationalized criteria were provided for PD and GAD in DSM-III. Here are brief summaries of the conditions provided. For PD, the DSM-III introduction reads:

> The essential features are recurrent panic (anxiety) attacks that occur at times unpredictably. . . . The panic attacks are manifested by the sudden onset of intense apprehension, fear or terror, often associated with feelings of impending doom . . .. Attacks usually last minutes, more rarely hours (American Psychiatric Association 1980, p. 230).

For GAD, DSM states:

> The essential feature is generalized persistent anxiety of at least one month's duration. . . . Although the specific manifestations of the anxiety vary from individual to individual, generally there are signs of motor tension, autonomic hyperactivity, apprehensive expectation and vigilance and scanning (American Psychiatric Association 1980, p. 232).

So, we now turn to the question of whether the distinction between PD and non-panic anxiety neurosis (later GAD) (and more broadly non-panic anxiety disorders) proved generative.

38.5 **Precipitants**

In a series of studies published over the last 50 years, a variety of precipitants have been identified that produced panic attacks in high proportions of individuals with PD. This is a large and complex literature that I can only survey briefly. I have tried to be representative in the studies reviewed. For us, the critical question is whether the PD versus GAD split (or less specifically the PD versus "other anxiety disorders" split) was "validated" by these studies.

The first of these precipitants studied was lactate. In 1967, Pitts and McClure described the infusion of lactate versus glucose into individuals with "anxiety neurosis" and controls (Pitts and McClure 1967). Thirteen of fourteen of the patients and two of the ten controls developed "anxiety attacks" after lactate infusion.

Rapee (1986) found that PD patients, compared to those with GAD, had a markedly greater distress and number of anxiety symptoms in response to voluntary hyperventilation. In an early review (1990) of the diagnostic utility of lactate in PD, the authors conclude:

> Analysis of lactate infusion studies to date suggests that patients with panic attacks are significantly more sensitive to lactate than are healthy controls or patients with other psychiatric disorders without panic attacks. However, the usefulness of lactate infusion is limited by the lack of standardized, objective criteria for lactate-induced panic and uncertainty as to the sensitivity and specificity of the test for current, clinically significant panic attacks (Cowley and Arana 1990, p. 277).

In 1992, Rapee and colleagues gave 5.5% CO_2 to 198 patients with anxiety disorders and 25 controls (Rapee et al. 1992). Using a liberal definition of a panic attack, the CO_2 produced attacks in 65% of patients with PD, 33% of patients with GAD, and 12% of controls. These differences were statistically significant. In 1995, Verburg et al. gave a much higher dose (35% CO_2) to patients with PD and GAD (Verburg et al. 1995). Their results were somewhat more mixed:

> Patients with panic disorder experienced a significantly stronger increase in subjective anxiety than patients with generalized anxiety disorder. However, increases in panic symptom scores were high in both groups.

In 2001, Kent et al. (including Klein as an author) studied the specificity of the panic response to 5–7% CO_2 inhalation in PD in comparison to major depression and premenstrual dysphoric disorder (Kent et al. 2001). They replicated the higher rate of panic attacks in the PD patients versus controls or those with depression. However, rates of panic attacks were also clearly elevated in those with premenstrual dysphoric disorder.

The cholecystokinin tetrapeptide (CCK) is also a relatively well studied "panicogen" in PD patients (Bradwejn and Koszycki 1994). However, in one small study, a CCK receptor agonist induced panic attacks in a high proportion of patients with

GAD similar to prior studies with PD patients (Brawman-Mintzer et al. 1997). The authors conclude:

> This suggests that individuals with generalized anxiety disorder may be similar to those with panic disorder with respect to enhanced sensitivity to the CCK-B receptor agonist challenge (Brawman-Mintzer et al. 1997, p. 702).

After reviewing this literature for some hours without much increasing clarity, I consulted with an expert who knows this research area very well. I asked, "How specific to PD versus other anxiety disorders are these various precipitating factors, especially lactate and CO_2?" The response was that while there are clearly "hints" in individual studies, the overall support is not as strong as one would expect based on Klein's theories.

38.6 Family and genetic data

In an early family study, Crowe et al found strong evidence that PD aggregated in first-degree relatives of PD probands (17%) versus controls (1.8%) (Crowe et al. 1983). More importantly for our purposes, the rates of GAD in the two groups of relatives did not differ significantly: 4.8 versus 3.6%, respectively. Mendlewicz et al. (1993) studied first-degree relatives of patients with PD and GAD. The risk for PD in relatives of PD, GAD, and control probands were, respectively, 13.2, 3.3, and 0.9%. The risks for GAD in these three groups of relatives were, respectively, 4.0, 8.9, and 1.9%. A substantial degree of familial specificity was seen.

In an early small sample twin study of anxiety disorders, Skre et al. (1993) found moderate specificity within twin pairs. In particular, PD was more common in cotwins of twins with PD (8/30 = 27%) than in cotwins of twins with GAD (0/12 = 0%). Pure GAD was more common in cotwins of twins with pure GAD (4/12 = 33%) than of PD (3/30 = 10%).

In by far the largest twin study of GAD and PD (n = 4938), Hettema et al. (2005) used structural equation modeling as applied to six anxiety disorders (GAD, PD, and four phobia subtypes). Their results were not consistent with the earlier family and twin studies as they demonstrated a substantial sharing of genetic risk factors for PD and GAD. These results were replicated in a large multivariate twin study from Norway where both PD and GAD loaded strongly on the same genetic factor for "axis I internalizing disorders" (Kendler et al. 2011).

38.7 Treatment

Focusing first on pharmacologic treatments (Ravindran and Stein 2010), a large body of evidence shows that tricyclic antidepressants (TCAs), especially imipramine, the agent first used by Klein, are effective for the treatment of PD. The evidence that TCAs are effective for GAD is much poorer but has been less well studied. The clinical consensus in these early years was that imipramine was much more effective for PD than for GAD.

SSRIs have been quite well studied in PD and all six major agents have been shown to be effective, with four being approved by the FDA. Of the serotonin and norepinephrine reuptake inhibitors (SNRIs), several are used clinically and one—venlafaxine—has been FDA approved for PD. SSRIs are also commonly used for GAD with two being approved by the FDA (paroxetine and escitalopram) and two of the SNRIs: duloxetine and venlafaxine. So the treatment specificity from the perspective of antidepressant treatment has decreased as the broader-spectrum SSRIs and SNRIs have replaced TCAs as the main line of treatment.

The benzodiazepines were, for many years, the mainstay of treatment for GAD when imipramine was the treatment of choice for PD. However, in recent decades the higher-potency benzodiazepines have been shown to be as effective as TCA or SSRIs in treatment of PDs (although with greater concerns about tolerance/addiction). There is good evidence for the efficacy of benzodiazepines for GAD but they are less frequently used long-term because of concerns about dependence.

Turning to psychotherapy, I will here focus on cognitive behavioral therapy (CBT) which has been the most studied form of psychotherapy. For PD, CBT has proved to be effective (Haby et al. 2006) and one of the popular methods, developed and manualized by Barlow's group at Boston University, combines interoceptive exposure, cognitive restructuring, and breathing retraining (Barlow et al. 2000). Here is a description of a similar approach:

> Treatment began with educational information and cognitive restructuring to address misappraisals of panic attacks and associated bodily sensations. Breathing retraining was taught as a coping technique especially for symptoms associated with overbreathing. During interoceptive exposure, participants repeatedly induced physical sensations associated with panic attacks (e.g., spinning, hyperventilating) to weaken conditioned emotional reactions and obtain corrective information designed to disconfirm `fearful misappraisals. Interoceptive exercises were extended to naturalistic activities that induced feared bodily sensations (e.g., sports, caffeine) and were incorporated into structured in vivo exposure. . . . (Craske et al. 2007, p. 1099).

CBT treatments have also been developed for GAD and shown to be effective (Covin et al. 2008). Here, however, the focus of the treatment is quite different. Two leading models are the "cognitive avoidance model" and the "intolerance of uncertainty" model. Both approaches focus on the key GAD symptom of the maintenance of worry. Here is a description of the second of these models:

> . . ., their conceptual model centers around the idea that individuals with GAD are much more intolerant of the uncertainty inherent in life . . . Intolerance of uncertainty is currently conceptualized as a dispositional characteristic that results from a set of negative beliefs about uncertainty and its implication . . . A unique element of this treatment is that clients are taught to separate their worry into two categories: those that are amenable to problem-solving and those that are not. The therapist helps the client to implement problem-solving strategies for the problems that can be changed, and worry exposure is used for those issues that the client cannot exert control over (Covin et al. 2008, p. 109).

A 2005 meta-analysis shows identical effect sizes for CBT trials for PD and GAD (0.64) (Haby et al. 2006). So for CBT, we have different methods developed for the treatment of PD versus GAD—focusing on the different key symptoms (panic versus worry)—but broadly similar efficacy.

38.8 Prediction by separation anxiety

From Klein's earliest work, it was noted that individuals who developed PD often had a developmental history of separation problems as a child. We are fortunate to have a recent meta-analysis of the large accumulated literature on the question of the association between a diagnosis of separation anxiety disorder and subsequent risk for PD and for "any" anxiety disorder (Kossowsky et al. 2013). Analysis of 25 studies showed aggregate odds ratios (ORs) for separation anxiety disorder and PD of 3.45 (95% CIs 2.37–5.03). Five studies examined the association between separation anxiety disorder and any anxiety disorder (three of which included PD). The aggregate OR for these studies was 2.19 (1.40–3.42). Given that this figure is likely biased upward by the inclusion of panic cases, this provides some evidence for the specificity of the association of separation anxiety and PD.

38.9 Imaging

This is a complex literature and space here is limited. fMRI findings in GAD have largely shown prefrontal cortex and anterior cingulate cortex hypofunction and deficient top-down control of subcortical centers during emotion regulation tasks (Mochcovitch et al. 2014). By contrast, the focus of much imaging work in PD has been on enhanced amygdala function with some evidence for enhanced threat responding in other areas such as the insula (D. Pine, personal written communication, 7/21/2015). So there is some evidence of distinct neural substrates to these two syndromes. But, this is of limited value in the absence of high-quality studies directly comparing patients from the two diagnostic groups.

38.10 Panic disorder as a progressive research programme

How well does the development of PD fit our picture of a progressive research programme? Our brief survey suggested that over time, the distinction between type 1 and type 2 DM has been repeatedly validated by advances in genetics, pathophysiology, clinical course, and treatment. For the PD–GAD distinction, the results are somewhat less clear cut. Since the distinction was first proposed by Klein in 1962 and made "official" by DSM-III in 1980, across a range of potential validators, PD was sometimes, but not always, shown to meaningfully differ from GAD. Observed differences were not always crisp. Across precipitants, genetic studies, and association with separation anxiety, the distinction between PD and GAD was evident but not complete. CBT treatments are effective for both conditions but with different foci of therapy. Imipramine might have been a specific treatment for PD but it does not appear to be the case for the SSRIs or SNRIs. Research into the neural substrates suggests some difference but definitive research is currently lacking.

Type 1 and type 2 DM are probably, at their root, etiologically distinct disorders that happened to share one common (albeit critical) symptom of excess sweet urine. Not unexpectedly, the etiologic nature of the psychiatric disorders of PD and GAD are far more difficult to pin down. My current educated guess is that they are partially separable syndromes but have shown shared etiological factors, being part of a broad spectrum of internalizing psychiatric disorders.

The generativity of the PD–GAD split might be most clearly seen in the development of different styles of CBT, in the research providing support for the stronger association of PD with childhood separation anxiety, and the preliminary evidence for different fMRI findings.

One interesting wrinkle in the PD–GAD story deserves brief comment. First-generation antidepressants may have been more selective anti-panic agents than second-generation antidepressants, with a broader spectrum of action, that successfully treat both PD and GAD. Does this mean that the validity of the PD–GAD distinction (at least with respect to treatment) has therefore declined over time? I am not so sure. Imagine we have two pathogenic bacteria which both produce bladder infections. Two quite different classes of antibiotics are developed which specifically only treat one infection or the other. Then a broad-spectrum antibiotic is discovered that treats both. What is more important for "validation" by treatment for different disorders—the current status of treatment or the prior evidence that agents could be developed that are specific for treating one disorder versus the other? I would lean toward the latter position, suggesting that the existence of classes of medications that have clearly different responses in PD versus GAD continue to provide evidence for the validity of the difference and hence the generativity of the distinction. But one could argue the other side.

38.11 **Subtypes of schizophrenia as a degenerative diagnostic system**

Lakatos also articulated a different potential fate for research programmes—degeneration. Such programs stopped generating new empirically testable (and at least sometimes verified) hypotheses. The participants tended to adopted a defensive posture and "circle the wagons around" to defend their enshrined beliefs or "hard core" assumptions underlying their paradigm, to use Lakatos's phrase.

Let me provide one potential psychiatric example of such a "program." When Kraepelin—the architect of our current psychiatric diagnostic system for psychotic disorders—first fully articulated his concept of dementia praecox (later renamed schizophrenia by Bleuler), he proposed three subtypes: hebephrenic, catatonic, and paranoid (Kraepelin 1902/1990). He provided rich clinical descriptions of these subtypes. They have been taught to generations of psychiatrists and medical students and have been the subject for many an exam question.

In recognition of their critical heritage, they were contained in every edition of DSM from the first up through the fourth. But systematic research with these subtypes, starting in the 1980s, began to run into problems. Follow-up studies revealed that the stability of the subtypes over time, while significant, was quite modest (Kendler et al. 1985). Family studies—critical validators for psychiatric illness—found little to no difference in the patterns of illness in the families of the different subtypes of schizophrenia (Kendler et al. 1988, 1994). A number of studies appeared suggesting that catatonia was not specific to schizophrenia (Braff et al. 2013). Interest in the field shifted to deficit or negative symptom schizophrenia which did not map well onto the subtypes (Crow 1980, Andreasen and Olsen 1982, Carpenter et al. 1988). Furthermore, subtypes were not helpful in predicting treatment.

Then in 2013, Braff et al. published a paper entitled, "Lack of use in the literature from the last 20 years supports dropping traditional schizophrenia subtypes from DSM-5 and ICD-11" (Braff et al. 2013). The senior author—Carpenter—was the chair of the DSM-5 Psychotic Disorders Work Group. This paper reviewed the empirical limitations emerging from the literature on schizophrenia subtypes and then did something novel—looked at the use of these subtypes in the schizophrenia literature. They found:

> A review of published articles reveals over the last 20 years (1990, 2000, 2010) the use of traditional subtypes in the [schizophrenia] literature has fallen from 27.7% to 9.8% to 6.5% (Braff et al. 2013, p. 751).

On the basis of these lines of evidence, the paper ends with this conclusion:

> Dropping subtypes in DSM-5 and ICD-11 schizophrenia classification is justified by the lack of stability, validity, heterogeneity reduction, and practical utility in the scientific literature (Braff et al. 2013, p. 753)

If we were to describe a degenerative diagnostic paradigm, would the traditional subtypes of schizophrenia provide a working model? While infused with clinical tradition, as psychiatric research geared up in the 1980s, these subtypes did not behave very well empirically. They did not provide the basis of meaningful differences that were beginning to be seen with other approaches to subdividing the schizophrenia syndrome. Their defenders were forced back onto the claim of clinical tradition. The DSM-5 Psychotic Disorders Work Group did not find the arguments of the defenders of these subtypes convincing and eliminated them from DSM-5.

38.12 **Iteration**

Where is the iteration in all this? In his essay on chemical constructs (Chang 2015), Chang suggests that they kept getting better over time. In this essay, I have focused more on whether the original dichotomies (type 1 versus type 2 DM, and PD versus GAD) were fruitful distinctions. It turns out that the diagnostic criteria for GAD changed quite a bit over the time period of this inquiry. In DSM-III, it required a minimum of 1 month duration with at least one symptom from three of four categories (motor tension, autonomic hyperactivity, apprehensive expectation, and vigilance and scanning) (American Psychiatric Association 1980). In DSM-III-R, 6 months were required, a greater focus on "excess anxiety and worry" was added, and at least 6 of 18 symptoms were required (American Psychiatric Association

1987). DSM-IV and DSM-5 markedly reduced the number of symptoms, now requiring at least 3 of 6 symptoms and everyone had to "find it difficult to control the worry" (American Psychiatric Association 1994, 2013). Some of these efforts were motivated by clarifying the differences between GAD and PD, and reducing the overlap of GAD and major depression.

Theoretically, we could examine whether these changes in GAD made it a better category and, in particular, made it more clearly different from PD in ways that were scientifically fertile. I am not optimistic that we yet have the data to address this question with confidence.

This brings us back to epistemic iteration as a possible model for psychiatric nosologic change. As I have written elsewhere (Kendler 2009, 2012), one fruitful way to articulate the goals of revisions of psychiatric nosology (as done by the DSM and ICD systems) is within the framework of epistemic iteration as articulated by Chang (2004). From this perspective, our task is to require any changes to improve the validity of the disorder and so develop a "spiral of improvement" for psychiatric nosology.

It is easy to see in general outline how the focus of this essay—progressive validation—could be integrated with the epistemic iteration. This might be clearest in an example. Assume a broad psychiatric category A was divided on the basis of preliminary validity studies into two disorders B and C. One way to increase the likelihood of a path of progressive validation of this distinction would be to permit this division to be re-examined at each subsequent iteration of the diagnostic manual. Are there ways in which the diagnostic criteria of disorders B and C could be improved to reduce overlap and generate further insights into their etiology and treatment? Although further conceptual development is needed, we can see important ways in which progressive validation and epistemic iteration are related and help provide fruitful ways to conceptualize the goals of psychiatric nosology.

38.13 **Conclusions**

What have we gained in our view of the validity of psychiatric disorders by taking a temporal perspective, as advocated by Lakatos and Chang? Prior validation approaches as used in DSM-IV and, especially, DSM-5 have been synchronic—snapshots of results typically taken out of temporal context. To paraphrase this approach, we might say, "A disorder is valid if it performs well on key validator categories with good studies from a range of research groups."

A diachronic approach looks at the question somewhat differently. Here we might say that a diagnostic concept is valid when a line of inquiry which employs it is successful in continuously producing new knowledge and is, in Lakatos's framework, generative. As Chang writes from an historical review of key chemical constructs, "A classificatory concept that keeps playing an obviously non-idle role in various successful systems of practice will gain increasing credence" (Chang 2015). The flip side of this is obvious. An invalid diagnosis is one that fails to provide new useful information. Arguing for its validity then becomes a defensive exercise based on tradition. That closely resembles Lakatos's idea of a degenerative paradigm.

One obvious place where the diachronic and synchronic approach might differ is the situation of a disorder that has been well researched and performed well in various tests of its validity but for whatever reasons, the research field has moved on and is not examining it much. This happens (I suspect) more in psychiatry than some of the harder sciences where diagnoses can move into and out of fashion. From a synchronic perspective, the diagnosis looks valid—tables of validators look good, etc. But would we conclude from a diachronic perspective that it is no longer generative?

What about a disorder that was well validated by older kinds of methods (e.g., family history, twin studies, personality) but then a few studies emerge using newer methods (molecular genetics or fMRI) where the diagnosis does not perform well. Here the synchronic method would probably still look pretty good, especially if the older validating studies substantially outnumbered the new studies. However, the diachronic method would weight the more recent studies more strongly and might conclude a real loss of validity. Which perspective is likely better?

I do not think there are any easy answers to this question. But I do think, standing on the shoulders of Lakatos and Chang, considering a diachronic or historical view of validity of psychiatric disorders adds a valuable perspective to our discipline and its nosology. Further conceptual and empirical efforts will be needed to determine the value to psychiatry of a diachronic approach to diagnostic validation.

References

American Psychiatric Association. (1952). *Diagnostic and Statistical Manual of Mental Disorders*, 1st edn. Washington, DC: American Psychiatric Association.

American Psychiatric Association. (1968). *Diagnostic and Statistical Manual of Mental Disorders*, 2nd edn. Washington, DC: American Psychiatric Association.

American Psychiatric Association. (1980). *Diagnostic and Statistical Manual of Mental Disorders, Third Edition* Washington, DC, American Psychiatric Association.

American Psychiatric Association, (1987). *Diagnostic and Statistical Manual of Mental Disorders*, rev. 3rd edn. Washington, DC: American Psychiatric Association.

American Psychiatric Association. (1994). *Diagnostic and Statistical Manual of Mental Disorders*, 4th edn. Washington, DC: American Psychiatric Association.

American Psychiatric Association. (2013). *Diagnostic and Statistical Manual of Mental Disorders*, 5th edn. Washington, DC: American Psychiatric Association.

Andreasen, N.C. and **Olsen, S.** (1982). Negative v positive schizophrenia. Definition and validation. *Archives of General Psychiatry*, **39**, 789–794.

Barlow, D.H., Gorman, J.M., Shear, M.K., and **Woods, S.W.** (2000). Cognitive-behavioral therapy, imipramine, or their combination for panic disorder: A randomized controlled trial. *JAMA*, **283**, 2529–2536.

Berrios, G.E. (1996). *The History of Mental Symptoms: Descriptive psychopathology since the nineteenth century.* New York: Cambridge University Press.

Bradwejn, J. and **Koszycki, D.** (1994). The cholecystokinin hypothesis of anxiety and panic disorder. *Annals of the New York Academy of Sciences*, **713**, 273–282.

Braff, D.L., Ryan, J., Rissling, A.J., and **Carpenter, W.T.** (2013). Lack of use in the literature from the last 20 years supports dropping traditional schizophrenia subtypes from DSM-5 and ICD-11. *Schizophrenia Bulletin*, **39**, 751–753.

Brawman-Mintzer, O., Lydiard, R.B., Bradwejn, J., et al. (1997). Effects of the cholecystokinin agonist pentagastrin in patients with generalized anxiety disorder. *American Journal of Psychiatry*, **154**, 700–702.

Carpenter, W.T., Jr., **Heinrichs, D.W.**, and **Wagman, A.M.** (1988). Deficit and nondeficit forms of schizophrenia: the concept. *American Journal of Psychiatry*, **145**, 578–583.

Chang, H. (2004). *Inventing Temperature: Measurement and scientific progress.* New York: Oxford University Press.

Chang, H. (2015). The rising of chemical natural kinds through epistemic iteration. Unpublished.

Cheta, D., Dumitrescu, C., Georgescu, M., et al. (1990). A study on the types of diabetes mellitus in first degree relatives of diabetic patients. *Diabète Métabolisme*, **16**, 11–15.

Covin, R., Ouimet, A.J., Seeds, P.M., and **Dozois, D.J.** (2008). A meta-analysis of CBT for pathological worry among clients with GAD. *Journal of Anxiety Disorders*, **22**, 108–116.

Cowley, D.S. and **Arana, G.W.** (1990). The diagnostic utility of lactate sensitivity in panic disorder. *Archives of General Psychiatry*, **47**, 277–284.

Craske, M.G., Farchione, T.J., Allen, L.B., et al. (2007). Cognitive behavioral therapy for panic disorder and comorbidity: more of the same or less of more? *Behavior Research Therapy*, **45**, 1095–1109.

Crow, T.J. (1980). Molecular pathology of schizophrenia: more than one disease process? *British Medical Journal*, **280**, 66–68.

Crowe, R.R., Noyes, R., Pauls, D.L., and **Slymen, D.** (1983). A family study of panic disorder. *Archives of General Psychiatry*, **40**, 1065–1069.

Decker, H.S. (2013). *The Making of DSM-III: A diagnostic manual's conquest of American psychiatry.* Oxford: Oxford University Press.

Haby, M.M., Donnelly, M., Corry, J., and **Vos, T.** (2006). Cognitive behavioural therapy for depression, panic disorder and generalized anxiety disorder: a meta-regression of factors that may predict outcome. *Australian and New Zealand Journal of Psychiatry*, **40**, 9–19.

Hettema, J.M., Prescott, C.A., Myers, J.M., et al. (2005). The structure of genetic and environmental risk factors for anxiety disorders in men and women. *Archives of General Psychiatry*, **62**, 182–189.

Himsworth, H.P. (1936/2013). Diabetes mellitus: its differentiation into insulin-sensitive and insulin-insensitive types. *International Journal of Epidemiology*, **42**, 1594–1598.

Kendler, K.S. (2009). An historical framework for psychiatric nosology. *Psychological Medicine*, **39**, 1935–1941.

Kendler, K.S. (2012). Epistemic iteration as a historical model for psychiatric nosology: promises and limitations. In K.S. Kendler and J. Parnas (eds.) *Philosophical Issues in Psychiatry II: Nosology*, pp. 303–322. Oxford, UK: Oxford University Press.

Kendler, K.S. (2013). A history of the DSM-5 Scientific Review Committee. *Psychological Medicine*, **43**, 1793–1800.

Kendler, K. S., Aggen, S. H., Knudsen, G. P., Roysamb, E., Neale, M. C., and Reichborn-Kjennerud, T. (2011). The Structure of Genetic and Environmental Risk Factors for Syndromal and Subsyndromal Common DSM-IV Axis I and All Axis II Disorders. *American Journal of Psychiatry*, **168**, (1) 29–39.

Kendler, K.S., Gruenberg, A.M., and **Tsuang, M.T.** (1985). Subtype stability in schizophrenia. *American Journal of Psychiatry*, **142**, 827–832.

Kendler, K.S., Gruenberg, A.M., and **Tsuang, M.T.** (1988). A family study of the subtypes of schizophrenia. *American Journal of Psychiatry*, **145**, 57–62.

Kendler, K.S., McGuire, M., Gruenberg, A.M., and **Walsh, D.** (1994). Outcome and family study of the subtypes of schizophrenia in the west of Ireland. *American Journal of Psychiatry*, **151**, 849–856.

Kent, J.M., Papp, L.A., Martinez, J.M., et al. (2001). Specificity of panic response to CO(2) inhalation in panic disorder: a comparison with major depression and premenstrual dysphoric disorder. *American Journal of Psychiatry*, **158**, 58–67.

Klein, D.F. (1964). Delineation of two drug-responsive anxiety syndromes. *Psychpharmacologia*, 5, 397–408.

Klein, D.F. (1969). *Diagnosis and Drug Treatment of Psychiatric Disorders*. Baltimore, MD: Williams & Wilkins.

Klein, D.F. and **Fink, M.** (1962). Psychiatric reaction patterns to imipramine. *American Journal of Psychiatry*, **119**, 432–438.

Kossowsky, J., Pfaltz, M.C., Schneider, S., et al. (2013). The separation anxiety hypothesis of panic disorder revisited: a meta-analysis. *American Journal of Psychiatry*, **170**, 768–781.

Kraepelin, E. (1902)./1990. *Psychiatry, A Textbook for Students and Physicians* (*Psychiatrie*, 6th edn, Vol. **2**, trans. Sabine Ayed). Canton, MA: Science History Publications.

Lakatos, I. (1970)., Falsification and the methodology of scientific research programmes. In I. Lakatos and A. Musgrave (eds.) *Criticism and the Growth of Knowledge*, pp. 91–197. London: Cambridge University Press.

Mandal, A. (2015). Diabetes pathophysiology. 12-9-2015. Retrieved January 11, 2016. http://www.news-medical.net/health/Diabetes-Pathophysiology.aspx

Mochcovitch, M.D., da Rocha Freire, R.C., Garcia, R.F., and **Nardi, A.E.** (2014). A systematic review of fMRI studies in generalized anxiety disorder: evaluating its neural and cognitive basis. *Journal of Affective Disorders*, **167**, 336–342.

Pitts, F.N., Jr. and **McClure, J.N.,** Jr. (1967). Lactate metabolism in anxiety neurosis. *New England Journal of Medicine*, **277**, 1329–1336.

Rapee, R. (1986). Differential response to hyperventilation in panic disorder and generalized anxiety disorder. *Journal of Abnormal Psychology*, **95**, 24–28.

Rapee, R.M., Brown, T.A., Antony, M.M., and **Barlow, D.H.** (1992). Response to hyperventilation and inhalation of 5.5% carbon dioxide-enriched air across the DSM-III-R anxiety disorders. *Journal of Abnormal Psychology*, **101**, 538–552.

Ravindran, L.N. and **Stein, M.B.** (2010). The pharmacologic treatment of anxiety disorders: a review of progress. *Journal of Clinical Psychiatry*, **71**, 839–854.

Robins, E. and **Guze, S.B.** (1970). Establishment of diagnostic validity in psychiatric illness: its application to schizophrenia. *American Journal of Psychiatry*, **126**, 983–987.

Skre, I., Onstad, S., Torgersen, S., et al. (1993). A twin study of DSM-III-R anxiety disorders. *Acta Psychiatrica Scandinavica*, **88**, 85–92.

Verburg, K., Griez, E., Meijer, J., and **Pols, H.** (1995). Discrimination between panic disorder and generalized anxiety disorder by 35% carbon dioxide challenge. *American Journal of Psychiatry*, **152**, 1081–1083.

Wellcome Trust Case Control Consortium. (2009). Genome-wide association study of 14,000 cases of seven common diseases and 3,000 shared controls. *Nature*, **447**, 661–678.

Chapter 39

Comments on "Progressive validation of psychiatric syndromes: The example of panic disorder"

Kenneth F. Schaffner and Kathryn Tabb

39.1. Introduction

In Chapter 38, Kenneth Kendler explores the implications of adding a temporal dimension to the notion of "diagnostic validation" in the area of psychiatry. The general idea is that validation has traditionally been considered synchronically—addressing the best evaluative evidence available at a specific time or within a short time-slice. Kendler examines how we might assess the diagnostic validity of psychiatric disorders if we look at the disorder diachronically. Kendler bases his approach on suggestions made by Hasok Chang about diachronically assessing some chemical concepts such as "element" and "acid" (Chang 2015). But Kendler also relies on the approach to "research programmes" developed by Imre Lakatos (Lakatos 1970). Lakatos's analysis is also diachronic, and Lakatos once remarked "the methodology of research programmes does not offer instant rationality" (Lakatos 1978, p. 6). Kendler's main example is to develop a series of validators that can be applied to distinguishing between two psychiatric disorders: generalized anxiety disorder (GAD) and panic disorder (PD).

Kendler compares this case to a touchstone example, one that virtually all would agree represents diachronic progress: the distinction between type 1 (juvenile) diabetes and type 2 (late-onset) diabetes. Initially both types were thought to be the same form of diabetes, but Kendler describes how advances in research and treatment differentiated them, leading to extraordinary improvements in diagnosis and patient care for diabetics.

After outlining this example, Kendler turns his attention to the proposal made in the 1960s by Donald Klein that panic attacks or PD might *not* be a part of a general anxiety neurosis (termed GAD in DSM-III) (Klein and Fink 1962). Kendler asks if the attempt to make this distinction into two separate disorders represents part of, in Lakatos's terms, a "progressive research programme" or rather a "degenerating" one. It is here that Kendler turns to some details of Lakatos's theory of research programmes. While we agree Lakatos is an appropriate philosophical resource to draw on here, we want to emphasize the relevance of an aspect of Lakatos's account of research programmes that we believe is neglected in Kendler's analysis but is crucial to any application of that account to the question of progress in psychiatry: positive and negative heuristics.

39.2 Lakatos and his research programmes

We see a Lakatosian research programme as one of a family of global metascientific constructs, the most famous of which is a Kuhnian paradigm, later called by Kuhn a "disciplinary matrix," a term that ultimately did not stick.[1] There are other global metascientific constructs, and most of them do have diachronic features. Toulmin (1972) introduced a notion of *conceptual* evolution in a *discipline*, Laudan subsequently proposed the term "research tradition," and Kitcher developed the notion of a scientific "practice." One of us in a similar vein developed the notion of a "temporally extended theory" in order to adequately describe the kinds of changes that occurred in the battle in immunology between the instructive theory and the subsequent and still dominant clonal selection theory of the immune response (Schaffner 1993).[2] Each of these constructs would have different advantages or disadvantages for the scholar looking for a framework with which to assess psychiatric change.

A Lakatosian research programme captures, among other elements, the temporal dimension of a paradigm but introduces a somewhat different internal dynamic structure than other temporal approaches to scientific development. A research program is constituted by methodological rules—"some tell us what paths of research to avoid (*negative heuristic*), and others what paths to pursue (*positive heuristic*)" (Lakatos 1970, p. 132). A research program also contains a "hard core"—in general this contains the essential hypotheses of a theory—and a "protective belt," a set of auxiliary hypotheses "which has to bear the brunt of tests and get adjusted and readjusted, or even completely replaced, to defend the hard core." The negative heuristic instructs us not to subject the hard core to falsification. For Lakatos, an excellent example of a research programme was Newton's gravitational theory.

39.3 Lakatos's heuristics and the value issue

Kendler describes several aspects of a Lakatosian research programme, but only implicitly cites Lakatos's notion of negative and positive heuristics. These surrogates for heuristics appear in outline in Kendler's account as a series of validator

[1] In point of fact, Lakatos came to his ideas as a reaction to Kuhn's critique of Popper's falsificationist philosophy, but leavened by Duhem's analysis of the difficulties of falsifying hypotheses.

[2] Also see some discussion of this temporally extended theory concept in connection with the dopamine hypothesis of schizophrenia in Kendler and Schaffner (2011).

topics, such as family and genetic data, treatment, and imaging. These validators are in fact part of the standard practices, approaches, and methods that are accepted by the psychiatric research community, and which guide research protocols and the selection of explanatory targets. Heuristics are, however, difficult to characterize, and the grounds for holding, abandoning, and adapting positive heuristics are controversial, as Kuhn noted in different terms when he discussed trying to specify criteria for paradigm change (more about Kuhn on this topic a bit later.) A particularly vexing issue is identifying the values that are involved both explicitly in the two forms of "heuristics," as well as in the "hard core" as opposed to the more changeable "protective belts." Kendler concludes that to assess if a research programme is *better* from the epistemic iterative perspective we need, as Chang also notes, to see if it is "getting better over time." But this means that we must assess the shifting standards for "better" through an analysis of that aspect of the Lakatosian program that Kendler does not avail himself of: the heuristics.

Kendler himself has written a landmark article on the importance of the appeal to values to determine what form of a disorder construct is better (if not best) (Kendler 1990). In that article Kendler distinguished between "little questions" such as the relative risk of schizoaffective disorder in first-degree relatives of an affected population versus "big questions." Big questions include such topics as "the best criteria set for anorexia nervosa." And big questions require answers that are not obviously part of the "scientific method" involving only "empirical" matters—rather they involve "informed value judgments" (Kendler 1990, p. 972).

We interpret Lakatosian negative and positive heuristics as guiding Kendlerian "big questions" and by implication as involving a set of value judgments that are (often implicitly) appealed to in setting priorities for scientific research and assessing the empirical impact of scientific data. The negative heuristic also establishes where to fix the distinction between the hard core and the protective belt, and *which* hard core to provisionally accept as being research-worthy. The positive heuristic, as Lakatos wrote, involves a series of policy decisions:

> Few theoretical scientists engaged in a research programme pay undue attention to "refutations." They have a long-term research policy which anticipates these refutations. This research policy, or order of research, is set out—in more or less detail—in the positive heuristic of the research programme. The negative heuristic specifies the "hard core" of the programme which is "irrefutable" by the methodological decision of its proponents; the positive heuristic consists of a partially articulated set of suggestions or hints on how to change, develop the "refutable variants" of the research programme, how to modify, sophisticate, the "refutable" protective belt. The positive heuristic of the programme saves the scientist from becoming confused by the ocean of anomalies. The positive heuristic sets out a programme which lists a chain of ever more complicated models simulating reality: the scientist's attention is riveted on building his models following instructions which are laid down in the positive part of his programme (Lakatos 1978, p. 49).

Earlier we mentioned that Lakatos was strongly influenced by the tension between Popper and Kuhn. Kuhn also struggled with this issue of values in scientific choice and progress, writing, "it should be easy to design a list of criteria that would enable an uncommitted observer to distinguish the earlier from the more recent theory time after time" (1977, p. 205). Kuhn then provides a list of such criteria, suggesting that the most useful might be "accuracy of prediction, especially quantitative prediction; the balance between esoteric and everyday subject matter; and the number of different problems solved" (1977, p. 206). Kuhn also indicated what he saw as less useful though still important criteria, suggesting "simplicity, scope, and compatibility with other specialties." This is not yet a complete list, but Kuhn thought the project was doable and might provide a sense of irreversible direction to the scientific process of development—of progress. Nonetheless he continued to be skeptical of the application of such criteria, and reiterated that skepticism, even after refining a list of criteria of theory choice in Chapter 13 of his later book *The Essential Tension* (Kuhn 1977).

Kuhn's list of criteria might be seen as outlining a set of values that could be merged with an account of positive and negative heuristics. In terms of amplifying the notion of a positive heuristic further along these lines, attention might well be paid to what Laudan termed the "logic of pursuit" (Laudan 1977). There has been some recent discussion of such a "context of pursuit"; for a discussion and citations see Seselia and Strasser (2014). If that merged and amplified account were developed in still more detail, it might then assist in the determination of the progressiveness or degeneration of a research programme.

39.4 **Conclusion**

In summary, what we would like to see as Kendler further develops a Lakatosian approach to epistemic iteration is a more explicit analysis of the values that are employed in analogues of Lakatos' positive and negative heuristics. We might expect, for example, that in some contexts there will be an emphasis on "clinical utility" with its various component values (see First 2005). In other contexts scientific validity will trump (see Tabb and Schaffner, Chapter 41 of this volume). Values and their application will thus be key, and more needs to be said about them in an explicit way to assess the "big questions" about various validators used in the GAD–PD example. While establishing whether certain epistemic, social, or other sorts of values should be privileged in evaluating scientific change is an enormous challenge, there are resources Kendler can draw on. Philosophers working in the feminist epistemology tradition have done work on precisely this question—which sort of values are to be privileged, which should be repressed, and on what grounds? (see, e.g., Kincaid et al. 2007). Philosophers have also wrestled with how the question of values uniquely impacts psychiatric inquiry (see, e.g., Sadler 2005).

Attention to how the "hard core" of each diagnostic entity is determined is also needed. A related point is whether we can we stand back far enough to assess whether the set of validators used are the right ones "in the long run." For example, did psychiatry take the wrong turn when it began to focus on drug response as a key factor in contrast to more phenomenological assessments of patient progress? Kendler's focus on "treatment" seems to genuflect to the chemical over the phenomenological, perhaps in response to the sort of positive heuristic that Lakatos's account can help characterize. If the turn towards biomedical explanation is the right way forward for psychiatry, a stronger and more explicit defense using Lakatos's machinery might help make a case for it, especially given the persistence of critics who see this direction as degenerative.

References

Chang, H. (2016). The rising of chemical natural kinds through epistemic iteration. In C. Kendig (ed.) *Natural Kinds and Classification in Scientific Practice*, pp. 33–46. London: Routledge.

First, M.B. (2005). Clinical utility: a prerequisite for the adoption of a dimensional approach in DSM. *Journal of Abnormal Psychology*, **114**, 560–564.

Kendler, K.S. (1990). Toward a scientific psychiatric nosology. Strengths and limitations. *Archives of General Psychiatry*, **47**, 969–973.

Kendler, K.S. and **Schaffner, K.F.** (2011). The dopamine hypothesis of schizophrenia: An historical and philosophical analysis. *Philosophy, Psychiatry, and Psychology*, **18**, 41–63.

Kincaid, H., Dupré, J., and Wylie, A., eds. (2007). *Value-Free Science? Ideals and illusion*. New York: Oxford University Press.

Klein, D.F. and **Fink, M.** (1962). Psychiatric reaction patterns to imipramine. *American Journal of Psychiatry*, **119**, 432–438.

Kuhn, T.S. (1977). *The Essential Tension: Selected studies in scientific tradition and change*. Chicago: University of Chicago Press.

Lakatos, I. (1970). Falsification and the methodology of scientific research programmes. In I. Lakatos and A. Musgrave (eds.) *Criticism and the Growth of Knowledge*, pp. 91–196. London: Cambridge University Press.

Lakatos, I. (1978). *Philosophical Papers*. Cambridge: Cambridge University Press.

Laudan, L. (1977). *Progress and its Problems: Toward a theory of scientific growth*. Berkeley, CA: University of California Press.

Sadler, J. (2005). *Values and Psychiatric Diagnosis*. Oxford: Oxford University Press.

Schaffner, K.F. (1993). *Discovery and Explanation in Biology and Medicine*. Chicago: University of Chicago Press.

Seselia, D. and **Strasser, C.** (2014). Epistemic justification in the context of pursuit: a coherentist approach. *Synthese*, **191**, 3111–3141.

Part IV

Descriptive to etiologic and living document

Section 14

Descriptive to etiologic in psychiatric nosology

Chapter 40

Introduction to "Causal pathways, random walks and tortuous paths: Moving from the descriptive to the etiological in psychiatry"

Josef Parnas

The chapter by Kathryn Tabb and Kenneth Schaffner is a detailed analysis of the dilemmas involved in the ambition to convert descriptive classification into thicker etiology-based categories of mental disorders. They offer a thoughtful examination of some of the major theoretical perspectives often employed in schizophrenia research (i.e., purely behavioral accounts, phenomenological psychopathology, genetics, and models with a strong cognitive focus). In this review by Tabb and Schaffner, it appears that these different conceptual frameworks do not result in establishing clear natural kind categories in psychiatric nosology.

Instead, Tabb and Schaffner introduce the concept of robust patterns which

> do not refer to a discrete sort of entity that exists in the world. Rather they are better seen as heuristics, categories that grow out of our best empirical theories in response to our practical needs.

Many of the considerations put forward by Tabb and Schaffner echo the problems addressed in the chapter by Eric Turkheimer (Chapter 5 in this volume).

From a clinical perspective the existence of 300–400 mental disorders in the fifth edition of the *Diagnostic and Statistical Manual of Mental Disorders* (DSM-5) is of course beyond any practical or scientific grasp. Epidemiological studies have shown that at least Danish psychiatrists are happy with about 15–20 categories for diagnostic purposes (Munk-Jørgensen et al. 2010). Among those categories schizophrenia, major depression, melancholia, and bipolar disorder are perhaps examples of robust patterns.

Reference

Munk-Jørgensen P., **Najarraq Lund M.**, and **Bertelsen A.** (2010). Use of ICD-10 diagnoses in Danish psychiatric hospital-based services in 2001–2007. *World Psychiatry*, **9**, 183–184.

Chapter 41

Causal pathways, random walks, and tortuous paths: Moving from the descriptive to the etiological in psychiatry

Kathryn Tabb and Kenneth F. Schaffner

41.1 Introduction

Over the last decades a consensus position has formed among psychiatrists and philosophers that progress in psychiatric nosology consists in the validation of descriptive categories through the discovery of underlying causal mechanisms (Andreasen 1995, Murphy 2006, Hyman 2010, Tsou 2015). Etiological means of investigation resembling those popular in the hard sciences have therefore come to be considered psychiatry's state of the art (First et al. 2002). There is enthusiasm for the notion that instead of aimlessly changing course in response to sociopolitical, commercial, and clinical trends, psychiatric classifications can be made to more closely track underlying causal mechanisms through proper iterative processes (Kendler 2009, 2012).

Our general task is to offer a philosophical assessment of attempts to redraw nosological topographies on the basis of causal roadmaps. We believe that the sort of complete causal explanations that constitute bottom-up reductions appropriate for describing some closed physical systems are not a viable aim for psychiatry. As a result, simply validating current diagnostic categories is not a straightforward project. In what follows we emphasize that decisions must be made every step of the way—the best categories will not "fall out" of psychiatric consensus, which can merely reveal patterns in thinking about psychopathology. At times these patterns may suggest that a nosological category be revised to accommodate new biomedical discoveries; at times the experience of clinicians may lead to the dismissal of such results as irrelevant to the project of healing.

This view is deflationary compared to a common approach taken by philosophers of psychiatry that treats diagnostic categories as *kinds* constituted by symptom clusters with underlying causal mechanisms. This approach optimistically—and we believe preemptively—grants psychiatric constructs some of the appealing properties attributed to the objects of study of the hard sciences (see Chang, Chapter 29 of this volume). Even when underlying causal mechanisms are not known, positing that psychiatric kinds are natural kinds or, more flexibly, what Richard Boyd has called homeostatic property cluster kinds (Boyd 1999, Cooper 2007, Sin 2007, Tsou 2008, Kendler et al. 2010) suggests that investigation should take the symptom clusters offered up by psychiatric nosology as a given and proceed by validating them through the discovery of their underlying causal mechanisms.

The lack of biomarkers, endophenotypes, genetic predispositions, or other sorts of validators for psychiatric classifications can encourage pessimism about whether insights from cognitive science, neuroscience, genetics, and other fields can successfully justify our diagnostics in this manner; more specific discussion on this point will be presented later in this article. Work in philosophy of psychiatry has demonstrated the challenges of providing truly integrative explanations in psychiatry across different levels of description (Sullivan 2014). One of us has previously demonstrated why in some cases the validation of current diagnostic classifications may be unrealistic, without good reason to think that the descriptive categories of psychiatric nosology, drawn up in response to clinical, sociological, political, and industrial need, will be appropriate starting points for biomedical research (Tabb 2015, also cf. Hyman 2010). Other critics have argued that the psychiatric kinds picture imports a hard-nosed reductionism from the basic sciences that may not be appropriate to medicine, especially psychiatry (Andreasen 2007, Parnas et al. 2013).

Our aim is to take an alternative approach utilizing some conceptual tools from the philosophy of science. We argue that diverse theoretical frameworks in psychiatry can work in tandem in the form of what we will call *robust patterns*. As opposed to natural or homeostatic property cluster kinds, robust patterns do not refer to a discrete sort of entity that exists in the world. Rather they are better seen as heuristics, conceptual tools that grow out of our best empirical theories in response to our practical needs. Rather than being settled by an authoritative body such as the American Psychiatric Association, patterns that emerge across diverse psychiatric research studies may be recognized by anyone with access to the data. While these patterns may not be immediately relevant in the clinic, where the entrenched framework dominated by the *Diagnostic and Statistical Manual of Mental Disorders* (DSM) may remain the most useful for the classification and treatment of patients on the basis of observational signs and symptoms, they can be compared, contrasted, and integrated to productively guide psychiatric research. It is therefore important to distinguish them from diagnostic categories in our analyses of psychiatry as a medical science.

We argue that the clinical perspective can guide the selection between competing theories by recognizing patterns in the absence of explanations integrating levels of analysis. Robust patterns do not represent etiological entities in a way that will satisfy those hungry for natural kinds in psychiatry. Rather than being metaphysical kinds, they bear a closer resemblance to what have been called "epistemic hubs" (Kutschenko 2011)—pragmatic concepts that integrate our best theories into useful heuristics. That said, our position is not anti-realistic. Robust patterns emerge from the phenomena, and while the choice of which patterns to focus on is underdetermined, some are more in line with our intentions toward the phenomena than others, and some better represent the phenomena than others. In other words, we will argue that although the phenomena of psychiatry shape its nosological landscape, which tortuous path psychiatric researchers take is ultimately a choice, and we need to assess such choices carefully on the basis of our best theories and epistemic values.

Our term *robust pattern* is a portmanteau that applies two philosophical terms to psychiatry: Daniel Dennett's *real patterns*, and William Wimsatt's theory of *robustness*.[1] Dennett developed the notion of a "real pattern" to describe those mental items which are important cognitively but which are ontologically ambiguous; they can neither be "vindicated along with the viruses [n]or banished along with the banshees" (1991, 27). The subject of Dennett's analysis is intentional states, but it can be seen as offering up a general ontology of patterns (Haugeland 1993). Unlike natural kinds, insofar as patterns "are 'by definition' a candidate for pattern *recognition*" (Dennett 1991, p. 32), they are defined in terms of the perspective of the observer, rather than their structure alone. To speak of patterns is to recognize that there are many possible grounds for delineating entities in the world on the basis of our diverse theoretical frameworks, but that only some will be meaningful.

Wimsatt's robustness, meanwhile, emphasizes that while our drawing of these delineations is the result of our perceptual and cognitive capacities, this need not suggest anti-realism—we may grant that some patterns are more robust than others due to stuff in the world, and that this robustness can guide decisions about boundaries. Wimsatt calls "robust" those objects of investigation whose existence and character are determined using a variety of independent means (2007, p. 43). To define psychiatric categories as robust patterns is to recognize that when conceptualizing psychiatric phenomena, the diverse data resulting from varied means of investigating psychopathology are best assessed together; not only so that all the pertinent information can be brought to bear on the challenge of constructing the best nosological system, but also so that the perspectives of different stakeholders are taken into account. It is to focus on utility as well as validity as a desideratum for nosology—and to suggest that, for all intents and purposes, the distinction is not as significant as some have suggested (Jablensky 2016, Schaffner 2016).

In order to illustrate the scope of the problem and motivate our preferred solution, we begin with a brief summary of a descriptive core example from DSM-5, schizophrenia. We then ask what rationale has been provided for relying on its clustering of descriptive symptoms, and ask whether there are alternatives proposed in the recent literature that could endorse a different clustering. We explore whether alternative perspectives on the disorder might provide a more robust

---

[1] In a manuscript entitled "Brain disorders? Not really ... why network structures block reductionism in psychopathology research," Denny Borsboom, Angélique Cramer, and Annemarie Kalis apply Dennett's theory of real patterns in support of a network model of psychopathology. While similar (and complementary), our analyses developed independently.

disease pattern, leading to etiologically-informed substitutes for classical descriptive schizophrenia in the research setting. Our alternative examples are drawn from recent research on cognitive aspects of schizophrenia, represented by the work of Michael Green and more etiologically by David Lewis' group; more briefly, the phenomenological, self-oriented accounts by Josef Parnas and McGorry's group; and the etiological speculations by the Psychiatric Genetic Consortium (PGC) group based on genome-wide association studies (GWAS).

We will conclude by considering the ontological status of diagnostic categories viewed as robust patterns, using Dennett's analysis of "real patterns" in which he contrasts his "mild realism" with Jerry Fodor's "industrial strength realism" and the reductionistic approach to mental objects promoted by Paul Churchland. Churchland's picture, we suggest, is analogous to that of hard-nosed psychiatric reductionists, and falls prey to the same criticism: the lowest level may not be the one on which the patterns of interest are visible. Our critique of Churchland is supported by the recent research of Cori Bargmann and Eve Marder on the "connectome" and by critical analyses of the PGC work on the biology of psychiatric etiological pathways by Farrell, Sullivan, and others. Our view is ultimately pluralistic, but not integrated; employs an account of robustness that we think is viable for psychiatry; and uses a strongly prudential orientation drawn from the American pragmatist philosophical tradition.

41.2 Etiology from description? The case of schizophrenia

41.2.1 A descriptive account of schizophrenia and some alternatives

We take as paradigmatic of a descriptive approach to a standard psychiatric disorder the formulation of classical schizophrenia in the recent DSM-5. A brief summary of this disorder is characterized in DSM-5 by listing five descriptive reported symptoms and observed signs:

1 delusions
2 hallucinations
3 disorganized speech (e.g., frequent derailment [ideas slip off track] or incoherence)
4 grossly disorganized or catatonic [motor problem] behavior
5 negative symptoms, i.e., diminished emotional expression or avolition [inability to initiate or persist in goal-directed activities].

DSM-5 adds that for a diagnosis, "two (or more) of the above need to each be present for a significant portion of time during a 1-month period (or less if successfully treated) and also states that "at least one of these must be (1), (2), or (3)" (American Psychiatric Association 2013, p. 99). In addition, social/occupational dysfunction must be present, and the symptoms need to be evident, though with some waxing and waning, for a six-month period (there are also additional exclusion conditions, and time-course descriptions of different types of durational forms of the disorder found in those afflicted).

Questions have periodically arisen in the psychiatric literature about whether the collection of symptoms listed above really identify *one* psychiatric disorder or are a motley mix of several rather different unusual and disturbing experiences (Bentall 1993, Ritsner and Gottesman 2011). One approach to seeking objective confirmation of a common pathology underlying the typical DSM clustering was pursued by Kendler using latent class analysis (LCA; Kendler et al. 1998) to seek categories underlying clusters of reported symptoms, signs, and history items in a large group of psychiatric patients (in this case, probands in the well-known Roscommon Family Study Irish psychiatric registry). LCA (and other statistical clustering approaches) had been used before for similar psychiatric classification purposes, and Kendler et al. (1998) provide nine additional citations to other similar studies. In general, LCA creates non-observational, higher-level or "latent" classes based on a collection of observable symptoms and signs in the population of interest.

This 1998 LCA analysis based the resultant latent classes on 21 signs and symptoms, of which 19 came from the standard list in the OPCRIT instrument (see website at: http://sgdp.iop.kcl.ac.uk/opcrit/). Representative OPCRIT items included "persecutory delusions" and "pressured speech." An additional seven items were constructed to increase coverage and limit computational demands. Examples of these composite symptoms are the merging of OPCRIT's "third-person auditory hallucinations" and "running commentary voices" into *Schneiderian hallucinations*; and compiling "abuse/accusatory/persecutory voices" and "other (non-affective) auditory hallucination" into *other auditory hallucinations*. The LCA generated six classes of psychiatric disorders, of which two fit well: class 1 with the classic schizophrenia of Kraepelin and Bleuler, and a class 2 with the classical and current picture of major depression. These results thus support the traditional DSM view of schizophrenia.

More recently Derks and colleagues have used a similar approach and reported that:

> We combined factor analysis and latent class analysis to analyze variation in Comprehensive Assessment of Symptoms and History lifetime-rated symptoms in 4286 subjects.... Variation in 5 continuous dimensions (disorganization, positive, negative, mania, and depression) was accounted for by the presence of 7 homogeneous classes (Kraepelinian schizophrenia, affective psychosis, manic-depression, deficit nonpsychosis, depression, healthy, and no symptoms). Eighty-five percent of the schizophrenia patients was assigned to the Kraepelinian schizophrenia class . . . (Derks et al. 2012, p. 495).

Neither of these studies, however, is definitive, and Kendler has expressed doubts about the implications of his own 1998 study (personal communication).

41.2.2 Non-behavioral accounts

In the past two decades, several quite different approaches to characterizing schizophrenia, as well as identifying an underlying pathological process in schizophrenia, have developed in the psychiatric literature. In addition to the operational DSM approach just summarized, there has been an active research program based on phenomenological types of analysis, represented by Parnas and his colleagues (Parnas et al. 2005, Parnas 2008, 2011), as well as by the work of Nelson in the McGorry group (Nelson et al. 2009, 2012, 2014). Northoff's group has also investigated schizophrenia using this approach, and recently wrote that "schizophrenia is a disturbance of the self, of which the attribution of agency is a major component" (Robinson et al. 2016). They also provided a review of current theories of sense of agency, including neuroscience-oriented analyses of the "resting state" of the brain.

In what can be characterized as the general etiological area of recent research on mental disorders, including schizophrenia, the PGC has been publishing general and putatively causal pathways that have substantial genetic support from their GWAS investigations. In their major schizophrenia GWAS article in July 2014, they stated that they had identified 108 loci related to schizophrenia, and that these results tended to focus on glutamergic synapses and calcium channel function, as well as support some type of immune function disorders affecting schizophrenia (Ripke et al. 2014). Then in their February 2015 article, the PGC wrote (Network and Pathway Analysis Subgroup of Psychiatric Genomics 2015):

> Genome-wide association studies (GWAS) of psychiatric disorders have identified multiple genetic associations with such disorders, but better methods are needed to derive the underlying biological mechanisms that these signals indicate. We sought to identify biological pathways in GWAS data from over 60,000 participants from the Psychiatric Genomics Consortium. We developed an analysis . . . [of] three adult psychiatric disorders: schizophrenia, major depression and bipolar disorder. Histone methylation processes showed the strongest association, and we also found statistically significant evidence for associations with multiple immune and neuronal signaling pathways and with the postsynaptic density. Our study indicates that risk variants for psychiatric disorders aggregate in particular biological pathways and that these pathways are frequently shared between disorders.

These pathway suggestions are what we might term *pathway sketches* since they suggest types of causal influences in a very abstract way. Much more specificity would be needed to begin to fill in identified genes or loci, and other biological entities' actions, and indeed such efforts are underway. The PGC's 2014 study indicated that the strongest genomic region associated with SCZ risk was the immunologically-related major histocompatibility complex (MHC). Sekar et al. (2016) have published an analysis of a gene in that region responsible for the complement component 4 (C4), suggesting that overproduction of this C4 protein has a pathological effect on the synaptic pruning important in brain development. This study has been widely praised, though it will need additional replication and further elucidation (Ruzzo and Geschwind 2016). In addition, it is very important to note that all these GWAS results are obtained by using, as inclusion criteria, the ancestors to the DSM-5 diagnostic criteria (e.g., DSM-IV and also ICD-10).

A still different approach to schizophrenia, focusing on more cognitive deficits, surfaced in the psychiatric literature beginning roughly in the 1990s (Green 2001). This cognitive focus has been the main driver of the more etiological work of David Lewis and his group at Pittsburgh, which has received major praise from the former head of the U.S. National Institute for Mental Health (NIMH), Thomas Insel. Insel wrote that the Lewis investigations into schizophrenia

> provides something this field really needed: a framework for linking observations at the molecular, cellular and systems levels. We haven't had a story that crossed those levels of explanation before. And his story, whether it pans out in all its details or not, is invaluable for doing that (Dobbs 2010).

In the next section we will briefly describe Lewis' approach to schizophrenia, and will contrast it with descriptive and more clinically relevant analyses of schizophrenia later in this paper.

41.2.3 The Lewis model of schizophrenia

This model is as situated within a broader context of evolving concepts of schizophrenia, including the additional attention since the 1990s to cognitive dimensions (such as disturbances in memory) of the disorder just noted. A number of investigators now see these deficits as a "core domain" of schizophrenia, perhaps underlying a number of aspects of the disorder, though they are not as dramatic as the traditional hallucinations and delusions. An important aspect of the Lewis model is that it provides etiological mechanisms and pathways that generate effects on human brain gamma-frequency oscillations, now believed to be one of the key underlying factors in brain function and dysfunction. The Lewis model has contributed to the increased attention paid recently to the neurotransmitters glutamate and GABA, which are believed to be as relevant to schizophrenia today as was dopamine originally (Kendler and Schaffner 2011). The Lewis approach also intercalates with an overlapping etiological model developed by Harrison and Weinberger (2011), though for lack of space this chapter cannot delve into that model. In addition, the Lewis model is much more detailed and specific than are the "pathway sketches" proposed by the 2015 PGC article, though the Lewis model might turn out to be an implementation of the PGC's neuronal signaling pathways, and thus receive GWAS support.

The attention to gamma oscillations as perhaps a key factor in schizophrenia is quite recent. A useful recent review article summarizes some of this work as follows:

> There has been a fascinating convergence of evidence in recent years implicating the disturbances of neural synchrony in the gamma frequency band (30–100 Hz) as a major pathophysiologic feature of schizophrenia. Evidence suggests that reduced glutamatergic neurotransmission via the *N*-methyl-D-aspartate (NMDA) receptors that are localized to inhibitory interneurons, perhaps especially the fast-spiking cells that contain the calcium-binding protein parvalbumin (PV), may contribute to gamma band synchrony deficits, which may underlie the failure of the brain to integrate information and hence the manifestations of many symptoms and deficits of schizophrenia (Woo et al. 2010).

This review article adds further that gamma oscillation disturbances might affect important *developmental* aspects of the schizophrenia pathophysiology, as well as introduce "excitotoxic or oxidative injury to downstream pyramidal neurons, leading to further loss of synapses and dendritic branchings," both in prodromal and early phases of the disorder. It should also be noted that gamma oscillations have been considered related to the "binding problem" of consciousness, whereby multiple sense streams are bound into one common perception (Merker 2013).

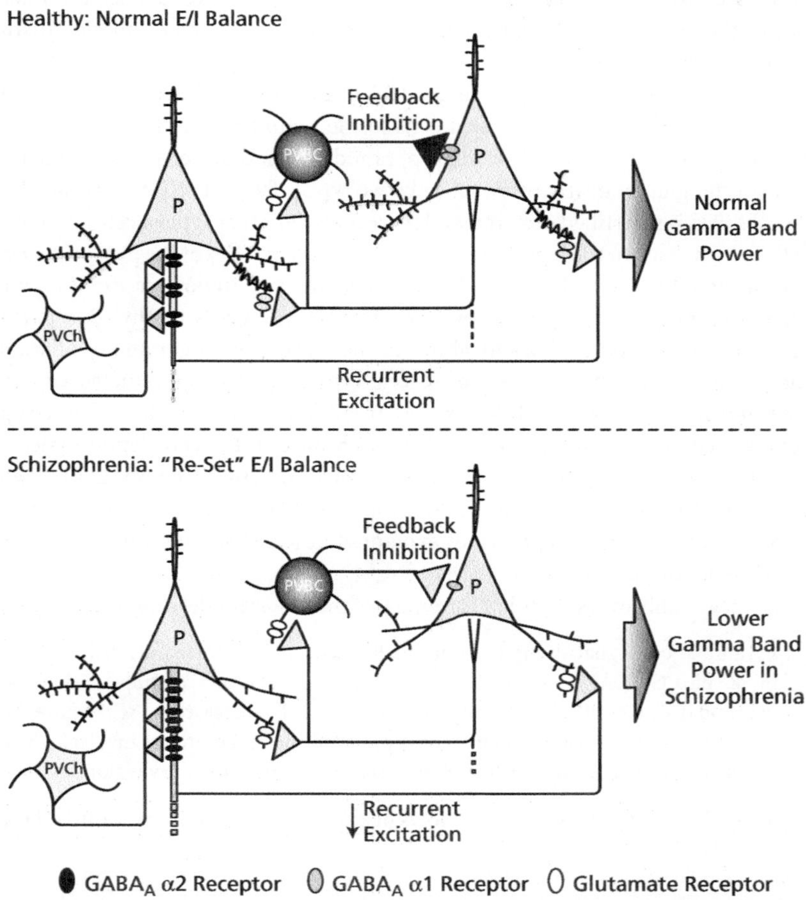

Lower recurrent excitation between P neurons	Lower feedback inhibition from PVBC neurons	Greater P neuron depolarization from PVCh neurons
• Smaller dendritic arbor • Fewer dendritic spines	• Reduced GABA synthesis • Increased suppression of GABA release • Fewer GABA$_A$ α1 receptors • Reduced chloride influx	• Reduced GABA re-uptake • More GABA$_A$ α2 receptors

Figure 41.1 Alterations in disordered cells in schizophrenia leading to gamma band power changes. See text for explanation.

Reprinted from *Trends in Neurosciences*, 35 (1), David A. Lewis, Allison A. Curley, Jill R. Glausier, and David W. Volk, Cortical parvalbumin interneurons and cognitive dysfunction in schizophrenia, pp. 57–67, Copyright (2012), with permission from Elsevier.

The extent to which gamma oscillation pathologies can be identified with standard schizophrenia symptoms is still under discussion and requires further research. The review article just cited, however, does provide a number of references that support these connections, stating that "gamma abnormalities have been found to be associated with various symptom domains of schizophrenia, such as hallucinations, thought disorder, disorganization, and psychomotor poverty" (see Woo et al. 2010, p. 3 for references). As noted above, the Lewis model is one of the more detailed models that can account for gamma oscillation disturbances in schizophrenia.

The central element in the Lewis model is the circuit that involves these inputs from the parvalbumin (PV) basket cells to the brain's pyramidal neurons using the neurotransmitter GABA, though pyramidal cells themselves use the neurotransmitter glutamate (there are actually two types of basket cells that we need not discuss in this simplified account, and there is also another type of cell, chandelier cells, which assist in the regulation of the oscillatory activity of the pyramidal neurons as noted briefly below.) In addition, there are two important input regulating receptor types for glutamate, one termed the NMDAR (*N*-methyl-D-aspartate receptor) and introduced briefly above in the discussion of gamma oscillations, these being under the influence of several type(s) of schizophrenia susceptibility genes including *NRG1*. There is also an additional glutamate receptor type, abbreviated as AMPAR (α-amino-3-hydroxy-5-methyl-4-isoxazolepropionic acid receptor), which mediates fast synaptic neurotransmission (the NMDA receptor is the main molecular mechanism controlling memory function, but a balance between both types of receptors may explain some features of pyramidal cell oscillation regulation).

A considerably oversimplified summary of the Lewis model might be:

> Pyramidal cell signal strength ↓ (via smaller cells and decreased dendritic spines in SZ) plus NMDAR ↓ → PV basket cell activity ↓ (as feedback compensation) → pyramidal cell oscillation activity still insufficiently increased = schizophrenic symptoms (the types of symptoms varying depending on the circuits involved, thus memory in some areas and decreased tone sensitivity in the auditory region).

Figure 41.1, from the Lewis group, shows healthy and schizophrenic brains (Lewis et al. 2012).

41.3 **Robust patterns**

Let us take stock of the various approaches to schizophrenia that we have outlined. Based on the type of empirical clustering of symptoms and signs represented by the Kendler and Derks analyses, it can be argued that these at least weakly support the use of the DSM's characterization of schizophrenia both as a research tool, as we noted in connection with the recent GWAS findings, and as a diagnostic option for patients reporting and displaying the problems listed in the DSM-5. However, the support is characterized as "weak" since there are schizophrenia symptoms that are seen as important in the cognitive and phenomenological approaches that are not mentioned in the DSM-5, such as those targeted by Lewis, and there is no consensus on the etiological underpinning that might allow for further developments using the classical types of validators. These classical validators have been discussed elsewhere (Schaffner 2012, Kendler 2013).

In this chapter, for reasons of space, we will not be able to comment on the phenomenological analysis approach represented by the research of Parnas, Nelson, and Northoff. However, we wish to note that it offers another novel direction for research both in terms of patient diagnosis using the "Examination of Anamolous Self-Experience" scale, as well as a neuroscience-based research program, as noted in the earlier citations. Due to its attention to those phenomenological aspects of schizophrenia such as ipseity disturbance, which are neglected by the DSM framework, it may suggest a pattern in clinical data that is distinct from the DSM's. Given that our focus here is on the viability of reductive biomedical explanations, however, we will focus on contrasting the DSM descriptive approach with the Lewis approach, which represents a well-received molecular–genetic–pathophysiological model. The Lewis model brings together a group of cognitive disturbances associated with schizophrenia, provides a series of empirical tests for these cognitive problems, and offers a detailed, complex, and well-supported etiological analysis combining genetic and neuroimaging modalities. It provides a model that a number of investigators can and do pursue, and is consistent with the NIMH turn toward a distinctive set of criteria for research on mental disorder, the Research Domain Criteria (RDoC). However, much more specificity would be needed to begin to fill in identified genes or loci, cell types, and the actions of other biological entities. The Lewis group continues to add such specificity, and recently reported a study showing that the neuropathology of schizophrenia includes a lower number of excitatory synapses on the PV interneurons (Chung et al. 2016).

Akin to the "theory of everything" heralded and lambasted as a goal for physics, we might imagine this framework expanding into a causal model for schizophrenia that would constitute a complete explanation for the disorder. Philosophers of the life sciences, however, have long recognized that the complexity of biological systems may simply not allow for this sort of completeness. In the early 1970s, Wimsatt introduced a philosophical analysis of such frustratingly complex systems, to counter what he a saw as the bias in the literature "towards theoretical monism" despite

> an obvious plurality of large, small, and middle-range theories and models, which overlap in unclear ways and which usually partially supplement and partially contradict one another in explaining the interaction of phenomena at a number of levels of description and organization (Wimsatt 1972/4, p. 67).

Given the wealth of contributions from different scientific, psychological, and social-scientific fields toward the understanding of psychiatric disorders, Wimsatt's analysis is germane to the challenges facing contemporary psychiatry. He gives compelling arguments for assessing the complexity of scientific phenomena in order to allow for a reappraisal of the appropriateness of theoretical monism versus a more pluralistic approach.

Wimsatt offers an account of the *boundaries* of scientific objects and their internal processes in terms of what Kaufman (1971) has called *decompositions*, similar to the pathway sketches introduced above. He uses Kaufman's concept of boundaries to argue that when different theoretical viewpoints—about "what the system is doing"—on the same system yield decompositions with spatially non-coincident boundaries, it suggests the system is complex. Wimsatt gives an example comparing decompositions of a fruit fly and a piece of granite; for figure see Wimsatt (2007, p. 183). A piece of granite can be decomposed into subregions on the basis of chemical composition, crystalline form, tensile strength, electrical conductivity, and thermal conductivity. These different theoretical frameworks will produce loosely coincident boundaries, giving granite that property Wimsatt calls robustness—the "coincidence of boundaries" that indicate different theoretical approaches confirming the existence of the same phenomenon (Wimsatt 2007, p. 353). The robustness of the results of different theoretical approaches to the granite is in contrast with the results when different biological approaches are applied to the fly. Here anatomical, physiological, biochemical, genetic, and functional frameworks will result in radically different decompositions. The fly, in Wimsatt's terms, has "substantial 'descriptive complexity.'"

How can we use the notion of robustness to think about psychiatric kinds? Once we recognize that mental disorder is nefariously complex, it becomes clear that, if we want to reconceive psychiatric nosology in biological terms, which cluster of signs and symptoms we favor as diagnostic will depend on which pathway sketch or sketches we focus on. If we want to take into account the diversity of different pathway sketches offered up for a condition like schizophrenia, we will focus on those signs and symptoms that represent a robust medical object; that is, an object whose boundaries are delineated by a significant number of those sketches. So, for example, taking patients displaying symptoms of psychosis, we may consider how the space of signs and symptoms is subdivided into diagnoses by potential etiological accounts—in terms of a genetic predisposition, a problem of circuitry, or a specific environmental risk factor, for example. It may be that for some psychiatric categories, like Alzheimer's disease, diverse theoretical frameworks neatly draw boundaries around the clinical population picked out by our best clinical manuals. For others, like schizophrenia, the variation among the decompositions suggests a complexity that belies any optimism about locating a single causal pathway for everyone sharing the diagnosis, in which case a compromise must be necessary: Which theoretical decomposition do we favor? Which boundaries, and their associated pathways, do we choose?

Wimsatt points out that systems with profound descriptive complexity often have high degrees of *interactional complexity*, in which causal interactions within the system cross over between decompositions at the descriptive level. This interactional complexity can be used as a measure of the viability of using any given theoretical framework to predict the behavior of the system, other things being equal. As Wimsatt notes, when a system is both descriptively and interactionally complex, the researcher looking for a causal pathway is required to consider a bewildering array of relationships between different subsystems at different levels of analysis, rather than the same subsystems at different levels. It is on account of this particular sort of overwhelming complexity that biological and social scientists claim "no one perspective appears to do justice to their objects of study, or, somewhat more obscurely, that their systems are unanalyzable into component parts" (Wimsatt 2007, p. 186). In such cases, Wimsatt continues, scientists may feel that there is no way of privileging the decomposition of any one theoretical framework over any other. In the psychiatric setting, we may imagine that while a neuroscientist might think that a given biomarker should confirm a diagnosis of schizophrenia, a phenomenologist might focus on a disturbance in the perception of ipseity. While each level contains explanatory information, taken as a whole the interactions between levels in this type of system are inconclusive as to the boundaries of the disorder. It is here we believe Dennett's notion of a pattern can help.

In his influential 1991 article "Real Patterns," Dennett addresses an old question from philosophy of mind: "Are there really beliefs?" Dennett argues that such metaphysical concerns might be overblown for mental items, which function in our ontologies not as entities nor as constructions but as *compressions* of more complex data sets that do important work in our theories of mind. Rather than taking a metaphysical approach to the question of the existential status of our beliefs, Dennett argues, we should take a scientific one, which focuses on the predictive utility of adopting certain patterns as scientific objects. Dennett accepts Arthur Fine's "natural ontological attitude" or NOA (pronounced "Noah"). As one of us (Schaffner 2012) has noted, Fine disarms the critic who worries that acceptance of this view would lead to an anti-scientific relativism, writing that "it seems to me that both the realist and the antirealist [instrumentalist] must toe what I have been calling "the homely line." That is, they must both accept the certified results of science as on a par with the more homely and familiarly supported claims" (Fine 1984, p. 96) such as "the existence and features of everyday objects" (Fine 1984, p. 95). Fine proposes to call this acceptance of scientific truths the "core position." He then suggests that the realists' so-called addition to the core amounts to little more than "a desk-thumping, foot stamping shout of 'Really!'" (Fine 1984, p. 97). Fine's positive suggestion, NOA, "is the core position itself, and all by itself" (Fine 1984, p. 97). From this perspective any invoking of "the external world" is just another gesture toward an inscrutable and inaccessible "something out there." According to Fine, such an appeal cannot and will not justify any legitimate form of realism.

We see this NOA view as salutary and as clearing up a lot of muddy thinking that is based on strong habits and metaphysical confusion, though that it "marks a revolutionary approach to understanding science," as Fine writes (Fine 1984, p. 101), might be too strong a claim. We refer to Fine's NOA view because the conceptualization of patterns as "real" in his sense is important for the pluralistic approach we are endorsing. Dennett defines a pattern as any "candidate for pattern *recognition*" (1991, p. 31), that is, any description of a series in which the information required to describe the series has been compressed. Dennett uses two kinds of examples, the first a set of dot patterns akin to QR codes (which he calls "frames") from which various simplified extractions that he dubs "barcodes" can be extracted. Such barcodes are more "efficient" albeit "inexact" ways of capturing the information in the frames. His second set of examples comes from Conway's

Game of Life. One important question about pattern-based models like Conway's is which is the "right level" of abstraction, scale of compression, or representation to focus on to find interesting and useful "patterns." For Dennett, the "intentional stance" in humans is a "stupendous" compression in contrast to the details of a supercomputer's processes, say in chess: in the intentional stance, most of us interpret the behavior of opponents by treating them as rational agents whose behavior is governed by mental states including beliefs and desires, rather than computing their every possible move. The same could be said of the neurobiological events occurring in the enormously complex parallel processors of the brain and yielding nosological intuitions in psychiatry.

Dennett argues that the language of thought, or mentalese, is an extraordinarily efficient set of patterns for getting around in the world and interacting with other persons. Analogously, we can think of diverse sorts of theories about psychopathology—from clinicians, researchers, service users, and other interested parties—as similarly subject to compression within our nosological categories, both those codified in the DSM and those implicitly at work in the research setting. All of these sources add data, and the job of the nosologist is to separate patterns from the noise. However, while diverse compressions can be advantageous, there is no absolute "best" pattern. Dennett's realism is a mild one, insofar as being a pattern depends on being recognized, an intentional act reliant on the perceptual capacities of the observer. *Real patterns*, therefore, depend on the phenomena available for discovery but nonetheless have a "deeply pragmatic source" (1991, p. 36). Despite this, such patterns can be priceless for scientific discovery. When intellectual patterns are perceived—like those created by Wimsatt's composites—such "fanciful interpretations (or what W. V. Quine would call 'analytical hypotheses') may uncover a goldmine" (Dennett 1991, p. 41). Some patterns are better than others because they are based on real or at least projectable relationships. But we select them not on the basis of this metaphysical character but due to their usefulness. To take Dennett's example,

> It is undeniable that astrology provides its adherents with a highly articulated system of patterns that they think they see in the events of the world. The difference, however, is that no one has ever been able to get rich by betting on the patterns, but only by selling the patterns to others (1991, p. 50).

The "reality" of patterns can thus be determined by their "profit," or pragmatic utility; thus Dennett considers the theoretical claims of astronomy more "real" than those of astrology.

We believe that Wimsatt's robustness satisfactorily characterizes the sort of "realness" that interests Dennett, without dipping into metaphysical waters that are deeper than our pragmatic purpose. It is useful to think of psychiatric kinds as robust because when we group patients together on the basis patterns drawn from of different theoretical frameworks, the resulting taxonomic boundaries can overlap more or less precisely, requiring an intentional choice on the grounds of utility. A Wimsattian decomposition can be at many different levels of aggregation, for example genetic, and a genetic decomposition might result in a different set of groupings of patients than if we used cellular pathophysiology, or some higher-level, more clinical, classifiers. When diverse decompositions overlap significantly they create a robust psychiatric kind, and we have reason to be optimistic that some of the interactional complexity between theoretical frameworks can be resolved in ways that will allow for prediction and manipulation. However, as both Wimsatt and Dennett's work suggests, distinct frameworks may give rise to distinct patterns that stand in relations of significant tension since each can have value under different perspectives—see Kendler's (1985) discussion of schizotypy an example of this phenomenon. For clinical purposes, psychiatry's manifest images—the patterns most obviously observable in the clinic, what we may call "folk" psychiatry—may be more important than those based in biology. For the purposes of laboratory research, other patterns, drawn from part–whole decompositions, may be more viable. We can anticipate that such diverse patterns will ultimately converge (or might be replaced by other more convergent patterns), but we must also acknowledge that descriptive and interactional complexity will endure. As Wimsatt notes, to suggest "that if our theories are successful, then they should produce descriptions of systems according to which the systems are interactionally simple [puts] the conceptual cart before the phenomenal horse."

41.4 Applications and conclusions

Having devoted the immediately preceding section to philosophical matters, primarily making use of philosophical tools of Wimsatt and Dennett, let us return to the accounts of schizophrenia that we sketched in section 41.2. Our task now is to draw some lessons for current debates about psychiatric description and etiology in light of our philosophical discussion. First, we summarize how the notion of robust patterns can be usefully applied to the task with which we were charged, the possibility of moving from the descriptive to the etiological in psychiatry. A second arena for application is necessarily very abbreviated, but it involves a number of difficult and deep philosophical issues concerning validity, the topic of extensive debate in recent meetings of this Copenhagen group. Space permits only the briefest of comments on this second, broader theme.

41.4.1 Robust patterns in schizophrenia

What do the varying accounts of schizophrenia suggest to us in the light of our philosophical analyses above? What we see are several different theoretical frameworks offering up various pathway sketches, which give rise to different nosological patterns: the traditional DSM operationalist account, a phenomenological analysis that focuses on self-images and a perception of "ipseity" that does not figure in the DSM, and a variety of biomedical attempts to explain the causes of schizophrenia at a variety of descriptive levels, such as the cognitive disability-based and etiologically-implemented Lewis analysis. This survey points to differing delineations that may have some yet-to-be-well-characterized overlaps forming a pattern. In our section 41.2, we only looked closely at the two levels of the cognitive Lewis model, but suggestions for the phenomenological ipseity model have been published (Nelson et al. 2014). The DSM analysis explicitly eschews an etiological component, but it can be noted that it is the DSM (and related ICD) criteria from DSM-IV that were largely the basis of the GWAS etiological proposals, since it was that set of schizophrenia criteria that were used to select the patient populations that the PGC analyzed and used to speculate on three etiological pathway sketches. Therefore, the GWAS studies can be seen as contributing to the robustness of the DSM's characterization of schizophrenia.

We have two proposals. The first, trading on the extensive complexity shown by different decompositions of schizophrenia, is that rather than compromising for the sake of consistency, clinicians and laboratory investigators should place their bets on the *most robust* model that each can defend as reliable and preliminarily valid *for their particular purposes*, and then deploy it extensively to see if they become "rich," to use the Dennett payoff term, by contributing to a robust pattern. This approach temporarily sacrifices reliability across the diverse subfields of psychiatric research and puts a premium on predictive and therapeutic utility. It is is consistent with the Wimsattian complexity we noted in section 41.3, as well as Dennett's suggestion that we allow for multiple patterns and see which are satisfactory in meeting our criteria of success.

Our second proposal here is that where there are reasonably strong overlaps in the classifications that result from different theoretical approaches such that a pattern forms, these overlaps should be taken as a sign that the pattern is a valuable one. An example from our review in section 41.2 using the Lewis theory could be a more tractable set of instruments to assess cognitive deficits, a symptom that is already clinically very significant. If those instruments produced specific results, they could allow this type of symptom to appear in the schizophrenia diagnostic criteria in a future DSM-5.X. However, it is important to note that a strong etiological analysis *may still not ultimately* be useful as a clinical guide. This view mirrors Dennett's critique of Paul Churchland's reductionistic and eliminativist thesis regarding "folk psychology":

> If the "pattern" is scarcely an improvement over the bit map, talk of eliminative materialism will fall on deaf ears—just as it does when radical eliminativists urge us to abandon our ontological commitments to tables and chairs (Dennett 1991, p. 51).

The analogue of this argument in the psychiatric domain is that phenomenological descriptions similar to the DSM model might well be more useful, and not easily replaceable, even by a suite of well-supported pathway sketches such as RDoC envisions. For example, the Kendler and Derks articles referred to in section 41.2 suggest that up to 85% of patients seen clinically for schizophrenia will fit into this neo-Kraepelinian paradigm despite its lack of attention to cognitive deficits.

41.4.2 **Broader concluding reflections**

Betting on any of the etiological pathway sketches summarized above at the expense of attention to broader psychopathological patterns may be problematic. In the past two years, there has been considerable interest in the various BRAIN projects, from a (controversial) billion-dollar EU initiative, to the more modest but still extensive (approximately 100-million dollar) U.S. effort to map and understand the brain at the neurophysiological level(s). Significant advances are being made in understanding and representing the brain, but some comments by one of the U.S. leaders of the BRAIN Initiative, Cori Bargmann, writing with neuroscientist Eve Marder, should be attended to. One of their examples comes from the connectivity diagram of the stomatogastric ganglion (STG) of the Jonah crab, *Cancer borealis*. Discussing the extensive variation of neuromodulation in neurotransmitters and neurocircuit effects, due to neuromodulation, the process by which neural activity is regulated by controlling the physiological levels of one or more classes of neurotransmitters, they write:

> Many years of work on the effects of neuromodulators on the STG have revealed that the functional connections that give rise to a specific circuit output are specified, or in fact "configured," by the neuromodulatory environment. Every synapse and every neuron in the STG is subject to modulation; the connectivity diagram by itself only establishes potential circuit configurations, whose availability and properties depend critically on which of many neuromodulators are present at a given moment. Under some modulatory conditions, anatomically "present" synaptic connections may be functionally silent, only to be strengthened under other modulatory conditions. Likewise, modulators can qualitatively alter the neurons' intrinsic properties, transforming neurons from tonic spiking to those generating plateau potentials or bursts. These effects of neuromodulators can activate or silence an entire circuit, change its frequency and/or the phase relationships of the motor patterns generated (Bargmann and Marder 2013).

This suggests an important caveat to us. "Drilling down" to the specific circuits, cells, and molecules undergirding psychopathology, especially given their unstable and shifting temporal character, may well lead to an analogous problem to that Dennett forecast for Churchland. There may not be any payoff at these "bit levels" due to unmanageable complexity, and much more might be accomplished in terms of diagnosis, prognosis, and useful interventions at more abstract, functionally emergent levels.

Of course there will not be a single answer here across the field. "Drilling down" might be shown in certain cases to be a very successful strategy. For example, this type of success happened in physics in the nineteenth century when the search for lower-level causes in optics yielded Maxwell's electromagnetic theory, the backdrop for radio and TV today. Chemical valence was ultimately explained by quantum mechanics, though complexity there often requires higher-level information to model chemical structures and reactions. In biology, Seymour Benzer pushed phage genetics down to the Watson–Crick model, with great success, and against the prognostications of Max Delbruck who thought that "paradoxes" and strong emergence would prohibit such a reductionist program. So attempts such as the Lewis model may succeed, and unify portions of schizophrenia with cellular and circuit processes. In that case, we will have etiology, and hopefully clinical advances both in diagnosis and in therapeutic interventions, based on these robust cross-level interactions. Our analysis leads us to believe, however, that progress will not occur through such reductionistic efforts easily, and certainly not through them *only*. Time, and much more research, will tell.

References

American Psychiatric Association (2013). *Diagnostic and Statistical Manual of Mental Disorders, 5th edn*. Arlington, VA: American Psychiatric Association.

Andreasen, N. (1995). The validity of psychiatric diagnosis: new models and approaches. *American Journal of Psychiatry*, **152**, 161–162.

Andreasen, N. (2007). DSM and the death of phenomenology in America: an example of unintended consequences. *Schizophrenia Bulletin*, **33**, 108–12.

Bargmann, C.I. and **Marder, E.** (2013). From the connectome to brain function. *Nature Methods*, **10**, 483–490.

Bentall, R. (1993). Deconstructing the concept of "schizophrenia." *Journal of Mental Health*, **2**, 223–238.

Boyd, R. (1999). Kinds as the workmanship of men: realism, constructivism, and natural kinds. In J. Nida-Rümelin (ed.) *Rationalität, Realismus, Revision: Proceedings of the Third International Congress, Gesellschaft für Analytische Philosophie*, pp. 52–89. Berlin: de Gruyter.

Chung, D.W., Fish, K.N., and **Lewis, D.A.** (2016). Pathological basis for deficient excitatory drive to cortical parvalbumin interneurons in schizophrenia. *American Journal of Psychiatry*, **173**, 1131–1139.

Cooper, R. (2007). *Psychiatry and the Philosophy of Science*. Durham, UK: Acumen Press.

Dennett, D.C. (1991). Real patterns. *Journal of Philosophy*, **88**, 27–51.

Derks, E.M., Allardyce, J., Boks, M.P., et al. (2012). Kraepelin was right: a latent class analysis of symptom dimensions in patients and controls. *Schizophrenia Bulletin*, **38**, 495–505.

Dobbs, D. (2010). Schizophrenia: the making of a troubled mind. *Nature*, **468**, 154–156.

First, M.B., Bell, C.C., Cuthbert, B., et al. (2002). Personality disorders and relational disorders: a research agenda for addressing crucial gaps in DSM. In D.J. Kupfer, M.B. First, and D.A. Regier (eds.) *APA Research Agenda for DSM-V*, pp. 123–199). Washington, DC: American Psychiatric Association.

Green, M.F. (2001). *Schizophrenia Revealed: From neurons to social interactions*. New York: Norton.

Hyman, S. (2010). The diagnosis of mental disorders: the problem of reification. *Annual Review of Clinical Psychology*, **6**, 155–179.

Haugeland, J. (1993). Pattern and being. In B. Dahlbom (ed.) *Dennett and His Critics*, pp. 53–69. Cambridge, MA. Blackwell Publishers.

Jablensky, A. (2016). Psychiatric classifications: validity and utility. *World Psychiatry*, **15**, 26–31.

Kendler, K.S. (1985). Diagnostic approaches to schizotypal personality disorder: a historical perspective. *Schizophrenia Bulletin*, **11**, 538–553.

Kendler, K.S. (1990). Toward a scientific psychiatric nosology. Strengths and limitations. *Archives of General Psychiatry*, **47**, 969–973.

Kendler, K.S. (2009). An historical framework for psychiatric nosology. *Psychological Medicine*, **39**, 1935–1941.

Kendler, K.S. (2012). The dappled nature of causes of psychiatric illness: replacing the organic-functional/hardware-software dichotomy with empirically based pluralism. *Molecular Psychiatry*, **17**, 377–388.

Kendler, K.S. (2013). A history of the DSM-5 Scientific Review Committee. *Psychological Medicine*, **43**, 1793–1800.

Kendler, K.S., **Karkowski, L.M.**, and **Walsh, D.** (1998). The structure of psychosis: latent class analysis of probands from the Roscommon Family Study. *Archives of General Psychiatry*, **55**, 492–499.

Kendler, K.S. and **Schaffner, K.F.** (2011). The dopamine hypothesis of schizophrenia: an historical and philosophical analysis. *Philosophy, Psychiatry, and Psychology*, **18**, 41–63.

Kendler, K.S., **P. Zachar** and **C. Craver**. (2010). What kinds of things are psychiatric disorders? *Psychological Medicine*, **41**, 1143–1150.

Kutschenko, L.K. (2011). How to make sense of broadly applied medical classification systems: introducing epistemic hubs. *History and Philosophy of the Life Sciences*, **33**, 583–602.

Lewis, D.A., **Curley, A.A.**, **Glausier, J.R.**, and **Volk, D.W.** (2012). Cortical parvalbumin interneurons and cognitive dysfunction in schizophrenia. *Trends in Neuroscience*, **35**, 57–67.

Merker, B. (2013). Cortical gamma oscillations: the functional key is activation, not cognition. *Neuroscience and Biobehavioral Reviews*, **37**, 401–417.

Murphy, D. (2006). *Psychiatry in the Scientific Image*. Boston, MA: MIT Press.

Nelson, B., **Fornito, A.**, **Harrison, B.J.**, et al. (2009). A disturbed sense of self in the psychosis prodrome: linking phenomenology and neurobiology. *Neuroscience and Biobehavioral Reviews*, **33**, 807–817.

Nelson, B., **Parnas, J.**, and **Sass, L.A.** (2014). Disturbance of minimal self (ipseity) in schizophrenia: clarification and current status. *Schizophrenia Bulletin*, **40**, 479–482.

Nelson, B., **Thompson, A.**, and **Yung, A.R.** (2012). Basic self-disturbance predicts psychosis onset in the ultra high risk for psychosis "prodromal" population. *Schizophrenia Bulletin*, **38**, 1277–1287.

Network and Pathway Analysis Subgroup of Psychiatric Genomics Consortium. (2015). Psychiatric genome-wide association study analyses implicate neuronal, immune and histone pathways. *Nature Neuroscience*, **18**, 199–209.

Parnas, J. (2008). Varieties of phenomenology: on description, understanding, and explanation in psychiatry. In K.S. Kendler and J. Parnas (eds.) *Philosophical Issues in Psychiatry*, pp. 239–278. Baltimore, MD: Johns Hopkins University Press.

Parnas, J. (2011). A disappearing heritage: the clinical core of schizophrenia. *Schizophrenia Bulletin*, **37**, 1121–1130.

Parnas, J., **Moller, P.**, **Kircher, T.**, et al. (2005). EASE: examination of anomalous self-experience. *Psychopathology*, **38**, 236–258.

Parnas, J., **Sass, L.** and **Zahavi, D.** (2013). Rediscovering psychopathology: the epistemology and phenomenology of the pyschiatric object. *Schizophrenia Bulletin*, **39**, 270–277.

Ripke, S., **Neale B.M.**, **Corvin, A.**, et al. (2014). Biological insights from 108 schizophrenia-associated genetic loci. *Nature*, **511**(7510), 421–427.

Ritsner, M.S. and **Gottesman, I.G.** (2011). The schizophrenia construct after 100 years of challenges. In M.S. Ritsner (ed) *Handbook of Schizophrenia Spectrum Disorders, Volume I Conceptual Issues and Neurobiological Advances*, pp. 1–44. Dordrecht: Springer.

Robinson, J.J., **Wagner, N.F.**, and **Northoff, G.** (2016). Is the sense of agency in schizophrenia influenced by resting-state variation in self-referential regions of the brain? *Schizophrenia Bulletin*, **42**, 270–276.

Ruzzo, E.K. and **Geschwind, D.H.** (2016). Schizophrenia genetics complements its mechanistic understanding. *Nature Neuroscience*, **19**, 523–525.

Sin, J. (2007). *Essays in the Philosophy of Psychiatry.* PhD dissertation, University of Massachusetts.

Schaffner, K.F. (2012). A philosophical overview of the problems of validity for psychiatric disorders. In K.S. Kendler and J. Parnas (eds.) *Philosophical Issues in Psychiatry II: Nosology*, pp. 167–189. Oxford, UK: Oxford University Press.

Schaffner, K.F. (2016). Variation and validation: the example of schizophrenia. *World Psychiatry*, **15**, 39–40.

Sekar, A., Bialas, A.R., de Rivera, H., et al. (2016). Schizophrenia risk from complex variation of complement component 4. *Nature*, **530**(7589), 177–183.

Sullivan, J.A. (2014). Stabilizing mental disorders: prospects and problems. In H. Kincaid and J.A. Sullivan (eds.) *Classifying Psychopathology*, pp. 195–208. Cambridge, MA: MIT Press.

Tabb, K. (2015). Psychiatric progress and the assumption of diagnostic discrimination. *Philosophy of Science*, **82**, 1047–1058.

Tsou, J. (2008). *The Reality and Classification of Mental Disorders: Issues in the philosophy of psychiatry.* PhD dissertation, The University of Chicago.

Tsou, J. (2015). DSM-5 and psychiatry's second revolution: descriptive vs. theoretical approaches to psychiatric classification. In S. Demazeux and P. Singy (eds.) *The DSM-5 in Perspective: Philosophical reflections on the psychiatric Babel*, pp. 43–62. Dordrecht: Springer.

Weinberger, D.R., and **Harrison, P.J.** (2011). *Schizophrenia*, 3rd edn. Chichester, UK: Wiley-Blackwell.

Wimsatt, W.C. (2007). *Re-engineering Philosophy for Limited Beings: Piecewise approximations to reality.* Cambridge, MA: Harvard University Press.

Woo, T.U., Spencer, K., and **McCarley, R.W.** (2010). Gamma oscillation deficits and the onset and early progression of schizophrenia. *Harvard Review of Psychiatry*, **18**, 173–189.

Chapter 42

Comments on "Causal pathways, random walks, and tortuous paths: Moving from the descriptive to the etiological in psychiatry"

Hasok Chang

42.1 Introduction

It might be taken as common sense that in psychiatry (and in medicine and science much more generally) it is good to move from the descriptive to the etiological. Our knowledge would thereby be made deeper, more secure, and more efficacious. But the matter is not so simple as that, as Kathryn Tabb and Kenneth F. Schaffner rightly point out in Chapter 41 of this book.

Tabb and Schaffner offer two proposals that I can readily agree with (section 41.4.1). First, practitioners should value the "*most robust* model that each can defend as reliable and preliminarily valid *for their particular purposes*, and then deploy it extensively to see if they become 'rich.'" Second, "reasonably strong overlaps" in patterns "should be taken as a sign that the representation is especially worth further pursuit." In fact, I agree so much with their pragmatist and pluralist orientations that I have very little to add in that regard. One question I have is whether their two proposals are really distinct from each other, as the notion of robustness (taken from Wimsatt), as the "coincidence of boundaries" (section 41.3), seems to be quite similar to the idea of "overlap." But this does not affect the validity of their proposal(s).

What I would like to add is a few more considerations intended to help sharpen and develop their proposals further. Some back-to-basics moves are useful here, I think, as is often the case in philosophy.

42.2 A realist worry about seeking the cause of non-existent things

One very basic point is that the move to the etiological only makes sense if the descriptive category in question is taken to be pointing at something real. What would be the wisdom in seeking the cause of something, if that something is not real? In most people's conceptions, the notion of a "cause" presumes a high degree of realism; it would make no sense to say that A causes B, if either A or B were non-existent. Therefore, an attempt to move to the etiological without first securing the reality of the descriptive category in question runs the risk of entering into a fruitless wild goose-chase. To stay with Tabb and Schaffner's principal example: if there is no real condition behind the label "schizophrenia," then what good does it do to spend a lot of money and time looking for its genetic, neurological, environmental, or any other kind of cause? If Bentall et al. (1988) and others are right that the concept of schizophrenia should be abandoned altogether, then the search for its etiology should also cease.

This consideration reveals an interesting and important tension among the enemies of the descriptive approach of the *Diagnostic and Statistical Manual of Mental Disorders* (DSM). On one side, some DSM opponents deny that the symptom-based DSM categories point to anything real. On the other side, other DSM opponents insist that the DSM categories should be understood in a reductive way by reference to material processes. These two positions are at least not straightforwardly compatible with each other.

I think there needs to be some patience concerning etiological work. There is probably some need for more descriptive work, to check if the descriptive categories will settle down well enough for etiological research to make sense. The stability of a concept does not guarantee its reality, but it should be regarded as an insufficient but necessary condition for reality. Another way to put the general point would be to say that a concept, a construct, or a measure should be shown to have a high degree of reliability at least, before we try to investigate its validity. This does not mean that all etiological work should be postponed, but it does mean that it needs to be entered into with care and circumspection.

There are two clarifications I must add at this point. The priority of descriptive over etiological work, which I am arguing for here, is a separate and complementary point to Tabb and Schaffner's argument that the descriptive categories may remain more *useful* than etiological ones for certain purposes. And my view that reliability needs to be established before validity is sought does not contradict their proposal that (predictive) validity within a given domain should be prioritized over broad cross-domain reliability (section 41.4.1).

42.3 **Epistemic iteration and evolving meaning**

The foregoing discussion is too crude. In order to introduce more subtlety, let us think not in terms of existence, but of meaning. Any attempt to *redefine* a category is necessarily based on an acceptance of the meaningfulness of that category to begin with. And if there is a reasonable *debate* going on about definitions, that means there must be some degree of agreement about the basic meaning of the category. So when one says to another "schizophrenia isn't *this*, it's *that*," that means there is some prior agreed notion of "schizophrenia" that allows an agreed identification of at least a sufficient number of clear cases. (This even applies to the statement "there is no such thing as schizophrenia" because otherwise the statement itself would be meaningless, unless what one means is that when people use the word "schizophrenia" they do not mean anything consistent.)

This means that any process of redefinition (as opposed to a complete obliteration of the concept) is a process of epistemic iteration (see my Chapter 29 in this book). Typically, there is something that we do commonly mean by the concept in question, which enables the whole discourse to begin with; that prior concept needs to be recognized and respected. In the case of schizophrenia, what is this starting point? It must be something like the DSM-IV or DSM-5 concept, or perhaps a core set of symptoms smaller and more vague than the list given in either of those DSM editions. And is it even possible that the old Kraepelin or Bleuler concept of schizophrenia still lives on, in an iteratively modified form, in our current concept of schizophrenia?

Similarly, seeking the etiology of a disease means accepting the cogency of the descriptive disease-category in question in a provisional way. Tabb and Schaffner rightly note that "it is the DSM (and related ICD) criteria from DSM-IV that were largely the basis of the GWAS etiological proposals, since it was that set of schizophrenia criteria that were used to select the patient populations" for the GWAS (section 41.4.1). However, if the etiological work is successful, it is very likely that the descriptive concept will be modified accordingly. This indicates that successful etiological work is, again, a process of epistemic iteration. An uncertain starting point is accepted in order to have some basis for inquiry; if the inquiry is successful, it is liable to introduce changes in its own starting point.

It is possible that later in the iterative process the descriptive notion would become wholly redefined and regulated by reference to its etiology. Such reversals of primitiveness or fundamentality are in fact quite common in epistemic iteration. For example, warmth might initially be defined through our bodily sensation, but later in the iterative development of the temperature concept, the thermometer (or even a theory) plays the definitive role, and our sensations are overruled or corrected if they do not agree with the verdict of the thermometer (see Chang 2004, pp. 47–48). So one day we may identify such clear genetic (or other) causes of schizophrenia that we make those traits definitive of the disease. That would change the very meaning of "schizophrenia," and what used to be considered perfectly good instantiations of it may be ruled as something else that only presents like schizophrenia, and perhaps be billed as "pseudo-" or "quasi-schizophrenia." In such cases of etiological triumph, the symptoms would be regarded only as, literally, symptoms (i.e., indications) of something that underlie them. But that would ultimately be a conventional choice, ruled by considerations of utility rather than truth, as Tabb and Schaffner note.

42.4 **The primacy of description**

Having noted the iterative aspect of the developmental process at issue, we can now tackle the question of whether and how one may sensibly go into the etiological, before the descriptive is secure. I would start with the rather obvious suggestion that etiological investigations should be directed to the most stable descriptive categories. This merely echoes Tabb and Schaffner's proposals. But there are some quandaries involved in putting this unexceptionable advice into practice. In trying to understand any complex phenomena, there are many relevant levels of description and a large number of inter-level connections that could be entertained. How does one know where to start in making multi-level investigations, which are bound to be unmanageable unless one has some clear guidelines at the outset? My sense is that it would be more plausible to start with thorough descriptive work at each level aimed at revealing the most stable descriptive categories, which would then constitute plausible variables for multi-level models.

In this context, I believe that it would be advisable to take another look at latent class analysis (LCA), which seeks "categories underlying clusters of reported symptoms, signs and history items in a large group of psychiatric patients"; on the basis of the clustering of observable factors, LCA "creates non-observational, higher level or 'latent' classes" (section 41.2.1). Tabb and Schaffner note that no definitive results have been obtained by this method as yet, and that Kenneth Kendler, who had led a pioneering LCA study published in 1998, "has expressed doubts about the implications" of that study (section 41.2.1). But might a slightly different approach not have some promise? What if we took all the various descriptive symptoms and signs of mental illnesses, and asked which of these are found most reliably correlated with each other, and then sought etiological explanations for those clusters? Finding etiological explanations, in practice, would mean finding connections between the symptom clusters and similar property clusters to be found at other levels (such as genomics and neurophysiology) that are generally considered to be realms in which causes of mental traits and events lie. However, it is not necessary to subscribe to reductionist materialism here, and the causes of symptom clusters may also be sought in event clusters in the upbringing of the person, or property clusters in the environment. Another valid way to see the general situation would be that we are generally seeking inter-level connections, whether or not it is plausible to interpret them as causal/etiological. The contrast between the descriptive and the etiological may be somewhat misplaced. Etiological thinking is not opposed to descriptive thinking; rather, etiology concerns a particular type of linkage between the description of symptoms and the description of factors existing at another level.

Taking sufficiently successful descriptive work as a precondition for launching etiological work can lead to a mode of investigation that is both focused and systematic at once. Such a method of proceeding would be in clear contrast to the aimless search for connections exemplified by GWAS, which I think amounts to an over-hasty attempt to find useful inter-level connections without sufficient descriptive preparation at each level. Another interesting contrast is with the kind of premature theorizing seen in the Lewis line of work on schizophrenia, which starts from a seemingly unjustified sense that cognitive deficits form the "core domain" of schizophrenia, which is then linked up with gamma-frequency oscillations in the brain (section 41.2.3). We can also avoid the one overly restrictive feature that I see in Tabb and Schaffner's proposals, namely their seemingly exclusive concern with how different analytical frameworks divide up populations (section 41.3). Conceptual clusters consisting of biochemical processes, intercellular interactions, etc. may not easily map on to sets of whole individual organisms in which they take place. Generally speaking, an open-minded search for inter-level connections among stable descriptive clusters would seems to be a reasonable way forward.

References

Bentall, R.P., Jackson, H.F., and **Pilgrim, D.** (1988). Abandoning the concept of schizophrenia: some implications of validity arguments for psychological research into psychotic phenomena. *British Journal of Clinical Psychology*, **27**, 303–324.

Chang, H. (2004). *Inventing Temperature: Measurement and scientific progress.* New York: Oxford University Press.

Section 15

Progress in psychiatric research

Chapter 43

Introduction to "What is progress in psychiatric research?"

Kenneth S. Kendler

Stephan Heckers is well qualified to take on the task of this essay—to try to define progress in psychiatric research. He was educated in Germany and hence is able to read the primary sources of the most relevant historical material in the original language—since the modern paradigm of psychiatric research is largely a product of late nineteeth-century German neuropsychiatry. He studied philosophy before deciding to go into medicine and then psychiatry. He has been a biologically oriented researcher with a focus on schizophrenia but is also interested in "big picture" questions about our field.

The history of psychiatry is particularly rich (although some might say chaotic) in the number of research paradigms that have been proposed to organize scientific efforts. In my view, that is because so many levels of science are of relevance to risk for psychiatric disorders. And, as we often see in science, each subfield is naturally inclined to see its discipline as instantiating the most important approach—the key to understanding psychiatric illness. And so we have orientations that focus on, among other areas, molecular neuroscience, systems neuroscience, neuropsychology, personality, psychodynamic processes, cognitive constructs, and social and cultural factors.

Hecker's focus, however, is narrower—largely on an exposition and then evaluation of the dominant Kraepelinian paradigm that has had its greatest impact in the areas of severe psychiatric illness (especially schizophrenia and major mood disorders) that were the major foci of Kraepelin's nosologic theorizing.

He lucidly outlines the three key elements of Kraepelin's paradigm:

- Clinical features, experiment, and anatomy are validators of psychiatric diagnoses.
- Validators of psychiatric diagnoses converge on natural disease units.
- There is a hierarchy of validators, with course and outcome being the most important.

He notes the rapid growth of potential validators for psychiatric diagnoses with the latest iteration—using a framework of antecedent, concurrent, and predictive validators—playing a rather important role in the fifth edition of the *Diagnostic and Statistical Manual of Mental Disorders* (DSM-5).

Heckers then gives us a concise typology of the four broad negative responses to the Kraepelinian paradigm, which I might briefly summarize as:

- Validators don't converge.
- It should only be symptoms.
- Person not diagnosis centered" (aka idiographic rather than nomothetic).
- Brain up rather than symptoms down.

Heckers is overall more positive and feels that Kraepelin's paradigm is still of substantial value but in need of some refinement. He focuses on the central concept of validators and proposes to determine the strength of evidence for each validator for each diagnosis, and to build a consensus for the value for particular validators. He quite correctly notes that the strengths of individual validators are likely not constant across some disorders. This complexity has not been recognized in traditional discussions about the application of validators to DSM decisions. The question of the value of individual validators is of great interest and sits, as I have suggested in the past, at a crossroads between science and values. That is, the value of an individual validator is inextricably linked with the question: what do we want this diagnosis to do? If our goal is to focus on predicting treatment response versus maximal correlation with molecular genetic markers, we might not end up with the same diagnostic criteria. But how do we chose between these two perspectives? Is this in any sense an empirical question or is it solely one of values?

Heckers ends up broadly endorsing Kraepelin. He writes:

> Kraepelin's paradigm still has great value today. It has been the main engine of the psychiatric research agenda for more than 100 years.

Hecker's essay is a thoughtful bird's eye view of the field of psychiatry circa 2015 given by an individual who works both in the trenches as a clinician and as a researcher and is able to step back and look at the broad historical trends of our field and the conceptual issues underlying them.

Chapter 44

What is progress in psychiatric research?

Stephan Heckers

44.1 Introduction

Psychiatric research emerged from the enlightened viewpoint of the natural sciences in the middle of the nineteenth century (Schmitt 1983). Psychiatrists defined diseases in their patients and began to study the mechanism of illness in the laboratory. This was a clear departure from the work of the alienists, who had taken care of the mentally ill in asylum settings that typically contained little to no medical research infrastructure. It also started the debate about the scientific status of psychiatry. Brain researchers argued for psychiatry as a clinical neuroscience discipline, but most clinicians had little interest in reducing abnormal mental states to the brain (Engstrom 2004). This debate continues today (Luhrmann 2001).

Here I review progress in the understanding and explanation of psychiatric disorders. Scientific progress is normative: through a competition of paradigms we improve our understanding of nature. The scientific method of hypothesis testing includes failures and temporary setbacks, but, in the long run, we are making progress. The usually iterative process can be disrupted by innovation, which often accelerates the scientific discovery. Less frequent are radical departures from the status quo, when an entirely new paradigm reshapes the scientific discourse.

The nosology developed by Emil Kraepelin in the last century of the nineteenth century was the first and remains the most influential paradigm change in psychiatric research (Heckers 2008). In this chapter I review how our current research strategy continues to be shaped by Kraepelin's paradigm and what attempts have been made to change, replace, or reject it. I conclude that progress in psychiatric research will depend on a new strategy for psychiatric research. I will not review the full spectrum of psychiatric research, but focus mainly on psychotic disorders. Kraepelin formulated his scientific agenda in response to his evolving nosology of psychotic and affective disorders: the former was defined by a chemical etiology and a neural disease mechanism, whereas the latter was defined by longitudinal observations of mood swings (depression and mania).

44.2 The current research paradigm

Psychiatric researchers are still living in a Kraepelinian world (Berrios and Hauser 1988, Jablensky 2007). We have changed the names of his two main diagnostic constructs: dementia praecox is now known as schizophrenia and manic-depressive illness as bipolar disorder. And we do no longer support his conservative politics and naturalist philosophy (Engstrom 2004, Hoff 1995). But we continue to embrace his nosology, which is built on three main axioms:

- Clinical features, experiment, and anatomy are validators of psychiatric diagnoses.
- Validators of psychiatric diagnoses converge on natural disease units.
- There is a hierarchy of validators, with course and outcome being the most important.

In addition, Kraepelin's paradigm follows the medical model, which rests on the notion that the unique experience of a person can be reduced to a clinical diagnosis. In technical terms, a psychiatric researcher can replace the idiographic approach to the individual patient with a nomothetic approach to the definition of cases. Here I briefly review the relevance of Kraepelin's paradigm for current psychiatric research.

Kraepelin's choice of validators (clinical features, experiment, and anatomy, see Figure 44.1a) is shaped by his own experiences as a psychiatric researcher (Kraepelin 1987). Early in his career, he worked in the anatomical laboratory of Bernhard von Gudden. But he recognized that he was not suited for work in the morgue and at the microscope and he moved on to experimental psychology. He joined the laboratory of Wilhelm Wundt, who established the first academic department of psychology at Leipzig University in the 1870s (Steinberg 2001). He continued to support anatomical and experimental research throughout his career: he hired Alois Alzheimer to establish an anatomical laboratory in his department and he pursued psychological experiments himself (Hippius et al. 2008).

With the development of new research methods, better diagnostic approaches, and successful treatments, the list of validators grew. Robins and Guze extended Kraepelin's list of validators to five: Clinical description, laboratory studies, delimitation from other disorders, follow-up study, and family study (Robins and Guze 1970). Kendler updated the list and grouped them into antecedent, concurrent, and predictive validators (Kendler 1980, 1990) (Figure 44.1b). These validators remain the foundation of our psychiatric classification system and serve as benchmarks for any changes of the fifth edition of the *Diagnostic and Statistical Manual of Mental Disorders* (DSM-5) (Appelbaum, Chapter 47 in this book).

Clinical features are essential for any psychiatric research agenda. Even biological psychiatry, which has reduced the role of psychopathology (Andreasen 2007), begins with the definition of psychiatric signs and symptoms. Among the clinical features, course and outcome have a unique status (Heckers 2014). The longitudinal assessment of signs and symptoms adds antecedent risk factor and outcome predictors to the traditionally cross-sectional definition of psychiatric disorders. For example, the clinical features of depression, mania, or psychosis can be assessed in a clinical interview. But through longitudinal assessments we have defined bipolar disorder and schizoaffective disorder, which provide a better prediction of course and outcome than the cross-sectional diagnosis of a single episode (Goodwin and Jamison 1990).

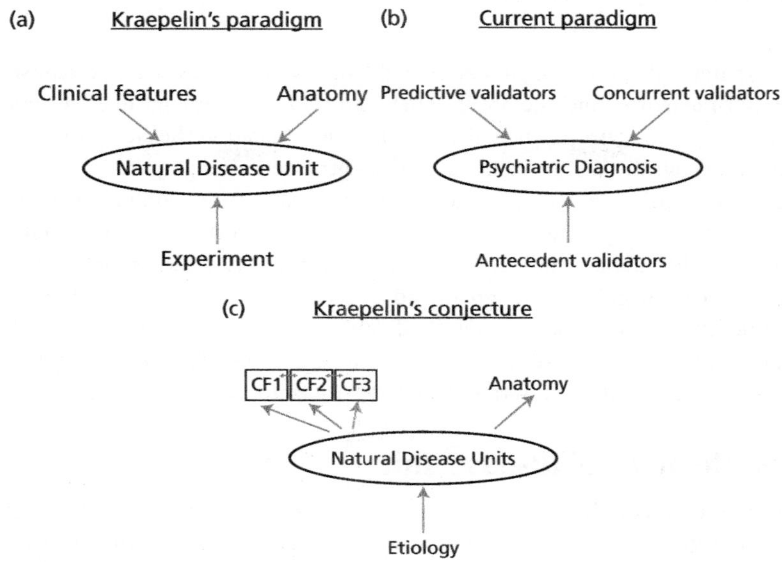

Figure 44.1 Psychiatric research paradigms.

Figure 44.1a Kraepelin's paradigm

Kraepelin defined psychiatric disorders based on their clinical features. But he proposed that anatomical and experimental studies will converge on the same diagnostic construct that he termed natural disease unit ("natürliche Krankheitseinheit").

Figure 44.1b Current paradigm

The current psychiatry research paradigm has taken an "atheoretical" stance: different sets of validators converge on diagnostic constructs. Ideally, the evidence is strong for all validators, but that is rarely the case. For DSM5, some validators were ranked higher than others (see text).

Figure 44.1c Kraepelin's conjecture

Kraepelin proposed the natural disease units as an epistemological tool for psychiatry research. The direction of the arrows indicate the underlying structure (compare to figures 1a and 1b, where the validators point to the diagnostic construct).

Etiological factors (e.g., genes or environmental stressors) generate a disease process in the brain. Anatomical methods (e.g., neuroimaging, post-mortem) can detect the structural and functional abnormalities in the brain that are the consequences of the etiological factors. At the same time, clinical features are the observable signs of an abnormal mental state caused by the etiological factors. While Kraepelin did identify distinct clinical features (CF1, CF2, CF3) for most psychiatric disorders, he did not propose any interactions between these clinical features (see: Borsboom chapter in this book).

Kraepelin proposed the following abnormalities for dementia praecox (now known as schizophrenia): An autointoxication by a yet unknown chemical substance (etiology) leads to selective destruction of pyramidal cells in the upper three layers of the cerebral cortex (anatomy), leading to several clinical features, of which avolition and poor outcome are the defining features.

Experimental approaches to psychopathology were already firmly established during Kraepelin's time (Steinberg 2001). This tradition was continued for many years by clinical neuropsychologists and has culminated in the current research agendas of cognitive neuroscience and psychiatric neuroimaging.

Using Kraepelin's paradigm of describing clinical features, conducting experiments, and studying anatomy we have made progress. Post-mortem research has identified reliable abnormalities in the brains of psychiatric patients (Berretta et al. 2015). Molecular genetics has greatly advanced the psychiatric research agenda (Kendler 2013). Finally, a more nuanced appreciation of non-genetic factors has come from studies of environmental biological (e.g., drugs of abuse, diet) and non-biological (e.g., psychological trauma, stress) risk factors of mental illness.

44.3 **The natural disease unit**

The central axiom of Kraepelin's scientific agenda is his claim that the three validators converge (Figure 44.1c). He conjectured that validators of a psychiatric diagnosis converge because they share a common biological substrate. Kraepelin defined psychiatric disorders as natural entities that can be discovered with the scientific method. In the end, nature will reveal the disorders to the clinicians and researchers who search for them. Rather than simply testing for a statistical relationship of validators with a diagnostic construct, this view asserts that the *natural disease uni*t defines the brain correlates and clinical features of a psychiatric condition. This is indicated in Figure 44.1c by the reversal of the arrows in Figure 44.1a: they are now pointing away from the natural disease unit.

Kraepelin's paradigm allows for a research strategy of "divide and conquer." As long as we can operationalize the diagnosis of a psychiatric disorder, we can then study the etiology, disease mechanism, course, and outcome. For example, a post-mortem researcher or a geneticist can make progress by studying just the biological sample of a person, without getting lost in the details of the person's experiences. The first-person experience or the phenomenology of psychiatric disorders are no longer essential for the scientific inquiry. This sets Kraepelin apart from many psychiatrists who remain conflicted and ambivalent about the value of psychiatric diagnoses in the care of their patients (Luhrmann 2001, Ghaemi 2003). It allowed Kraepelin to articulate a strong vision for psychiatry research (Hippius et al. 2008). No other psychiatric research agenda has generated the same degree of enthusiasm and support.

44.4 **Hierarchy of validators**

Kraepelin also formulated a hierarchy of validators. Most clinicians will focus on the clinical features of a psychiatric disorder. Researchers, on the other hand, may focus on one aspect of the disorder (e.g., genetics, clinical trials, neuroimaging) and develop a highly specialized expertise about psychiatric disorders.

Kraepelin considered course and outcome to be the primary validator of psychiatric disorders. Such a hierarchy of validators is a value judgment, with implications not only for the research agenda, but also for the patient and society at large. A rank order of psychiatric diagnoses, based on course and outcome, limits the patient's autonomy for the conditions defined by poor outcome. This hierarchy contributes to the stigma of mental illness. The recovery movement of psychiatric patients can be seen as a rejection of such a hierarchy and the paternalistic viewpoint of psychiatry (Frese et al. 2009).

There have been various responses to Kraepelin's paradigm. Here I distinguish proposals to change, but hold on to, the nosology, from those that reject it.

44.5 **Changing the paradigm**

Eugen Bleuler was concerned about a nihilistic attitude associated with the term *dementia praecox* and suggested *group of schizophrenias* as an alternative (Bleuler 1911, Scharfetter 2005) With this change of names, Bleuler also challenged two of Kraepelin's core axioms. First, patients with the same clinical features can have markedly different course and outcome of their illness. Second, he moved the primary focus from course and outcome to the clinical features and their psychological explanation. His four As (affect, ambivalence, association, autism) were an initial effort to bring order to psychiatric nosology by clinical observation, not through experiments and post-mortem studies. After his retirement, Kraepelin acknowledged some of these concerns and expressed his own doubts about the ability to distinguish schizophrenia from bipolar disorder (Kraepelin 1920). But he never abandoned his scientific agenda of studying *natural disease units*.

Social dysfunction remains one of the defining criteria of schizophrenia (criterion B in the DSM-5). There have been several prominent proposals to define a more severe subtype of schizophrenia, based on clinical features, laboratory data, and family history. In fact, Guze and Robins, who introduced Kraepelin's paradigm into American psychiatry, concluded that poor-outcome schizophrenia is separate from the rest of schizophrenia (Robins and Guze 1970). Other prominent examples of this approach are the deficit syndrome of schizophrenia (Carpenter et al. 1988) and the Kraepelinian subtype of schizophrenia (Keefe et al. 1991).

Over the years, the term schizophrenia became associated with the stigma that Bleuler wanted to avoid. For example, the Japanese Psychiatric Association voted in 2002 to replace the name schizophrenia with "integration disorder" (*togo shitcho sho*) (Sato 2006, Lieberman and First 2007).

In addition to name changes, several new entities were defined to compete with the prominent role of schizophrenia in psychiatric nosology. Kasanin introduced "schizoaffective disorder" in 1933 to characterize a group of high-functioning outpatients, who presented with the clinical features of schizophrenia, but also struggled with mood symptoms and did well in the long run (Kasanin 1933). While the reliability of this diagnosis is weak, it has been embraced by patients and clinicians as a less malign diagnosis for a psychotic person and by geneticists, who see great value in the broader phenotype for gene discovery (Hamshere et al. 2009, Heckers 2009).

An even more fundamental reconceptualization of the current psychotic/mood disorder dichotomy came from Leonhard's classification of non-affective and affective psychoses (Leonhard 1957). He defined several intermediate conditions based on their clinical presentation, course, outcome, and family history.

These attempts of changing diagnostic labels or replacing simple dichotomies with a more complex nosology do not challenge Kraepelin's research agenda. They remain committed to the idea that psychiatric disorders can be validated by clinical features, experiment, and anatomy.

44.6 **Rejecting the paradigm**

Kraepelin's "natural disease unit" paradigm was never universally accepted. Here I distinguish four different viewpoints in psychiatric research that reject his research agenda. The first position challenges the idea of the natural disease unit; the second asserts that clinical features should be the sole object of inquiry in psychiatric research. The third and fourth positions replace the diagnosis at the center of the scientific inquiry with either the person or the brain.

The most fundamental rejection of Kraepelin's paradigm is the notion that validators do not converge. Hoche (1912) made this argument early and became Kraepelin's main critic in German psychiatry. He favored a symptom-based research agenda and wrote that Kraepelin was "barking up the wrong tree" with his natural disease units (Hoche 1912). If validators do not converge, then we need to redesign psychiatric research and need to identify a principal validator (or at least a limited set). For the clinician Hoche, this was the syndrome of clinical signs and personal experiences. For molecular geneticists, it has become the genetic risk factor, which can be linked to more than one disorder (Craddock and Owen 2005).

Another fundamental rejection of the current research agenda can be summed up with the axiom: "There are only symptoms." Richard Bentall made this case for psychotic disorders (Bentall 2005). He accepts that symptoms such as delusions or hallucinations can be studied scientifically (including studies of their neural mechanism), but he insists that such research cannot establish a diagnostic class (Bentall 2006). Related to this is the growing concern that we cannot easily separate mental illness from the spectrum of normal mental states and behavior (van Os and Linscott 2012).

Beyond these two challenges is the fundamental rejection of any research that focuses on cases rather than persons. It is one of psychiatry's goals to understand the human condition, and many practitioners and some researchers see the individual person at the center of any psychiatric research agenda (Luhrmann 2001). Psychiatric phenomenology has focused on the first-person experience and has developed sophisticated models (including specialized terminology) to study it scientifically. For some, the phenomenological perspective is superior to any other in the understanding and explaining mental illness (Jaspers 1913, Parnas and Bovet 1995) Other have concluded that several perspectives are needed to capture psychiatric problems and that a person cannot be reduced to a diagnosis (McHugh and Slavney 1983).

Finally, some psychiatric researchers want a revolution. They have become impatient with the laborious and slow process of validating psychiatric diagnoses. They argue that we need to study the brain first, before we can explain normal and abnormal mental states. In short, psychiatry needs to be replaced by clinical neuroscience (Reynolds et al. 2009). This has been developed as a research agenda, with implications for study design and setting priorities for research (Cuthbert 2015).

44.7 **Hypothesis testing and experimental designs**

Kraepelin's paradigm has been challenged and rejected, but it has not been replaced. We continue to design experiments and studies based on the dogma of the natural disease unit.

How can we advance psychiatric research? What experiments and study designs are needed to refine or replace the current paradigm? Here I briefly review several approaches to strong hypothesis testing. They have focused on the clinical features, outcome, and etiology of a psychiatric disorder. With each of these efforts, one set of validators is studied in detail, which then yields a dichotomous or dimensional definition of subtypes. The diagnostic subtypes are then tested for their ability to increase of the validity compared to the original disorder.

The polythetic definition of many psychiatric disorders results in considerable clinical heterogeneity of patients within a diagnostic class. This has led some researchers to conclude that we need to define a more homogeneous subgroup of patients in order to uncover the etiology and disease mechanism (Figure 44.2). Examples for such an approach are Carpenter's deficit syndrome of schizophrenia (Carpenter et al. 1988) and Liddle's three-factor model of psychosis (Liddle et al. 1992).

A very powerful approach is the definition of subgroups based on treatment response. For example, two groups of patients with the same diagnosis,

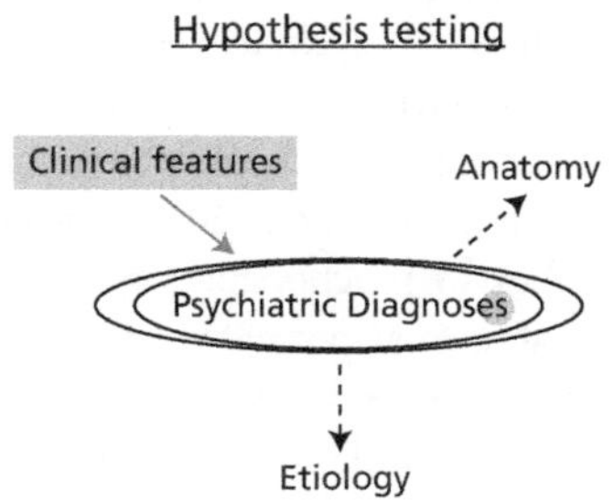

Figure 44.2 Hypothesis testing in psychiatric research.

There is no a-priori hierarchy of validators for psychiatric diagnoses: the different validators shown in Figure 44.1b have all equally strong connections to the diagnostic construct.

Figure 44.2 shows the process of testing hypotheses in psychiatric research that can increase the validity of the diagnoses. It shows only one of many examples: distinguishing clinical features into subgroups/subtypes. Similar figures could be shown for efforts to distinguish anatomical features or etiological factors.

The process of hypothesis testing shown here begins with a strong hypothesis that clinical features need to be separated into distinct subgroups (e.g., deficit and non-deficit schizophrenia, see Carpenter et al. 1988). Then the researcher has to work backwards to the diagnostic construct and explore different etiological pathways and anatomical patterns (please note that the grey arrow indicates the start of the search and the dashed arrows indicate the hypotheses). A possible outcome of such hypothesis testing can be the broadening or widening of the diagnostic construct (indicated by the two oval shapes), including the proposal to add additional diagnoses.

a treatment-responsive and a treatment-resistant group, can be studied for any difference in brain structure/function and genetic risk factors. Some have proposed that treatment response can be the defining feature of a diagnostic class (e.g., positive benzodiapzepine challenge test in patients with catatonia; Taylor and Fink 2003) or can dissect behaviorally similar phenotypes (e.g., panic disorder responds to imipramine, but generalized anxiety does not; Klein 1964).

Significant effort has been invested into the study of biomarkers that can define etiological subtypes. A compelling recent example is NMDA-receptor autoantibody encephalitis. Patients with such a condition can present with an acute and fulminant onset of psychosis, often with prominent psychomotor abnormalities (Kayser and Dalmau 2011). There is "face validity" for such a secondary psychosis syndrome: the acute onset of psychosis in a patient with a highly specific perturbation of NMDA receptors provides a compelling example for glutamatergic dysfunction as a mechanism of psychosis. Other well-known examples are drug-induced psychotic disorders and psychoses secondary to medical and neurological disorders (Coleman and Gillberg 1996).

44.8 **Where do we go from here?**

Psychiatric researchers need to embrace the complexity of their task. Progress has been slow, especially at the conceptual level of defining the nature of mental illness, resulting in polarized views of psychiatry (Eisenberg 1986).

One first step forward is the growing awareness that we have ignored the clinical complexity of psychiatric diagnoses. They need to be deconstructed at a more granular level (Andreasen 2007, Tamminga et al. 2010). This can be achieved through more dimensional approaches to psychopathology (Barch et al. 2013). Simple dichotomies (normal versus abnormal, present versus not present) are not sufficient to capture clinical phenotypes. We need to supplement current categorical assessments with dimensional rating in our daily clinical practice (Ritsner et al. 2013).

Second, we need to acknowledge that the strength of validators varies within and across psychiatric diagnoses. It is unlikely that the same hierarchy of validators will be appropriate for all psychiatric disorders. For example, cognitive disorders with clear evidence of neurodegenerative changes in the brain need to be studied differently than disorders that can be diagnosed in early childhood and yet differently than abnormalities of personal characteristics that lead to strive and suffering in adulthood.

Third, we need to develop a much broader definition of disease course and outcome. The clinico-pathological method of correlating clinical features with biological outcomes (including those defined at autopsy) remains a gold standard for medical, including psychiatric, research. But we have to develop more complex, multidimensional outcome measures that are relevant for daily living. This can include exciting new opportunities of defining phenotypes derived from electronic medical records (Hebbring et al. 2015) and the application of modern technology in the sampling and analysis of first-person experiences, using mobile technology (Marzano et al. 2015). This will be far superior to the current standard of assessing psychopathology during a clinic visit or a psychiatric hospitalization.

Fourth, we will continue to see remarkable progress in the study of genetic and non-genetic risk factors for the development of psychiatric disorders. Polygenic and environmental risk scores and their potential interactions will remain a fruitful area of investigations (Kendler 2016). We will have entered the era of personalized medicine (or precision medicine) when we can use such risk scores to predict the therapeutic benefit and adverse responses to treatment (Jameson and Longo 2015).

I propose these three steps for the evaluation of each psychiatric diagnosis:

1 Determine the strength of evidence for each validator.

2 Rank the strength of evidence for each diagnosis.

3 Build consensus for the value for validators.

Testing the strength of evidence is well established for some areas of medical research. For example, evidence-based medicine approaches are readily available for the assessment of therapeutic interventions. Randomized clinical trials are the gold standard and we can distill the evidence through structured reviews and meta-analyses. But how do we assess the evidence for other validators of psychiatric diagnoses? For example, it is not trivial to condense the vast clinical literature into quantitative measures of psychopathology. Different schools of psychopathology define the same person differently.

Even more challenging is the second step. We have not developed a metric to measure the strength of all validators. How can we evaluate the strength of evidence across all of psychiatric research? For example, the drug discovery researcher will use a different metric than a population health manager or a relative who wants to relate to the first-person experience of a person struggling with mental illness.

We need to ask some fundamental questions: Is there an a-priori hierarchy of validators? What values make us select one over the other? Is there one that is closer to causality?

We do not know the answers to these questions for many of the psychiatric diagnosis. We have to acknowledge that the rank order of validators and the strength of validators differs across diagnoses. For example, some diagnoses are more closely linked to changes in brain structure and function than others.

Finally, we need to build consensus in the evaluation of validators. Kraepelin's paradigm was shaped by the politics and philosophy of Imperial Germany (Engstrom 2004). We have abandoned this, but are still holding on to a paternalistic attitude towards patients. We need to embrace the input from patient advocacy groups to develop a model that allows for recovery and self-efficacy, yet holds on to the notion that psychiatric disorders can be studied scientifically (Ennis and Wykes 2013).

Several ongoing debates about the diagnostic criteria of psychiatric diagnoses in the DSM-5 are the result of conflicting value judgments regarding validators. Some value clinical utility more than any other feature of a diagnosis, whereas others prefer mechanistic models of etiology and disease progression. In addition, there is growing concern that access to clinical services needs to be taken into consideration when changing diagnostic criteria, since changes of diagnostic criteria can make a previously diagnosed person ineligible for services.

Kraepelin's paradigm still has great value today. It has been the main engine of the psychiatric research agenda for more than 100 years. It provides hope for a cure. At the same time, psychiatric movements and sects have moved away from a shared vision for psychiatric research (Havens 2005). We need nudges to bring psychiatric researchers together. Progress in psychiatric research will depend on our shared values.

References

Andreasen, N.C. (2007). DSM and the death of phenomenology in America: an example of unintended consequences. *Schizophrenia Bulletin*, **33**, 108–112.

Barch, D.M., **Bustillo, J.**, **Gaebel, W.**, et al. (2013). Logic and justification for dimensional assessment of symptoms and related clinical phenomena in psychosis: relevance to DSM-5. *Schizophrenia Research*, **150**, 15–20.

Bentall, R.P. (2005). *Madness Explained. Psychosis and human nature*. London: Penguin.

Bentall, R. (2006). Madness explained: why we must reject the Kraepelinian paradigm and replace it with a "complaint-orientated" approach to understanding mental illness. *Medical Hypotheses*, **66**, 220–233.

Berretta, S., **Heckers, S.**, and **Benes, F.M.** (2015). Searching human brain for mechanisms of psychiatric disorders. Implications for studies on schizophrenia. *Schizophrenia Research*, **167**, 91–97.

Berrios, G.E. and **Hauser, R.** (1988). The early development of Kraepelin's ideas on classification: a conceptual history. *Psychological Medicine*, **18**, 813–821.

Bleuler, E. (1911). *Dementia Praecox oder Gruppen der Schizophrenien*. Leipzig: Franz Deutike, p. 420.

Carpenter, W.T., Jr., **Heinrichs, D.W.**, and **Wagman, A.M.** (1988). Deficit and nondeficit forms of schizophrenia: the concept. *American Journal of Psychiatry*, **145**, 578–583.

Coleman, M. and **Gillberg, C.** (1996). *The Schizophrenias. A biological approach to the schizophrenia spectrum disorders*. New York: Springer.

Craddock, N. and **Owen, M.J.** (2005). The beginning of the end for the Kraepelinian dichotomy. *British Journal of Psychiatry*, **186**, 364–366.

Cuthbert, B.N. (2015). Research Domain Criteria: toward future psychiatric nosologies. *Dialogues in Clinical Neuroscience*, **17**, 89–97.

Eisenberg, L. (1986). Mindlessness and brainlessness in psychiatry. *British Journal of Psychiatry*, **148**, 497–508.

Engstrom, E.J. (2004), *Clinical Psychiatry in Imperial Germany: A history of psychiatric practice*. Ithaca, NY: Cornell University Press.

Ennis, L. and **Wykes, T.** (2013). Impact of patient involvement in mental health research: longitudinal study. *British Journal of Psychiatry*, **203**, 381–386.

Frese, F.J., 3rd, **Knight, E.L.**, and **Saks, E.** (2009). Recovery from schizophrenia: with views of psychiatrists, psychologists, and others diagnosed with this disorder. *Schizophrenia Bulletin*, **35**, 370–380.

Ghaemi, S.N. (2003). *The Concepts of Psychiatry*. Baltimore: Johns Hopkins University Press.

Goodwin, F.K and **Jamison, K.R.** (1990). *Manic-Depressive Illness*. New York: Oxford University Press.

Hamshere, M.L., et al. (2009). Genetic utility of broadly defined bipolar schizoaffective disorder as a diagnostic concept. *British Journal of Psychiatry*, **195**, 23–29.

Havens, L. (2005). *Psychiatric Movements. From sects to science.* Piscataway, NJ: Transaction Publishers.

Hebbring, S.J., et al. (2015). Application of clinical text data for phenome-wide association studies (PheWASs). *Bioinformatics*, **31**, 1981–1987.

Heckers, S. (2008). Making progress in schizophrenia research. *Schizophrenia Bulletin*, **34**, 591–594.

Heckers, S. (2009). Is schizoaffective disorder a useful diagnosis? *Current Psychiatry Reports*, **11**, 332–337.

Heckers, S. (2014). 'Future in psychopathology research. *Schizophrenia Bulletin*, **40** Suppl 2, S147–151.

Hippius, H. and **Möller, H-J.** (2008). *The University Department of Psychiatry in Munich.* Heidelberg: Springer.

Hoche, A.E. (1912). Die Bedeutung der Symptomenkomplexe in der Psychiatrie. *Zeitschrift für die Gesamte Neurologie und Psychiatrie*, **12**, 540–551.

Hoff, P. (1995), Kraepelin. Clinical Section—Part I. In G. Berrios and R. Porter (eds.) *A History of Clinical Psychiatry*, pp. 261–279. New York: New York University Press.

Jablensky, A. (2007). Living in a Kraepelinian world: Kraepelin's impact on modern psychiatry. *History of Psychiatry*, **18** (71 Pt 3), 381–388.

Jameson, J.L. and **Longo, D.L.** (2015). Precision medicine--personalized, problematic, and promising. *New England Journal of Medicine*, **372**, 2229–2234.

Jaspers, K. (1913). *Allgemeine Psychopathologie.* Berlin: Springer-Verlag (9th edn, 1973).

Kasanin, J. (1933). The acute schizoaffective psychoses. *American Journal of Psychiatry*, **90**, 97–126.

Kayser, M.S. and **Dalmau, J.** (2011). The emerging link between autoimmune disorders and neuropsychiatric disease. *Journal of Neuropsychiatry and Clinical Neurosciences*, **23**, 90–97.

Keefe, R.S., **Lobel, D.S.**, **Mohs, R.C.**, et al. (1991). Diagnostic issues in chronic schizophrenia: Kraepelinian schizophrenia, undifferentiated schizophrenia, and state-independent negative symptoms. *Schizophrenia Research*, **4**, 71–79.

Kendler, K.S. (1980). The nosologic validity of paranoia (simple delusional disorder). A review. *Archives of General Psychiatry*, **37**, 699–706.

Kendler, K.S. (1990). Toward a scientific psychiatric nosology. Strengths and limitations. *Archives of General Psychiatry*, **47**, 969–973.

Kendler, K.S. (2013). What psychiatric genetics has taught us about the nature of psychiatric illness and what is left to learn. *Molecular Psychiatry*, **18**, 1058–1066.

Kendler, K.S. (2016). The schizophrenia polygenic risk score: to what does it predispose in adolescence? *JAMA Psychiatry*, **73**, 193–194.

Klein, D.F. (1964). Delineation of two drug-responsive anxiety syndromes. *Psychopharmacologia*, **5**, 397–408.

Kraepelin, E. (1920). Die Erscheinungsformen des Irreseins. *Zeitschrift für die gesamte Neurologie und Psychiatrie*, **62**, 1–29.

Kraepelin, E. (1987). *Memoirs*, ed. H. Hippius, G. Peters, and D. Ploog. Berlin: Springer-Verlag.

Leonhard, K. (1957). *Aufteilung der endogenen Psychosen.* Berlin: Akademie Verlag.

Liddle, P.F., **Friston, K.J.**, **Frith, C.D.**, et al. (1992). Patterns of cerebral blood flow in schizophrenia. *British Journal of Psychiatry*, **160**, 179–186.

Lieberman, J.A. and **First, M.B.** (2007). Renaming schizophrenia. *BMJ*, **334**, 108.

Luhrmann, T.M. (2001). *Of Two Minds: The growing disorder in American psychiatry.* New York: Knopf.

Marzano, L., **Bardill, A.**, **Fields, B.**, et al. (2015). The application of mHealth to mental health: opportunities and challenges. *Lancet Psychiatry*, **2**, 942–948.

McHugh, P.R. and **Slavney, P.R.** (1983). *The Perspectives of Psychiatry.* Baltimore, MD: Johns Hopkins University Press.

Parnas, J. and **Bovet, P.** (1995). Research in psychopathology: epistemologic issues. *Comprehensive Psychiatry*, **36**, 167–181.

Reynolds, C.F., 3rd, **Lewis, D.A.**, **Detre, T.**, et al. (2009). The future of psychiatry as clinical neuroscience. *Academic Medicine*, **84**, 446–450.

Ritsner, M.S., **Mar, M.**, **Arbitman, M.**, and **Grinshpoon, A.** (2013). Symptom severity scale of the DSM5 for schizophrenia, and other psychotic disorders: diagnostic validity and clinical feasibility. *Psychiatry Research*, **208**, 1–8.

Robins, E. and **Guze, S.B.** (1970). Establishment of diagnostic validity in psychiatric illness: its application to schizophrenia. *American Journal of Psychiatry*, **126**, 983–987.

Sato, M. (2006). 'Renaming schizophrenia: a Japanese perspective. *World Psychiatry*, **5**, 53–55.

Scharfetter, C. (2005). *Eugen Bleuler 1857–1939. Polyphrenie und Schizophrenie.* Zürich: vdf Hochschulverlag AG an der ETH Zürich.

Schmitt, W. (1983). Das Modell der Naturwissenschaft in der Psychiatrie im Übergang vom 19. zum 20. Jahrhundert. *Berichte der Wissenschaftsgeschichte*, **8**, 89–101.

Steinberg, H. (2001). *Kraepelin in Leipzig.* Bonn: Edition Das Narrenschiff im Psychiatrie-Verlag.

Tamminga, C., Sirovatka, P.J., Regier, D.A., and van Os, J. (eds.) (2010). *Deconstructing Psychosis. Refining the research agenda for DSM-V.* Washington, DC: American Psychiatric Association Publishing.

Taylor, M.A. and **Fink, M.** (2003). Catatonia in psychiatric classification: a home of its own. *American Journal of Psychiatry*, **160**, 1233–1241.

van Os, J. and **Linscott, R.J.** (2012). 'Introduction: The extended psychosis phenotype—relationship with schizophrenia and with ultrahigh risk status for psychosis. *Schizophrenia Bulletin*, **38**, 227–230.

Chapter 45

Comments on "What is progress in psychiatric research?"

Derek Bolton

Dr Hecker's chapter provides a very helpful expert review of the major proposals, counter-proposals, and new directions for making progress in psychiatric research, specifically on schizophrenia, or psychosis more broadly conceived.

Overall I am left with the impression that in the history of research in psychiatry since Kraepelin there has been no shortage of theories on the nature of the phenomena and how to make progress in research. Progress itself is less abundant, signalled perhaps by the very fact of abundance of ideas, especially if we do not take into account the promise that is bound to be offered by new approaches. On the other hand it is early days and no doubt there is more progress to be made. This raises the central question of Heckers' chapter: what is progress in psychiatric research?

There are two broad ways of conceptualizing progress in any science: the first invokes the correspondence theory of truth, supposing that progress amounts to ever-increasing approximation of our models and theories to the way reality really is. The second way is more pragmatic, conceptualizing progress as ever-increasing power of prediction of our models and theories in the domains of interest. Progress can be defined in either way, but the former is more metaphysical, while the latter is the immediate concern of the scientist, and is in any case the way that progress can be ascertained and measured. Increasing power of prediction is closely tied to intervention and technological application. Predictions of the form "if we do A, then, according to the theory, the result is B," enables production of the outcome B, provided that A is modifiable.

Technological application is a particularly important feature of progress in any health science. The health sciences are by definition *applied sciences*, intended to achieve improvement in health-related outcomes. So what are the broad headings of health-related outcomes that interest us? Here is one list of possible headings:

- natural course of a health condition
- outcome of the condition
- treatment of the condition—broadly understood to include cure, amelioration, or prevention of complications

- prevention of the condition—reduction of incidence in the population—drawing on etiological models
- adjustment of a person to having the condition
- improvement of quality of life of the person with the condition, whether objectively understood, or as appraised by the person, or both.

These various headings have an ordering of sorts, but they are not sequential, and they do not all have equal weight across all health conditions, complications to be considered further below. The broad outcomes of interest as above are all prefaced on the assumption that we have identified a health condition in the first place. Identification of a health condition involves defining a recognizable pattern of one or more symptoms and associated signs, with a history, a course, and a reasonably well-defined typical outcome, in the broad range from remission or cure through to death, with everything in between.

Identification of a health condition is presupposed by progress in health science in areas such as in the list above, and from this point of view it must seem radically disappointing that in the case of schizophrenia even this axiomatic groundwork is still contested 100 years or so after Kraepelin. It is salutary to note in this connection that many medical conditions bear the name of their discoverer, implying that much of the work in identifying the condition, together with approximations of course and outcome, can be accomplished in one working lifetime. I do not know—in these terms—whether it is sensible to expect a clear definition of a putative health condition after 100 years of trying by the best minds in the best research teams. This point does not of course apply uniformly across medicine or psychiatry but is perhaps particularly the case with schizophrenia. In the face of so much controversy, much of it due to the fact that proposed definite criteria for the condition face counter-examples, it may be that the most we can expect is a broad agreement on a broader construct such as "psychosis."

In any case, once we have achieved a viable definition of a particular health condition, we can then move on to the matters of progress as for example listed above. Always a particularly important player on this pitch is the model of infectious disease, applied with success in general medicine and—early on—in psychiatry. A key feature of this model is that clinical features and course are driven by a singular cause, accounting for practically all of the outcome variance. As it happened, the causes in the case of bacterial infections were modifiable, once antibiotics had been discovered. In addition, the source of the infecting bacteria, and their mode of transmission into the body, were identified, and were modifiable, leading to prevention on a public health scale. In short, biomedicine achieved every kind of success with bacterial infectious diseases, some with viral infective diseases, including treatment and prevention. The validators all converge—likely because there is a single primary cause.

With notable exceptions, particularly tuberculosis, bacterial infectious diseases tend not be chronic; typically they spontaneously remit, or cause deterioration, or they respond to antibiotics if available. To this extent their management did not include issues of adjustment and quality of life. These issues do arise, however, for chronic long-term conditions, which are not self-limiting and have not yet succumbed to complete treatment, and may never. The list of chronic long-term conditions is long, both medical and psychiatric. For these conditions, it is typically of the utmost importance how the person responds to having the condition, to the restrictions it imposes, to the secondary losses, and to the possible unwanted side effects of medication that ameliorates the condition or prevents complications. These issues of adjustment and quality of life involve complex interpretations: for example, whether the person regards the condition as an illness, or alternatively perhaps just part of life, and either way, whether the person focuses on the unfairness of fate, or finds a way of accepting; and also questions about treatment, such as how the person weighs the advantages and disadvantages of taking the medicine, with the advantages and disadvantages of carrying on as normal without it. Such issues are pervaded and affected by personal, family, and social meanings and causes. As such, they are outside the purview of biomedical contribution to clinical care, complementary to it. Similar considerations apply to quality-of-life issues. The recovery movement in mental health services, for example, emphasizes the importance of the person gaining autonomy in their life, to achieve outcomes that matter to them, notwithstanding the illness and need for treatment.

Progress in psychiatry research, as research in any branch of health applied science, has to be measured by the ways that it improves clinical care, broadly conceived as comprising a heterogeneous range of tasks, as sketched above, from improving public health through to supporting individuals with chronic health conditions. This broad range of tasks has to be underpinned by a correspondingly broad range of research programmes and methodologies. Issues concerning adjustment and quality of life, for example, warrant methodologies sensitive to attitudes and values of individuals and effects of social contexts. The development of interventions to improve population health rely essentially on aetiological models encompassing broad ranges of variables including genetic and environmental risk and protective factors. All kinds of research, however, and especially theories of aetiology, rely on valid identification of health conditions. While noting towards the end his paper that progress has been slow, especially at the conceptual level of defining the nature of mental illness, Heckers recommends several ways forward: acknowledging the complexity of psychiatric diagnosis, the variable strengths of diagnostic validators, and the need for broader understanding of disease course and outcome, including relevance to daily living. Heckers' analysis of the basic issue of disease identification and these recommendations are a sound basis for progress.

Section 16

After DSM-5

Chapter 46

Introduction to "DSM-5.1: Perspectives on continuous improvement in diagnostic frameworks"

Kenneth S. Kendler

In this clearly written and informative chapter, Paul Appelbaum provides a history of the planning for future revisions of the *Diagnostic and Statistical Manual of Mental Disorders* (DSM) after the publication of the fifth edition (DSM-5). He is ideally positioned to write this as he has played a central role in these processes. I too was a participant in these processes. In this brief introduction, I want to make three points that might provide some context for the upcoming essay.

I see the proposed changes in the process of nosologic revision as outlined by Appelbaum as departing from the way things were done during the DSM-5 process in two major ways. First, instead of doing a major review of the entire manual all at once, where all diagnostic areas are potentially up for revision, the post-DSM-5 process will consider individual proposals in an ongoing manner. Ideally, this will mean that the field can wait until diagnostic areas are "ripe for change" rather than consider all categories together in a lock-step manner. How well this will work remains to be seen. A critical element is who is going to propose changes and for what reasons. Individuals and groups have a wide range of motivations for seeking to change DSM categories. Some of them are more likely to result in beneficial changes than others. The original conception of the "Work Group on the Future of the DSM" was for the Steering Committee to both respond to proposals for changes from individuals outside the form DSM process and for the committee members themselves to survey the scientific field and select areas for consideration for change when research advances might make them ripe for diagnostic revision. As the committee has formalized its process, it became clear that the latter approach would ideally require additional resources to review the literature and prepare the needed materials. In the end, although such resources were not available, this does not mean that members of the Steering Committee could not propose changes. Rather, they would need to do that like any individual in the field using entirely their own time and resources.

So in the current system, the main impetus for change will likely come from members of the broad mental health community. Will there be groups of nosologically oriented researchers and clinicians who are willing to put the time into preparing the needed materials for changes that will in the long run benefit the field? As I have observed over decades, motivations for proposing changes in DSM are varied. Sometimes they are idealistic and for "the good of the field." However, rather often they have self-promotional elements. Individuals seek to enlarge or legitimatize a clinical area of interest or further a particular research goal. They have produced some research findings the importance of which would be substantially increased if it were "enshrined" in the DSM. There is also the plain narcissistic reward, in terms of prestige, for having made changes in the DSM.

This is not necessarily bad. Indeed, some have argued that the system of modern science is largely based on exactly this range of motivations (Hull 1990). We have the idealistic scientist and truth-seeker. But any honest observer of the modern biomedical research structure (at least in the United States and Europe) would conclude that self-promotional motivations play a strong role in much of our world. We strive for high-profile publications, large grants, and the associated rewards of academic life such as promotions and awards. It is a remarkable feature of the organization of science that we can take this broad array of individual motivations and turn them into a process that has been quite successful at advancing human knowledge. In part, this works through the process of peer review and replication. We do have the rogue scientist who takes short-cuts (i.e., cheating) to scientific status. But such aberrations have not (at least not yet) been frequent enough to derail the momentum of forward progress of this historically striking process of Western science.

In DSM, these forces will not work in quite the same way. Instead, we will have the review process of the Steering Committee and the appointed work groups. The hope is that these will prevent proposals that might benefit individuals or small clinical or research groups at the expense of the broader field from getting into the DSM. If these quality control structures do their job, then the motivations of the originators of the proposals for change should become irrelevant. Whether it be idealism or blatant self-promotion, only proposals with broad positive impact on the field should make it through. That is the hope.

The second major change from the DSM-5 is in the level of structure in the process. Until the appointment of the Scientific Review Committee (SRC), the DSM-5 was relatively unstructured. There were no widely accepted or enforced "criteria for changing criteria." While the "Guidelines for Making Changes to DSM-V" (aka the "Kendler–Kupfer criteria") (Kendler 2013) were officially introduced midway through the process (10/2009) they were in fact not widely followed nor were they enforced by leadership. As a result, individual work groups developed quite different cultures and a variety of approaches to the rationale for proposed changes. Some of the work groups were relatively data-driven but others proposed changes based largely on conceptual arguments. The contrast with the approach of the DSM Steering Committee is striking. As Appelbaum outlines, the first task of the DSM Steering Committee was to develop a clear structure and process. This is now completed and is much more thorough than was seen in any prior DSM revision. The hope is that this will lead to a standardization of the process across diagnostic categories. It also makes clear to the community at large, and specifically those making proposals for change, what the requirements are. From my many hours spent on DSM committees, I can assure you that we will be approached by many individuals who want "special deals." I once joked that "stringent criteria for change in DSM categories is what everyone wants for other people's proposals." For the integrity of the process, it is vital that everyone has to meet the same threshold.

Finally, on a slightly different note, while the framework of the SRC has been influential in shaping the approach of the DSM Steering Committee, it is noteworthy that there has been a broadening of the criteria for change. The SRC was very "validity focused." As outlined by Appelbaum, the DSM Steering Committee included three additional possible rationales: improving reliability, improving clinical utility, or reducing the deleterious consequences of the diagnostic category. In each case, the language includes the important caveat "without a reduction in validity." While we have a well-developed framework of validators and quite clear metrics for reliability, the two other criteria for change are more novel. The hope is that over the first few years of work, the operationalization of what constitutes adequate evidence for improvement of clinical utility or reduction in deleterious consequences will become clearer.

References

Hull, D.L. (1990). *Science as a Process: An evolutionary account of the social and conceptual development of science*. Chicago IL, University of Chicago Press.

Kendler, K.S. (2013). A history of the DSM-5 Scientific Review Committee. *Psychological Medicine*, **43**, 1793–1800.

Chapter 47

DSM-5.1: Perspectives on continuous improvement in diagnostic frameworks

Paul S. Appelbaum

47.1 Introduction

Since the mid-twentieth century, the *Diagnostic and Statistical Manual of Mental Disorders* (DSM) of the American Psychiatric Association (APA) has guided psychiatrists in the United States in categorizing the disorders experienced by their patients. With the publication of the third edition of the manual (DSM-III) in 1980, the influence of the DSM spread to many other parts of the world. A new edition of the DSM has appeared approximately every 10–20 years since DSM-I in 1952: DSM-II was published in 1968, DSM-III in 1980, DSM-III-R in 1987, DSM-IV in 1994, DSM-IV-TR (text revision only) in 2000, and most recently DSM-5 in 2013.

At least since DSM-III, these revisions have been multi-year efforts. Planning for DSM-5, for example, began in 1999, and the Task Force that oversaw its development was appointed in 2006 (Regier et al. 2013). Work groups of specialists (more than 160 specialists spread across 13 work groups in DSM-5) were appointed to review each of the diagnostic categories in specific sections of the manual (e.g., Mood Disorders, Somatic Symptom Disorders) to determine whether changes were indicated. In addition, proposals were considered for the creation of new diagnostic categories and, in some cases, for the removal of existing categories or the collapse of multiple categories into a single new diagnosis (e.g., autism spectrum disorder in DSM-5). Work group recommendations were posted for extensive public comment and review, and when finalized, were sent on to the Task Force for its consideration. Proposals for changes to DSM-5, the most recent revision, were subject to several additional layers of internal review by APA committees charged with considering their scientific validity and clinical (including public health) implications; input was also received from the APA Assembly, a representative body elected by APA members, and the entire review package was integrated by a DSM Summit Group, before presentation to the APA Board of Trustees, which had the final say over changes (American Psychiatric Association 2013).

If anything, this description of the revision process for DSM-5 understates the effort that went into the process. A series of 13 international conferences on specific issues related to psychiatric nosology (e.g., use of dimensional as opposed to categorical diagnoses) was held in the early stages of planning the revision (Regier et al. 2013), and six study groups were appointed to advise the Task Force on specific issues, such as gender and cross-cultural issues. At the end of the process, once the diagnostic criteria sets were approved by the APA Board of Trustees, the work groups, and a team of nosologists and writers generated the text of the DSM, which described the diagnostic features of each disorder, its epidemiology and natural history, considerations related to differential diagnosis, and other characteristics. The target date for publication of DSM-5 was pushed back several times to accommodate the work that needed to be done to ready the manual for publication.

Notwithstanding the enormous effort that went into DSM-5, the process was open to criticism on a number of grounds. The comprehensive review of each diagnostic category was time-consuming and costly, involving as it did assembling a large number of experts to evaluate potential changes. Extensive attention and effort was given to proposals for changes that were not incorporated into the final version of the document. Despite an effort to rely on data generated from clinical and epidemiological studies to justify changes in the manual, decisions were often based on expert opinion rather than data. Insofar as the process depended on work group members who had spent years studying particular diagnostic categories, and who often believed that there were small but meaningful differences among patients experiencing the same disorder, it incentivized the proliferation of diagnostic categories. (Frances and Widiger 2012) APA's funding of the process and ultimate financial benefit from sales of manuals and associated materials seemed to some observers to threaten the independence of the effort by allowing financial considerations rather than scientific ones to determine the cycle of revision. (Frances 2012) With the publication of DSM-5 behind it, in light of these concerns the APA decided to explore a new model for updating the nosologic framework for American psychiatry.

47.2 Continuous improvement as an alternative model

A more timely and efficient approach to updating psychiatric diagnoses so as to incorporate changes in understanding of particular disorders would eschew the periodic massive efforts that have characterized DSM revisions since the inception of the manual. In its place would be a process that focused on continuous improvement of particular diagnostic categories, when and if supported by advances in the field. The primary rationale for a continuous-improvement model is based on avoiding the kind of delays in the incorporation of new scientific knowledge that were inherent in a process involving periodic updating at intervals of a decade or more. Once adequate data were available to support revision of diagnostic criteria sets, or the addition or deletion of diagnostic categories, changes could be accomplished relatively rapidly. Conversely, pegging revision to scientific advances and requiring explicit supportive data should discourage changes when they are not well supported by evidence, a risk that attends any process that invites wholesale review and revision of the nosologic framework in its entirety. Continuous improvement of the DSM is enabled by online formats (online subscriptions to the DSM are now available) that allow instantaneous dissemination of changes at minimal cost.

To get this process off the ground, in the spring of 2013 APA appointed a Work Group on the Future of the DSM, charged with making recommendations to the Board of Trustees for the development of the DSM as a "living document." Although not everyone liked that term, since for some it connoted a rapidity of change at odds with the desire of many people in the mental health professions for a high degree of stability in diagnostic formulations, the charge to the work group made clear that it was to explore mechanisms for iterative updating of the DSM and consider the development of a process for transition to an entirely electronic format. The work group was made up of 12 APA members, all of whom had been involved in one way or another with the development of DSM-5, with consultation from David Kupfer, MD, who had been the chair of the DSM-5 Task Force, and a methodologist. As a former APA President and a member of the DSM-5 Summit Group, I was asked to chair the work group.

Over the course of the following year, the work group developed a report that was submitted to the APA Board of Trustees in March 2014 (Work Group on the Future of the DSM 2014). The report addressed both the principles that should guide an iterative revision process and a structure for governance of the process. It began by recognizing that, in general, stability in psychiatric diagnosis promotes consistency in clinical practice and research and is therefore desirable. Too rapid change can be disorienting for clinicians and can complicate research, since changes in the composition of diagnostic groups that may result from alterations in criteria sets make comparisons with previous studies more difficult and can disrupt longitudinal studies; in the latter case, a change in diagnostic criteria may require the addition of new survey items or create problems in comparability across the sample if the items required to evaluate the new criteria were not included in the earlier waves of assessment. However, the work group accepted that advances in the field may periodically require revision of the DSM diagnostic criteria and/or text, and since advances will occur at an uneven pace across disorders, changes to the DSM should be made incrementally and as warranted by advances in research. The work group noted that evolving models of online publishing made this approach feasible to an extent that would not have been the case just a few decades ago.

With regard to governance of the new process, the work group recommended the appointment of a Steering Committee, made up of persons with expertise in psychiatric nosology, psychiatric research, clinical psychiatry, and the DSM, with representation from the APA Board of Trustees and Assembly. Membership of the Steering Committee would not be limited to APA members, but could include persons with appropriate expertise from other clinical specialties and other mental health professions. The process of detailed review of proposals for change and drafting specific changes to the text and criteria sets would be given to a small number of review committees, which would cover broader areas of psychopathology than had been traditional for the DSM work groups. By enlarging the portfolio of the review committee and recruiting members with a wider perspective on the field, the work group hoped to avoid the dynamic sometimes seen in DSM work groups, in which subspecialists committed to ever-finer definitions of subcategories of illness drove a proliferation of diagnoses in psychiatry. The Board of Trustees endorsed the recommendations of the Work Group on the Future of the DSM, and charged the APA President with appointing a Steering Committee to move the process forward.

47.3 **Putting the pieces into place for continuous improvement**

In the spring of 2014, a 13-member Steering Committee was appointed, including 11 psychiatrists and 2 psychologists, along with a group of external liaisons comprising senior figures in the U.S. National Institutes of Health (NIH) institutes that relate most closely to psychiatry (National Institute of Mental Health, National Institute of Alcohol Abuse and Alcoholism, and National Institute of Drug Abuse) and in the World Health Organization's International Classification of Diseases mental and behavioral disorders section. I was asked to chair the Steering Committee; the vice-chairs are Kenneth Kendler, MD and Ellen Leibenluft, MD. Beginning with an organizational meeting in November 2014, the Steering Committee in monthly conference calls and occasional face-to-face meetings has focused on developing standards and procedures for consideration of proposals. A lesson learned from the DSM-5 process, which had rocky moments in its early phases, is that the creation of explicit criteria by which proposals for revisions can be judged and clear procedures for their review are essential for a coherent process. Hence, priority was given to these issues.

The Steering Committee envisioned three types of proposals for changes to the DSM-5: changes to an existing criteria set; addition of a new diagnostic category or specifier; deletion of an existing diagnostic category or specifier/subtype. In addition, the process will allow for correction of errors and clarification of confusing or misleading content. For each of these, the Steering Committee identified the criteria that must be met (DSM Steering Committee 2015).

Proposals for *changes to existing criteria sets* must provide substantial evidence that the proposed changes would markedly improve at least one of the following:

- validity of an existing diagnostic criteria set
- reliability of a diagnostic criteria set, without an undue reduction in validity
- clinical utility of a diagnostic criteria set, without a reduction in validity or reliability.

Alternatively, proposals must provide substantial evidence that:

- proposed changes would substantially reduce deleterious consequences associated with a diagnostic criteria set, without a reduction in validity.

For *additions of new diagnostic categories to the DSM*, often the most controversial of the potential changes, proposals must provide substantial evidence that they would accomplish all of the following:

- meet DSM-5 criteria for a mental disorder
- have strong evidence of validity
- have at least moderate reliability
- manifest substantial clinical value (e.g., identify a group of patients now not receiving appropriate clinical attention)
- avoid substantial overlap with existing diagnoses, and not be better conceptualized as a subtype of an existing diagnosis
- have a positive benefit/harm ratio (e.g., acceptable false positive rate; low risk of harm due to social or forensic considerations).

If the proposal is for the *addition of a new specifier or subtype to a DSM diagnosis*, it should provide substantial evidence that it:

- has strong evidence of validity (e.g., identifies patients with a common biological marker) and clinical utility (e.g., identifies patients who respond to the same treatment)
- can be applied reliably
- avoids substantial overlap with existing specifiers or subtypes.

Finally, since advances in the understanding of psychiatric disorders may warrant the elimination of diagnoses previously included in the *DSM*, proposals for *deletion of an existing category or specifier* must provide substantial evidence that it:

- has weak evidence of validity; and
- has minimal utility (e.g., is rarely used in clinical practice or research); or
- does not meet criteria for a mental disorder or is better conceptualized as a subtype of an existing diagnosis.

As should be clear from these criteria, the Steering Committee envisions that the revision process will privilege improvements in validity of diagnoses (criteria for which are discussed below), with the expectation that a process of what Chang has called "epistemic iteration" can be applied to psychiatric nosology (Chang 2007, Kendler 2009, 2012). If substantive changes to diagnostic criteria sets are limited to those that increase diagnostic validity (or, in the case of a proposal that would advance one of the other criteria for changes such as reliability, at least not decrease validity), over time the net effect should be convergence on a more valid diagnostic framework. Thus, even proposals that would increase the reliability with which diagnoses can be made or reduce deleterious consequences of particular criteria sets must not have negative effects on the validity of the diagnosis, and proposals for new diagnostic categories must offer strong evidence of validity. Conversely, weak evidence of validity paired with limited clinical utility will justify the removal of a category from the diagnostic manual.

Given the importance of evidence of improved validity to the continuous improvement process, the Steering Committee endorsed an explicit set of criteria for judging the validity of proposed changes. The set is a modification of the list of indicators of validity that were applied by the Scientific Review Committee during the development of DSM-5, in which validators fall into three categories: antecedent, concurrent, and predictive (Kendler et al. 2009). That is, the greater the validity of a diagnostic category, the more people who receive that diagnosis are likely to differ from other people with regard to variables that constitute risk factors for the condition, are related to the presentation of the disorder, and reflect the outcomes associated with the diagnosis. The validators identified by the Steering Committee were the following, with higher-priority validators indicated in italics:

- Antecedent validators include:
  - *familial aggregation and/or coaggregation (i.e., family, twin, or adoption studies)*
  - sociodemographic and cultural factors
  - environmental risk factors
  - prior psychiatric history
- Concurrent validators include:
  - cognitive, emotional, temperament, and personality correlates (unrelated to the diagnostic criteria)
  - *biological markers, e.g., molecular genetics, neural substrates*
  - patterns of comorbidity
  - *degree or nature of functional impairment*
- Predictive validators include:
  - *diagnostic stability*
  - *course of illness*
  - *response to treatment.*

Of course, it is very unlikely that any proposed change will be able to demonstrate improved validity according to all, or perhaps even most, of these indicators. Indeed, proposals may well be based on changes to criteria sets that improve some validators but weaken others. In many cases, although there may be data demonstrating improved performance of several validators, data may be lacking in other categories. Data regarding predictive validators (other than short-term treatment response), although arguably of greatest value for clinicians, will be the most difficult and expensive to collect, since medium-term to long-term follow-up studies will be required. Thus, decisions regarding revisions to the DSM will not be algorithmic, but some inevitably will involve consideration of the degree of improvement in some validators and trade-offs among validators that will reflect the judgment of the reviewers. Recognizing this, the Steering Committee indicated that greater weight would be given to the high-priority validators, that the strength of the data should be proportional to the magnitude of the proposed change (i.e., changes that are greater in magnitude should be supported by stronger data, encompassing a larger number of validators), and that data generally should come from more than one research group, thus encouraging independent verification of results before changes to the DSM are made on that basis. (DSM Steering Committee 2015)

47.4 **Procedures for consideration of revisions to the DSM**

Submissions of proposals for revisions will be web-based, with a dedicated portal for the purpose. Proposers will be required to provide information in a structured format, with supporting data, including descriptions of the reasons for the proposed change; magnitude of the change; impact of the proposed change on the validators listed above; extent to which the proposal would increase the reliability of an existing diagnosis or demonstrates that a new criteria set can be applied reliably; effect of the change on clinical utility; and impact on unintended deleterious consequences of an existing criteria set or consideration of potential negative consequences of a revised criteria set or new diagnosis. Inclusion of tables summarizing the literature review that supports the proposal will be encouraged.

Procedures adopted by the Steering Committee call for proposals to undergo initial review by the group to determine whether the evidence offered in support of the proposal appears likely to meet the criteria for approval. This decision can be analogized to the "probable cause" determination made by a judge under U.S. law to decide whether an arrest warrant or search warrant can be issued to the police; judges must determine, based on current evidence, whether there are reasonable grounds to believe that the person has committed a crime or, in the case of a search warrant, that probative evidence will be uncovered. However, the process recognizes that additional evidence may prove the person innocent or the search unnecessary. In the case of the DSM, the determination will focus on the likelihood that the proposal ultimately will be approved, without prejudging the final outcome, which will be affected by additional evidence gathered along the way. If necessary, the Steering Committee can reach out to experts in the area of the proposal for input.

On finding that the evidence in support of the proposal is likely to meet the criteria for approval, the proposal will be referred to one of six standing review committees, with each committee responsible for a broad area of psychiatric nosology. Standing committees, rather than ad hoc committees appointed for each proposal, offer the prospect of greater consistency in judgments across time. Conferring responsibility for broad areas of diagnosis on each committee means necessarily that the committees will not be dominated by area specialists; members may thus may be less likely to want to "have an impact" on a particular diagnosis by supporting changes. This builds into the process what the Steering Committee views as a desirable conservative bias.

The five committees approved by the APA Board of Trustees will cover respectively:

- intellectual disability, learning, communication, autism spectrum, and motor disorders
- schizophrenic spectrum, psychotic and bipolar disorders, and neurocognitive disorders
- depressive, anxiety, trauma, obsessive-compulsive, dissociative, and somatic symptom disorders
- personality, disruptive, impulse control, substance use, and paraphilic disorders
- feeding and eating, elimination, sleep-wake, sexual dysfunction, and gender dysphoria disorders.

This division of the field is necessarily arbitrary, as any other division would be. The Steering Committee intends to monitor the work of the review committees to determine whether there is a serious imbalance in workload or whether an adjustment in the division of responsibilities is indicated for other reasons.

Review committees are charged with considering the evidence in support of the proposed change, including reviewing the material submitted to insure completeness and accuracy of the conclusions drawn. In addition, the review committee will need to undertake whatever additional investigation is required (e.g., review of additional literature not cited in the proposal), and summarize its findings. A review committee can recommend acceptance or rejection of the proposal, or suggest revisions to the original proposal, as appropriate. The proposal will then return to the Steering Committee for a determination as to whether there is considerable evidence in support of the proposal, and whether public comment is therefore warranted. If that decision is made affirmatively, the proposal will be posted on the DSM website, with notice to the field, and comments invited for a fixed period of time. Based on the comments received, the Steering Committee will decide whether to return the proposal to the review committee for additional work, to approve the proposal, or to reject it. If approved, the proposal will then be submitted to the APA Board of Trustees for final approval.

Although considerable effort has been put into the development of these procedures, they are as yet untested. It seems likely that adjustments will be needed based on experience with actual proposals.

47.5 Challenges ahead

As this unprecedented process of ongoing, evidence-based revision of a nosologic framework rolls forward, there will be challenges, undoubtedly including some that cannot be anticipated at this early stage. The web portal for submission of proposals, www.dsm5.org, opened shortly before the end of 2016. Even at this point, however, it is possible to anticipate some of the issues with which the Steering Committee and others involved in the process will need to grapple. Foremost among them will be the need to steer a course between overly rapid revisions and excessive resistance to change. As noted above, changes in nosologic frameworks are destabilizing to clinicians, who are faced with learning and applying new criteria, and perhaps recategorizing existing patients; and to researchers, who may confront difficulties comparing data collected under different sets of diagnostic criteria and whose ongoing studies may be rendered abruptly out of date. Thus, changes should be made only when clearly warranted by the science and likely to have a positive impact on the field. However, there would be no point to the elaborate review process outlined above if, as implemented, it were so restrictive that almost no changes to diagnostic criteria could occur. The Steering Committee will need to calibrate its review to an optimal level of rigor, balancing the virtues of stability with the desirability of accepting change when warranted.

A related issue involves the Steering Committee's commitment not to reopen the debates of DSM-5 unless new evidence becomes available to warrant reconsideration. A number of highly contentious proposals were addressed in the DSM-5 revision process, the resolution of which left advocates for one perspective or another extremely disappointed (e.g., Morey et al. 2015). Several of these diagnostic criteria sets ended up in Section 3 of the manual denoted as "Conditions for Further Study." As explained in that section, "The [DSM] Task Force determined that there was insufficient evidence to warrant inclusion of these proposals as official mental disorder diagnoses . . .," but encouraged the collection of additional data so that a more valid and reliable determination could be made in the future about inclusion in the DSM. Among the conditions involved are attenuated psychosis syndrome, persistent complex bereavement disorder, suicidal behavior disorder, and in a slightly different category, an alternative model for the diagnosis of personality disorders. Were advocates for these and other approaches rejected for DSM-5 allowed simply to return to reargue their cases, the Steering Committee would become enmeshed in redoing the work of the DSM-5 Task Force—without any assurance that the decisions reached would be any more valid than the original ones. To avoid this outcome, and to maximize the likelihood that subsequent changes to the DSM will represent incremental movement towards a more valid diagnostic framework, the Steering Committee will expect substantial new data to be presented in support of proposals as a condition for their consideration.

That being said, it nonetheless seems clear that there will be some kinds of changes in the DSM for which new empirical data will not be necessary. The DSM, like any complex document crafted by human beings, is imperfect. In places, descriptions in the text suffer from a lack of clarity or ambiguity of meaning; there are places where inconsistencies or contradictions appear within the text or criteria; and there may be errors of omission or inadvertent inclusion that are identified. Changes focused on correcting these problems, in contrast to revisions aimed at altering criteria sets, are inherently conservative; that is, they are aimed at protecting the intended meaning of the document rather than changing it. The Steering Committee has set up a process whereby such problems can be corrected. In doing so, it will require that proposed revisions be non-trivial and useful to users of the manual, recognizing that any changes should only be made for the most persuasive reasons.

A particular challenge attends the process of pruning diagnoses that lack validity or clinical utility from the manual. Interest groups often coalesce around additions or modifications of diagnoses, seeking recognition of disorders that they have identified or experienced themselves. Only rarely does one see a similar effort addressing the removal of diagnostic categories. To the extent that diagnoses of particular disorders are found not to be clinically useful, they may simply be ignored. And more researchers are interested in making a mark by demonstrating the validity of a new category than the invalidity of an existing one. Hence, the Steering Committee itself may need to be proactive in stimulating proposals for deletions of disorders or it may need to initiate such proposals itself. (Proposals of any sort coming from the Steering Committee will be judged by the same standards applied to proposals from external sources.)

A final challenge we face is keeping an open mind about the process that we have established. Although we hope that it will work well, it seems likely that we will learn things along the way that could improve its functioning. The inevitable inertia that is part of any organizational structure will need to be resisted, so that the revision process too can be subject to the kind of iterative improvement that we hope to bring to the DSM. Given the importance of this effort to psychiatry, the other mental health disciplines, and the community of people with mental disorders, no less should be expected of us.

References

American Psychiatric Association. (2013). *Diagnostic and Statistical Manual of Mental Disorders*, 5th edn. Arlington, VA: American Psychiatric Association.

Chang, H. (2007). *Inventing Temperature: Measurement and Scientific Progress.* New York: Oxford University Press.

DSM Steering Committee. (2015). Format for submissions of proposed changes to the DSM. July 12.

Frances, A. (2012). DSM-5 costs $25 million, putting APA in a financial hole. *Huffington Post*, October 31.

Frances, A. and **Widiger, T.** (2012). Psychiatric diagnosis: Lessons from the DSM-IV past and cautions for the DSM-5 future. *Annual Review of Clinical Psychology*, **8**, 109–130.

Kendler, K.S. (2009). An historical framework for psychiatric nosology. *Psychological Medicine*, **39**, 1935–1941.

Kendler, K.S. (2012). Epistemic iteration as a historical model for psychiatric nosology: promises and limitations. In K.S. Kendler and J. Parnas (eds.) *Philosophical Issues in Psychiatry II: Nosology*, pp. 305–322. Oxford, UK: Oxford University Press.

Kendler, K.S., Kupfer, D., Narrow, W., et al. (2009). Guidelines for Making Changes to DSM-V. October 21. Available as supplementary materials to **Kendler, K.S.** (2013). A history of the DSM-5 Scientific Review Committee. *Psychological Medicine*, **43**, 1793–1800.

Morey, L.C., Benson, K.T., Busch, A.J., Skodol, A.E. (2015). Personality disorders in DSM-5: emerging research on the alternative model. *Current Psychiatry Reports*, 17, 24.

Regier, D.A., Kuhl, E.A., and Kupfer, D.J. (2013). The DSM-5: Classification and criteria changes. *World Psychiatry*, 12, 92–98.

Work Group on the Future of the DSM. (2014). Report of the Work Group on the Future of the DSM, February 3.

Chapter 48

How do we improve the DSM?

Stephan Heckers

48.1 Introduction

The fifth edition of the *Diagnostic and Statistical Manual of Mental Disorders* (DSM-5) is the latest effort of the American Psychiatric Association (APA) to define psychiatric diagnoses. The document is widely used as a guide by clinicians and researchers. Clinicians use it to formulate cases and decide about treatment plans. Researchers use it to guide their studies of disease mechanism and to develop new diagnostic procedures, treatments, and prevention strategies. Here I comment on the continuous improvement process of the DSM-5, as outlined by Paul Appelbaum, the chair of the 13-member DSM Steering Committee. I will focus on three aspects: the process of implementing changes, the scientific rationale to accept or reject proposals for change, and the aims and values guiding the continuous improvement process.

48.2 The process

In 2014, the APA appointed a Steering Committee to oversee the process of improving the DSM-5 document, which had been published one year earlier. This was a remarkable step. All prior editions of the DSM (from DSM-I in 1952 to DSM-IV-TR in 2000) had been considered as the ultimate document, reified as the psychiatric "bible" (Hyman 2010). But we are now fully aware that any nosology of psychiatric disorders is preliminary, in constant need of review and, if appropriate, revision.

Many are disillusioned with the classification of psychiatric disorders. Some had hoped that DSM-5 would be a paradigm change in psychiatry: moving from signs and symptoms of mental disorders to biological markers of brain disorders. The change did not occur, simply because the data for such a change were lacking. The hope for a biological reduction of complex mental states to abnormalities in the brain remains, but we have become much more realistic about the timeline for such a revolution in psychiatry. It has also become clear that any such revolutionary agenda needs to overcome considerable inertia, if not frank resistance, to changes of the DSM. At the most basic level, changes will be costly. Clinicians need to be retrained and researchers need to change recruitment criteria, with the potential risk that new data will be incompatible with previously collected datasets.

Appelbaum rightly points out that the process of continuous improvement needs to be a trade off between progress and stability. He compares it to the "probable cause" determination made by a judge. For the DSM improvement process, the Steering Committee needs to decide whether there is sufficient evidence to (1) change existing criteria sets, (2) add new diagnoses or specifiers and subtypes, or (3) delete an existing diagnostic category or specifier.

What are the incentives to make changes? There are many reasons why one would like to see changes in the diagnosis of a psychiatric disorder. Patient advocacy groups might want to change diagnostic criteria if they affect eligibility for services. On the other hand, payors and providers of healthcare services will be interested in changes to the reimbursement of such services. The legal community will be interested in the exact definition of mental disorders as they will use such diagnoses in court proceedings. Researchers will be interested in aligning psychiatric diagnoses with their research interests. Finally, the pharmaceutical and medical devices industry has a significant interest in the diagnosis of mental disorders as it affects the market for their products.

Who is eligible to suggest changes? The web-based DSM improvement effort as outlined by Appelbaum is open to everyone with relevant new data. This could include patients, providers, researchers, companies, and government agencies. While this appears to be an open process (and a refreshing change from the secrecy of prior DSM committees), it is clear that only few will have new data that are strong enough to change the DSM-5.

48.3 **The scientific rationale for change**

There are at least four reasons to change the existing classification of a psychiatric disorder: to increase validity, reliability, and clinical utility and to keep deleterious consequences at a minimum. I will briefly discuss the last three reasons and then focus on the list of validators as identified by the DSM Steering Committee, especially the six high-priority validators.

The reliability of psychiatric disorders has been a major focus of the DSM process. In fact, the increased reliability of psychiatric disorders can be considered the major success of the DSM. But while reliability is a prerequisite for validity, it does not get us closer to the disease mechanism. In fact, there is growing concern that the focus on reliability has led to the neglect of crucial information that can be gathered in the interaction between clinician and patient (Andreasen 2007). Any focus on reliability needs to consider that a mental illness can only be defined in the interaction with an individual person.

This also affects the clinical utility of a diagnosis. Imagine we have unlimited time to understand the unique life story of a person and can describe all aspects in great detail. This would allow us to define normal and abnormal mental states much more accurately. In clinical practice, however, we do not have the luxury of time and often do not have access to all of the information necessary to fully describe the mental state of a person. Diagnostic criteria need to take these limitations into consideration.

The deleterious consequence of a diagnosis (or a change thereof) is often not immediately clear. For example, homosexuality was removed from the DSM, largely in response to advocacy groups (Spitzer 1981). Any introduction of a new diagnosis (e.g., attenuated psychosis syndrome) needs to consider the stigma that is associated with a psychiatric diagnosis.

The DSM Steering Committee will consider all new data that can improve 11 antecedent, concurrent and predictive validators of psychiatric diagnoses (see Chapter 47 in this book). They have already defined six of them to be high-priority validators that will be given more weight in their probable cause determination of changes:

- familial aggregation and/or coaggregation (i.e., family, twin or adoption studies)
- biological markers, e.g., molecular genetics, neural substrates
- degree or nature of functional impairment
- diagnostic stability
- course of illness
- response to treatment.

It is not clear what defines a high-priority validator. Kendler has provided some evidence for this ranking, but it is likely that this hierarchy will change over time. Here I focus on the challenge to assess the strength of the evidence and the challenge to weigh disparate strengths.

48.4 **Two challenges**

The committee will have to assess the strength of the evidence. This may seem straightforward, but I doubt that it will be. Many had hoped that biological markers will be included in the DSM-5. Promising examples were laboratory tests, brain scans, and performance on standardized tests of cognition. But meta-analyses and systematic reviews revealed a more complex picture. In addition, the clinical utility of many biological markers is low, e.g., due to limited access to equipment and the need to train a large workforce in the collection and interpretation of data. It will require a significant and concerted effort of the research community and dedicated healthcare delivery systems to provide strong enough evidence for the inclusion of biological markers in criteria sets for psychiatric disorders.

But even if the committee could develop an accurate tool/instrument/procedure to assess the strength of the evidence, they are still relying on others to provide the data. For example, comprehensive data that document the course of illness and the long-term response to treatment are highly desirable datasets. It will be crucial for a successful continuous improvement process to nudge the research community towards such goals.

The committee will also need to manage the disparate strength of validators. Let's take as an example a psychiatric diagnosis that can be defined by a pleomorphic clinical presentation that shows a remarkably consistent response to treatment, but an unpredictable course of illness and little or no evidence for familial aggregation. Let's say we could even define a diagnostic drug test that uses treatment response as the defining, single criterion for the diagnosis. Would we consider such a diagnosis as a new entity (Taylor and Fink 2003)?

There is no simple metric that allows us to define a hierarchy of validators. We do not have an instrument or a procedure that allows us to compare the strength of evidence across the 11 (or 6 major) validators. There are many proposals for such a hierarchy, often influenced by strong biases, including personal or economic interests, to rank one validator (or a limited set), over others. It will be important for the committee not to make any premature decisions, but to apply Solomonic wisdom.

48.5 The aims and values

We can easily agree on the four aspects that need to be considered when deciding about changes of a psychiatric diagnosis: validity, reliability, clinical utility, deleterious consequences. But it will be more difficult to agree on their value. We need to acknowledge considerable differences between psychiatric diagnoses: some are more valid than others (Alzheimer's disease versus delirium), some are more reliable than others (schizophrenia versus schizoaffective disorder), some have great clinical utility despite unclear validity (e.g., personality disorders) and some might have deleterious consequences. We need to include an open discussion about the values of psychiatric diagnoses as we engage in the more technical aspects of a continuous improvement process.

We also need to keep our focus on the goal: reaching better outcomes through epistemic iteration. We need to trust the scientific progress as we change psychiatric diagnoses. Psychiatric movements and sects that reject the iterative process of science altogether are not helpful (Ghaemi 2003, Havens 2005). Critics of the current epistemology and nosology need to engage with psychiatric researchers and clinicians, rather than remaining on the sidelines. The continuous improvement process of the DSM will be a success as long as we keep an open dialogue, allow the input from patient and advocacy groups and welcome disruptive, even radical, changes to the DSM, if they are in the best interest of patients.

References

Andreasen, N.C. (2007). DSM and the death of phenomenology in America: an example of unintended consequences. *Schizophrenia Bulletin*, **33**, 108–112.

Ghaemi, S.N. (2003). *The Concepts of Psychiatry*. Baltimore, MD: Johns Hopkins University Press.

Havens, L. (2005). *Psychiatric Movements. From sects to science* Piscataway, NJ: Transaction Publishers.

Hyman, S.E. (2010). The diagnosis of mental disorders: the problem of reification. *Annual Review of Clinical Psychology*, **6**, 155–179.

Spitzer, R.L. (1981). The diagnostic status of homosexuality in DSM-III: a reformulation of the issues. *American Journal of Psychiatry*, **138**, 210–215.

Taylor, M.A. and **Fink, M.** (2003). Catatonia in psychiatric classification: a home of its own. *American Journal of Psychiatry*, **160**, 1233–1241.

Index

Note: *fn* indicates footnotes